Central Auditory Processing Disorders

New Perspectives

A Singular Audiology Text
Jeffrey L. Danhauer, Ph.D.
Audiology Editor

Central Auditory Processing Disorders

New Perspectives

Gail D. Chermak, Ph.D.
Professor and Chair
Department of Speech and Hearing Sciences
Washington State University
Pullman, Washington

Frank E. Musiek, Ph.D.
Professor of Otolaryngology and Neurology and
Director of Audiology
Dartmouth-Hitchcock Medical Center
Lebanon, New Hampshire

Guest Author:
Chie Higuchi Craig, Ph.D.
Professor
Department of Communication Sciences and Disorders
University of Wisconsin-Milwaukee
Milwaukee, Wisconsin

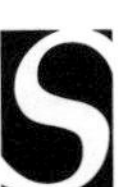

Singular Publishing Group, Inc.
San Diego · London

Singular Publishing Group, Inc.
401 West A Street, Suite 325
San Diego, California 92101-7904

19 Compton Terrace
London N1 2UN, U.K.

e-mail: singpub@mail.cerfnet.com
web site: http://www.singpub.com

Typeset in 10/12 Palatino by SoCal Graphics
Printed in United States of America by McNaughton and Gunn

Library of Congress Cataloging-in-Publication Data

Chermak, Gail D.,
Central auditory processing disorders / Gail D. Chermak, Frank E. Musiek ; guest author, Chie Higuchi Craig.
p. cm.
ISBN 1-56593-697-3
1. Word deafness. 2. Word deafness in children. I. Musiek, Frank E. II. Title.
RC394.W63C48 1997
617.8—dc21 97-4466
CIP

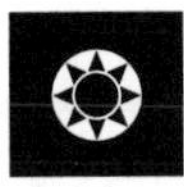

CONTENTS

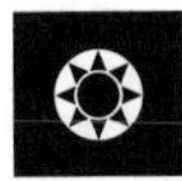

FOREWORD

Most of us take hearing for granted. That is, a sound occurs somewhere in the environment around us, and we, quite simply, "hear" it. The harsh reality is that a very large number of mechanical and neurobiological operations intercede between the arrival of those pressure waves at the eardrum and the conscious perceptual or linguistic elaboration of the sensory event. The mechanical operations are, of course, the reception and conduction of the vibrations through the outer and middle ears. The factors that influence the effectiveness of that sound transmission, the measurement of the extent to which the transmission might be impaired, and efforts at compensating for any such pathology traditionally have been the domains of audiology and otology. We have a long history of successful description of peripheral auditory function, diagnosis of peripheral pathologies, and successful audiological, medical, or surgical rehabilitation.

In part, this success story has been made possible by the fact that the essential functions of the outer and middle ears are relatively straightforward. Without wishing to be unnecessarily dismissive or trivializing of the complexities of peripheral auditory function (c.f., Pickles, 1988; Jahn & Santos-Sacchi, 1988), in the most comprehensive understanding of "hearing," there are not many active parts in the auditory periphery, and the parts themselves are not particularly complicated. This is not to say that we understand all there is to know about the middle ear; only that we know enough to recognize and measure a disorder when we see it and to intervene to achieve measurable improvement in hearing if the pathology is manageable.

A similar, if somewhat more preliminary, case might be made for the cochlea. In this instance, it is true that the details of cochlear function are still being worked out, often with considerable conceptual revolution. Such was the case with the abandoning of the notion of a "second filter"; we came to understand that basilar membrane tuning benefited from "active" cochlear processes, and we witnessed the discovery of the mechanisms that mediate those processes (e.g., Pickles, 1988). Nevertheless, the functions we ascribe to the cochlea, namely the spectral decomposition of the sound and the transduction of the mechanical signal into spike trains across appropriate sectors of the cochlear array, are, in principle, not all that complicated. It is partly for this reason that we now achieve considerable success at reintroducing hearing through the damaged cochlea in some patients by means of cochlear implants. With modern technology and instrumentation, it is simply not that difficult to spectrally decompose the incoming sound with an electronic (c.f. biological) device which then enables the selective electrical stimulation of the relevant sectors of the cochlear nerve array. Again, this is not to say that the fidelity of the process in implanted ears is even close to that of the normal ear; only that measurable and significant improvement in hearing can be achieved in some patients.

All of this is in marked contrast to the neurobiologically mediated components of hearing. There are millions of active parts, and the internal operations of each of them are extraordinarily complex. The neurons are active, dynamic, and plastic in their functions and connections. In ensembles, they "learn" through experience. Except under highly controlled laboratory conditions, access to the individual elements is almost impossible. The processes executed by these systems of neurons are massively more computational and complicated than simple conduction or transduction (Pickles, 1988; Popper & Fay, 1992).

By the same token, the auditory functions we ascribe to the central auditory system are also complicated and numerous. The business of detecting a sound, discriminating it along any of a host of dimensions, segregating it from the background, attending to it, recognizing it as familiar, comprehending its meaning—even conscious introspection about the qualities of the percept itself—are all functions of the brain. These are utterly different functions from those executed by the auditory periphery, and this is reflected in the fact that the language of our discourse about those functions has shifted, quite appropriately, from physics and engineering to neurobiology and psychology.

Similarly, the pathophysiologies that affect the central auditory system are fundamentally different from those that affect the periphery. It is because the functions and pathologies of the middle ear are mechanical that mechanical interventions to middle ear disease are effective. The operation of the brain is not built on this simple kind of mechanics; the individual neurons, and their interactions, are the products of fabulously rich and dynamic metabolisms which are only beginning to receive adequate description. Moreover, the architecture of the brain is highly parallel and distributed, so that it is not always easy to assign specific and unique functions to particular components. Such a system can be assaulted physically (as in the case of a space-occupying tumor), metabolically (perhaps in the disruption of a neurotransmitter-specific neuron system), or developmentally (perhaps by deprivation). The pathological processes themselves are highly individual, as are the sites or processes on which they operate, and thus the functions that they impair. It also is becoming increasingly clear that interference with a relatively low-level (e.g., perceptual) process can, in principle, lead to a kind of cascade error whose behavioral expression is of a high level (e.g., cognitive) problem.

What emerges from these kinds of considerations is that "hearing" is not a single sensory or perceptual skill (c.f., McAdams & Bigand, 1993; Moore, 1989). It is probably decomposable into many neurological or psychological processes that operate in serial and in parallel (Phillips, 1995). We, as normal listeners, may be aware only of the unity of our conscious auditory experience, but that unity actually emerges from separable processes operating in a highly intricate and dynamic network. Pathology can cut across that network, in strikingly individual fashions, to produce highly idiosyncratic patterns of impairment. This means that the tools we use to probe the integrity of central auditory processes have to be diverse and flexible; they have to be sensitive to the fact that there are many levels at which we "hear" things.

Similarly, the fashions in which we intervene to rehabilitate the listener with central impairment may not be like those we use for peripheral disorders. We may end up using strategies like selective amplification of some signal components—not to compensate for a sensitivity loss, but to increase the perceptual salience of elements that we wish to attract or engage the listener's attentive or other cognitive resources. Our interventions are unlikely to be mechanical, but they might take the form of intensive behavioral training, precisely to exploit some of the unique properties of the brain: its plasticity and trainability. And, simply because much of the intervention might be in the form of behavioral training, one needs a healthy awareness of the "metacognitive" factors that influence this training. It is clear, then, that to keep pace with both advances in basic science and the reality that the listener with hearing impairment often has an intact auditory periphery, clinical auditory science must expand its domain beyond the historical one of sound conduction through the middle ear and signal transduction in the cochlea.

Awareness of this issue is far from completely new. But if one traces the development of thinking about central auditory processing and its disorders (e.g., Keith, 1977; Pinheiro & Musiek, 1985; Phillips, 1995), one sees increasingly penetrating interrogations of hearing processes, couched in solid conceptual frameworks that seek to establish numerous and testable links between neuroscience and perception and cognition. The relevant domains of basic, experimental science are themselves still growing, and it is therefore no surprise that there are still matters of definition to resolve, or that the American Speech-Language-Hearing Association has only recently released its consensus statement on central auditory processing (1996).

Nor are we, as "auditory" professionals, alone in this regard; parallel developments can be seen in the visual sciences. Again there is a long history of description of peripheral visual function, its pathology, and successful optical corrections of that pathology. But conceptually, the process of successfully refracting an image onto the retina is a simple one compared to the neural processes executed on retinal output by the brain, and the psychological ones that emerge from them. Our comprehension of these processes is still growing, and will continue to do so for many years. Nevertheless, as in hearing, a clearer picture is emerging of how "seeing" something is a function with a complex architecture composed of specifiable subprocesses operating in serial and parallel (e.g., Farah, 1990; Farmer & Klein, 1995). It follows that the most competent understanding of the perceptual or cognitive elaboration of the visual stimulus will, of necessity, be a very multidisciplinary one.

In this book, Chermak, Musiek, and Craig have, in a single volume, provided students, researchers, and clinicians alike with a carefully balanced account of central auditory processing, its assessment, and approaches to management. From the outset, there is an appreciation that competent hearing is not just about absolute sensitivity, that there are whole tiers of processing levels above that of sound detection. The book takes for granted, and given the foregoing, quite appropriately so, the value of a multidisciplinary understanding of central auditory processing. Perhaps for the first time, we find a chapter on the basic neural science of the central auditory system backed by one on the cognitive science of spoken language processing. The chapters on central auditory assessment reveal a sensitivity to good psychological science in the development of the behavioral test battery and the value of electrophysiology as a complement to it. The chapters on intervention likewise lay out the theoretical foundations and reveal that successful intervention strategies are built on a solid comprehension of acoustics, neural, and psychological science.

The importance of pedagogical efforts like this one should not be minimized. It is precisely because the various research disciplines exploring "hearing" are themselves continuously providing new insights, that there is an onus on us to remain apprised of those developments. This is true in all sciences, of course, but it is especially true here because central auditory processing, as a field, is still very young and growing rapidly. With the increasing detection and/or recognition of listeners whose hearing impairment is of central origin, or reflects an impaired cognitive monitoring or elaboration of intact sensory processing, there is still greater need for volumes like this one to be available to clinicians and to teachers of clinicians. This book will not be the final word on central auditory processing and its disorders. It is, however, a highly positive step in the direction of collating the most recent evidence from the relevant fields and in encouraging clinicians and researchers to the optimistic view that understanding central auditory processing, its disorders and management, might be a tractable problem. For this, we are all indebted to the authors.

Dennis P. Phillips, Ph.D.
Dalhousie University
Halifax, Nova Scotia

References

Farah, M. J. (1990). *Visual agnosia. Disorders of object recognition and what they tell us about normal vision.* Cambridge, MA: MIT Press.

Farmer, M. E., & Klein, R. M. (1995). The evidence for a temporal processing deficit linked to dyslexia: A review. *Psychonomic Bulletin and Review, 2,* 460–493.

Jahn, A. F., & Santos-Sacchi, J. (Eds.). (1988). *Physiology of the ear.* New York: Raven Press.

Keith, R. W. (Ed.). (1977). *Central auditory dysfunction.* New York: Grune & Stratton.

McAdams, S., & Bigand, E. (Eds.) (1993). *Thinking in sound. The cognitive psychology of human audition.* Oxford: Oxford University Press.

Moore, B. C. J. (1989). *An introduction to the psychology of hearing* (3rd ed.). London: Academic Press.

Phillips, D. P. (1995). Central auditory processing. A view from auditory neuroscience. *American Journal of Otology, 16,* 338–352.

Pickles, D. O. (1988). *An introduction to the psychology of hearing* (2nd ed.). London: Academic Press.

Pinheiro, M. L., & Musiek, F. E. (1985). *Assessment of central auditory dysfunction. Foundations and clinical correlates.* Baltimore: Williams & Wilkins.

Popper, A. M., & Faye, R. R. (Eds.). (1992). *The mammalian auditory pathway: Neurophysiology.* New York: Springer-Verlag.

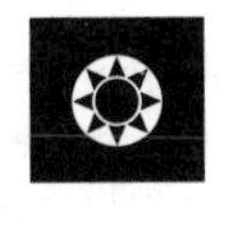

PREFACE

The perspectives contained in this volume evolved over the last decade in concert with our increasing understanding of the neurobiology of central auditory processing and its linkage with language and cognitive systems. This linkage, coupled with the recognition that central auditory processing disorders underlie functional deficits observed in diverse clinical populations, has caused misunderstandings about the nature of central auditory processing disorders and their diagnosis and treatment. We recognize that the complex linkages among central auditory processing, language, and cognition present challenges for assessment and diagnosis, challenges we see as surmountable. Moreover, we see the many opportunities these linkages offer to design effective intervention programming and thereby minimize the potential impacts of central auditory processing disorders on communication, learning, and social functions.

The information presented in this book is intended to help professionals improve the prospects for a better quality of life for children and adults with central auditory processing disorders and their families. Through our clients and their devoted families, we have come to understand and gain great compassion for the struggles they face in overcoming this disability with its potential for such pervasive and serious impact. Unfortunately, because central auditory processing disorders have not been well understood, clients, particularly, school-age children, have not received the support services they truly need to succeed. Perhaps readers of this book will rectify this unfortunate circumstance. Specifically, we will have met our objectives in writing a comprehensive volume on central auditory processing disorders only if these disorders are identified and diagnosed more efficiently and lead to more effective intervention for individuals across the life span.

Encompassing theory, assessment, and management, with special consideration for preschool-age children, school-age children, and older adults, we trust that this book will serve the range of professionals from different disciplines responsible for clinical, educational, and rehabilitative service delivery to this population. Specifically, we expect audiologists, speech-language pathologists, teachers, university faculty, neuropsychologists, neurologists, pediatricians, otolaryngologists, family physicians, school nurses, and school administrators will find this book useful in their professional practices. Believing strongly in the value and necessity for self-help, we also hope that the information provided here will encourage the active involvement of individuals with central auditory processing disorders and their families in designing and implementing their own treatment programs. Of tantamount importance, we hope this book helps students in professional education programs gain the theoretical and clinical knowledge they will need to serve this challenging population.

We attempt to provide current theoretical and clinical perspectives to guide assessment and intervention for central auditory processing disorders across the life span. In the first chapter, we begin by presenting a definition and clinical profile of central auditory processing and central auditory processing disorders based on scientific and clinical evidence. A brief historical overview is given to orient the reader to the nearly 50 years of scientific and clinical developments in central auditory processing disorders. A model of central auditory processing that recognizes the reciprocal relationships between auditory perception and more global linguistic and cognitive processes is developed. The spectrum of clinical populations presenting symptoms associated with central auditory processing disorders is explored along with the common and diverse threads that link and differentiate them. In considering secondary metacognitive deficits associated with deficient auditory perceptual processes, we suggest the need for comprehensive management programs integrating specific skills development and executive strategy training.

The remaining nine chapters of the book are divided into four sections covering basic science, assessment, intervention, and research needs and future directions. The basic science section is comprised of two chapters. A neurobiologic framework for assessment and management of central auditory processing disorders is presented in Chapter 2. In reviewing the neuroanatomy, physiology, and neurochemistry of the central auditory nervous system, linkages between neurobiology and central auditory processing and its attendant disorders are developed. The implications of key concepts in neuroscience (e.g., maturation, sensory stimulation, plasticity) for management of central auditory processing disorders are explored.

Spoken language processing is examined in Chapter 3, written by our good friend and esteemed colleague, Chie Higuchi Craig. Drawing on literature in spoken word recognition, auditory illusions, psycholinguistics, English as a second language, and clinical audiology, Chie examines the complex interactions between sensory-perceptual processes and non-modality-specific central resources for spoken language processing. She reviews models of real-time spoken language processing and illustrates their advantages in clinical assessment of everyday temporal processing of the dynamically changing speech signal. Finally, she highlights recent developments in real-time speech rate conversion technology that may herald a new generation of innovative management tools, as well as assessment paradigms.

Approaches to the identification and assessment of central auditory processing disorders are presented in the second section, comprised of Chapters 4, 5, and 6. Basic assessment and philosophical issues are discussed in Chapter 4. Following discussion of the importance of strict control of acoustic stimuli and the test environment, particularly in relationship to test efficiency, validity, and reliability, we examine issues pertinent to test selection, pass-fail criteria, test battery interpretation, and the appropriate role of both screening instruments and diagnostic tests and procedures in central auditory evaluation. Also considered are the diverse populations for whom central auditory testing may be appropriate, importance of patient history, and test materials and equipment.

The role of behavioral tests in assessing central auditory processes is discussed in Chapter 5. Tests are categorized according to the central auditory process(es) presumed to underlie performance. This taxonomy should inform test battery construction, as well as provide insight regarding functional deficits. Sensitivity and specificity of tests typical of the categories are reviewed, as are classic findings relative to site-of-lesion. Considerations for pediatric and geriatric populations are presented.

Electrophysiologic procedures and related physiologic measures (i.e., acoustic reflex and otoacoustic emissions) are considered in Chapter 6. Diagnostic indicators of central auditory nervous sytem pathology and central auditory processing disorders are reviewed following brief descriptions of the various procedures and sensitivity and specificity data. The chapter concludes with a discussion of the appropriate use and weighting of electrophysiologic procedures and behavioral tests in a diagnostic test battery.

The third section of the book focuses on intervention. Topics considered fundamental to intervention are described in Chapter 7, including discussion of efficacy, generalization, collaboration, multicultural considerations, and life span issues. The extent to which intervention can be customized as a function of differential diagnosis, age, and clinical profile is examined. The chapter concludes with a delineation of the theoretical foundation of our intervention approach. That foundation supports collaborative and ecological intervention which develops the client's auditory skills, metalinguistic skills, executive strategies, and self-regulatory processes. Auditory training and metalinguistic and metacognitive management strategies and techniques are presented in Chapter 8 along with special considerations for preschool-age, at-risk children, and older adult populations. Complementary interventions designed to enhance the acoustic signal and the listening environment are discussed in Chapter 9. Included is discussion of classroom acoustics, FM technology, instructional modifications, and the role of the speech-language pathologist in qualifying, assessing, and managing central auditory processing disorders.

The final section and final chapter of the book is devoted to discussion of research needs and future directions. In addition to recommendations for research needed to advance our understanding of central auditory processing disorders, we speculate about the technological, neuropharmacological, and behavioral approaches that may improve clinical service delivery and outcomes. A glossary of key terms used throughout the book with which the reader may be less familiar is also provided.

Significant scientific and technological advances have placed us at the threshold of truly understanding the nature of central auditory processing disorders. Although some longstanding questions remain and new questions continually arise, we have never been in better position to reaffirm central auditory processing disorder as an independent diagnostic category describing a neurobiologic disorder. Professionals responsible for the identification, assessment, and management of central auditory processing disorders must embrace these strong scientific and clinical foundations in assessing and managing these disorders, as well as in advocating on behalf of clients for educational, workplace, and public accommodations, and third party coverage for services. Researchers must collaborate with clinicians, accelerating our momentum in tackling the complex questions in basic and clinical sciences and advancing identification, assessment, and management strategies. So too, university educators must recognize central auditory processing disorders as a core disability area, designing and requiring course work and clinical experiences to develop knowledge competencies and skills. Together we shall continue to advance scientific understanding and clinical practice.

***To Mary Ellen, for sparking new possibilities,
and Isaac and Alina, for
inspiring my tomorrows. (g.d.c.)***

CHAPTER 1

CONCEPTUAL AND HISTORICAL FOUNDATIONS

It would be appropriate to begin a book on central auditory processing disorders with a definition of the subject matter. Unfortunately, one cannot simply turn to the dictionary to obtain this most basic grounding. A definition of central auditory processing disorder (CAPD) has proved elusive over the last 20 years as numerous authors and American Speech-Language-Hearing Association (ASHA) committees have attempted to define, at least operationally, this heterogeneous group of functional deficits (ASHA, 1990, 1992, 1996; Katz, Stecker, & Henderson, 1992; Keith, 1977, 1981b).

The difficulty in defining CAPD has stemmed from several factors. It results, in part, from the recognition that CAPD is not a label for a unitary disease entity, but rather a description of functional deficits (ASHA, 1996). Further, CAPD has been observed in a variety of clinical populations, including those associated with known lesions or pathology of the central nervous system (e.g., aphasia, Alzheimer's disease, traumatic brain injury) and others with suspected but unconfirmed central nervous system pathology or neuromorphological (i.e., neurodevelopmental) disorder (e.g., developmental language disorder, dyslexia, learning disabilities, attention deficit disorder) (Breedin, Martin, & Jerger, 1989; Chedru, Bastard, & Efron, 1978; Colson, Robin, & Luschei, 1991; Cook, Mausbach, Burd, Gascon,

Slotnick, Patterson, Johnson, Hankey, & Reynolds, 1993; Divenyi & Robinson, 1989; Efron, 1963; Elliott & Hammer, 1988; Ferre & Wilber, 1986; Gascon, Johnson, & Burd, 1986; Grimes, Grady, Foster, Sunderland, & Patronas, 1985; Jerger, Martin, & Jerger, 1987; Keith, Rudy, Donahue, & Katbamna, 1989; Keller, 1992; Mohr, Cox, Williams, Chase, & Fedio, 1990; Pillsbury, Grose, Coleman, Conners, & Hall, 1995; Robin, Tranel, & Damasio, 1990; Strouse, Hall, & Burger, 1995; Tallal & Piercy, 1974; Willeford, 1980). CAPD also has been reported in association with a history of chronic otitis media (Brown, 1994; Gravel & Wallace, 1992; Hall & Grose, 1993; Hall, Grose, & Pillsbury, 1994, 1995; Moore, Hutchings, & Meyer, 1991; Silva, Chalmers, & Stewart, 1986) and has been documented in older adults where neurologic changes, albeit not necessarily pathological, result from the aging process (Committee on Hearing, Bioacoustics and Biomechanics [CHABA] Working Group on Speech Understanding and Aging, 1988; Gulya, 1991; Stach, Spretnjak, & Jerger, 1990). The presence of CAPD in such diverse clinical populations has raised questions concerning the linkage between CAPD and the cognitive, linguistic, and social functions related to language learning and use. Although several frameworks have been proposed to explain this linkage (Campbell & McNeil, 1985; Tallal, Miller, & Fitch, 1993), unresolved theoretical differences persist, centered on whether central auditory processing deficits underlie or reflect language disorders (ASHA, 1996; Keith, 1981a, 1981c; Rees, 1973, 1981; Sloan, 1980a, 1986).

Notwithstanding theoretical differences regarding the linkages among the diverse clinical populations presenting overlapping symptomatology, auditory performance deficits associated with CAPD are well documented and include deficits in dichotic listening, selective attention, and temporal processing (Chermak, Vonhof, & Bendel, 1989; Jerger et al., 1987; Jerger, Johnson, & Loiselle, 1988; Musiek, 1983a; Musiek, Geurkink, & Keitel, 1982; Musiek & Pinheiro, 1987; Olsen, Noffsinger, & Kurdzeil, 1975; Speaks, Gray, Miller, & Rubens, 1975). Characteristically, individuals with CAPD experience difficulties comprehending spoken language in competing speech or noise backgrounds (Cherry, 1980; Jerger et al., 1987; Jerger et al., 1988; Musiek et al., 1982; Olsen et al., 1975). In addition, related performance deficits in understanding verbal directions, and auditory memory, as well as academic underachievement and reading difficulties, demonstrate the complex linkages between central auditory processing and more global cognitive and linguistic functions (Butler, 1983; Chermak & Musiek, 1992; DeConde, 1984; Musiek & Geurkink, 1980; Sloan, 1980a, 1986, 1992; Willeford & Burleigh, 1985).

DEFINITION

> Central auditory processes are the auditory system mechanisms and processes responsible for the following behavioral phenomena: sound localization and lateralization; auditory discrimination; auditory pattern recognition; temporal aspects of audition including, temporal resolution, temporal masking, temporal integration, and temporal ordering; auditory performance with competing acoustic signals; and auditory performance with degraded acoustic signals. (ASHA, 1996, p. 41)

Moreover, these auditory system mechanisms and processes generate electrical brain waves or auditory evoked potentials (i.e., auditory brainstem response, auditory middle-latency response, auditory late-latency response, and auditory event-related response) in response to acoustic stimuli.

Electrical brain activity, reflecting the responses of millions of brain cells to auditory events, encodes the spectral and temporal aspects of the auditory signal. The timing of activity within and across neural networks forms the basis of central auditory processing. Presumably, central auditory system mechanisms and processes affect nonverbal as well as verbal signals and influence various *higher* functions, including language and learning (ASHA, 1996; Phillips, 1993, 1995). Central auditory processes involve the deployment of nondedicated, global mechanisms of attention and memory in the service of acoustic signal processing (ASHA, 1996). Therefore, global neurocognitive mechanisms and processes such as attention and language representation are crucial to even the most basic auditory processing (e.g., discrimination and recognition). The deployment of these nondedicated, global mechanisms and processes in service of central auditory processing underlies the frequently observed clinical association between CAPD and disorders of language learning and use. Moreover, the involvement of these global processes complicates efforts to ascertain the nature of the relationship between CAPD and learning disabilities, language impairment, and attention deficit disorders.

In summary, CAPD refers to a deficit observed in one or more of the central auditory processes responsible for generating the auditory evoked potentials and the following behaviors: sound localization and lateralization; auditory discrimination; auditory pattern recognition; temporal aspects of audition including, temporal resolution, temporal masking, temporal integration, and temporal ordering; auditory performance with competing acoustic signals; and auditory performance with degraded acoustic signals. The processing deficit(s) may reflect a loss of function, disordered function, or release of function. CAPD results from dysfunction of processes dedicated to audition. CAPD also may co-exist with a more global dysfunction that affects performance across modalities (e.g., attention deficit, neural timing deficit, language representation deficit) (ASHA, 1996).

TYPES OF CENTRAL DYSFUNCTION

The behaviors observed in CAPD are presumed to correlate with underlying neurophysiological deficits or neuromaturational differences. Although the data are still inconclusive, Musiek and Gollegly (1988) posited three types of CAPD seen in children, particularly in association with learning disabilities. CAPD resulting from neuromorphological disorder may comprise the largest group, or some 65 to 70% of diagnosed CAPD. Underlying CAPD in this group would be areas of polymicrogyri (i.e., underdeveloped and misshapen cells) and heterotopias (i.e., misplaced cells), most likely in the left hemisphere and the auditory region (splenium) of the corpus callosum (Galaburda & Kemper, 1979; Musiek, Gollegly, & Ross, 1985). Some 25 to 30% of pediatric CAPD might be the result of maturational delay of the central auditory nervous system (Musiek, Kibbe, & Baran, 1984; Musiek et al., 1985). Neurologic disorders, diseases, and insults, including neurodegenerative disorders, might account for under 5% of CAPD diagnosed in association with learning disabilities (Musiek, Baran, & Pinheiro, 1992; Musiek et al., 1985). The latter category would also characterize acquired CAPD in adults.

Recent research employing brain imaging techniques, as well as postmortem studies, has begun to elucidate the probable sites of neuromorphological disorder thought to underlie CAPD and comorbid conditions, including attention deficits, learning disabilities, and dyslexia (Galaburda, 1989; Hynd, Semrud-Clikeman, Lorys, Novey, & Eliopulos, 1990; Lou, Henriksen, Bruhn, Borner, & Nielsen, 1989; Mann, Lubar, Zimmerman, Miller, & Muenchen, 1992). As will be discussed in Chapter 7, intervention may be customized, to some extent, consistent with our current understanding of the underlying differences in etiology and brain function, particularly as they relate to the patient's age, linguistic and cognitive competencies, and comorbid deficits.

MODEL OF CENTRAL AUDITORY PROCESSING

Models of central auditory processing reflect recent developments in cognitive neuroscience that underscore the highly complex, multistage, and interactive nature of central auditory processing (Chermak & Musiek, 1992). Stimuli are encoded as patterns of neural activity varying in temporal and spatial dimensions (Greenberg, 1996; Liberman, Cooper, Shankweiler, & Studdert-Kennedy, 1967). A network model, emphasizing the distributed nature of information processing within the nervous system, is replacing a pathway model in which information is thought to be processed in specific centers of the brain (Masterton, 1992). Consistent with the network model, perceptual responses to sensory stimuli are mediated across a large number of brain regions involving multiple serial, parallel, and distributed neural networks (ASHA, 1996; Ungerleider, 1995). These perceptual responses result from the activation, evaluation, and integration of multiple sources of information (Massaro, 1987). The essential role of neurotransmitters and molecular mechanisms triggered by sensory stimulation in facilitating central auditory processing also is becoming clear (Aoki & Siekevitz, 1988; Kalil, 1989; Musiek & Hoffman, 1990).

The emerging conceptualization of central auditory processing views information processing as neither exclusively bottom-up (i.e., data driven) nor top-down (i.e., concept driven). Rather, interactive networks operating on multiple sources of information provide constraints and corrections to guide pattern identification and interpretation (Churchland & Sejnowski, 1988; Elman, 1989, 1993; Elman & McClelland, 1986; Massaro, 1987; McClelland & Elman, 1986).

Top-down processes ensure the assimilation of lower order information consistent with the listener's experience and expectations; bottom-up processes ensure that the listener is alerted to novel information and information incompatible with ongoing hypotheses about the message (Neisser, 1976; Rumelhart, 1984). Extraction and analysis of lower level acoustic segments are guided by contextual processes, which in turn proceed with reciprocal input from bottom-up information sources (Cole & Jakimik, 1980; Cutler & Norris, 1988; Luce, 1986; Marslen-Wilson, 1987; McClelland & Elman, 1986). An active listener selectively attends, processes data, and imposes higher level constraints to construct the signal or message (Borkowski & Burke, 1996; Flavell, 1981; Gibson, 1966; Watson & Foyle, 1985).

The relative contribution of bottom-up and top-down processes is driven by the changing demands of the listening situation. The influence of top-down processes is more substantial when stimuli are presented in degraded form, including noisy environments and linguistically ambiguous contexts (Marslen-Wilson & Tyler, 1980; Neisser, 1976; Rumelhart, 1980, 1984; Warren & Warren, 1970). For persons with CAPD who routinely confront internal distortions that degrade the signal, top-down processing exerts a more significant influence in all listening situations, especially in noisy and reverberant environments and when coupled with complex linguistic and cognitive demands (e.g., classrooms). (See Chapter 9 for a discussion of means to enhance acoustic signal quality and the listening environment in classrooms.)

Implications for Intervention

This processing model guides the remediation efforts described in later chapters. A model of central auditory processing wherein central auditory processes interact in a complex manner with cognitive and linguistic processes under the control of an active listener suggests that remediation efforts focus on both basic skills (bottom-up) and executive strategy (top-down) training.

HISTORICAL PERSPECTIVE

Although reports of central auditory nervous system dysfunction in adults have appeared in the literature since the 1950s (Bocca, Calearo, & Cassinari, 1954; Bocca, Calearo, Cassinari, & Migliavacca, 1955), controversy has beset this poorly understood complex of functional deficits, particularly as observed in children. Unlike central auditory dysfunction in adults which results from identifiable neurologic pathology, the absence of remarkable neurologic findings in most children diagnosed with CAPD (Musiek et al., 1985) has fueled questions regarding the validity of this diagnosis (Cook et al., 1993; Gascon et al., 1986; Rees, 1973, 1981). Indeed, failure to define precisely this complex of functional deficits left the field floundering for identity and validation for over 20 years.

Use of the term CAPD with children to describe symptomatology similar to that observed in adults is rather recent. The earliest reports appeared in the late 1960s and 1970s (Chalfant & Scheffelin, 1969; Katz & Illmer, 1972; Manning, Johnson, & Beasley, 1977; Martin & Clark, 1977; Sweetow & Reddell, 1978; Willeford, 1977). It was not until a 1977 conference on CAPD in children (Keith, 1977) that this term became prominent, and interest in research on pediatric CAPD was stimulated (Manning et al., 1977; Martin & Clark, 1977; Sweetow & Reddell, 1978; Willeford, 1977). Since that time, numerous committees of the ASHA have been formed and conferences and symposia have been held to consider the nature of CAPD (ASHA, 1992, 1996; Katz et al., 1992; Keith, 1977, 1981b).

In recognition of the persistent controversies surrounding the definition, identification, assessment, and intervention for CAPD, ASHA convened a Task Force on Central Auditory Processing in 1993 to develop a consensus statement delineating the current status of research and the best practices related to the diagnosis and management of children and adults with CAPD. Since the authors were members of that task force, many of the perspectives presented in the 1996 consensus statement are reflected in this book.

Test Development

Adults

Recognizing the insensitivity of traditional auditory tests in assessing the central auditory nervous system (CANS), researchers developed behavioral tests composed of low redundancy materials, such as filtered speech, compressed speech, interrupted speech, and speech in noise to elucidate CANS dysfunction (Bocca, 1958; Bocca et al., 1954; Bocca et al., 1955; Calearo & Lazzaroni, 1957; Kurdzeil, Noffsinger, & Olsen, 1976; Morales-Garcia & Poole, 1972; Noffsinger, Olsen, Carhart, Hart, & Sahgal, 1972; Olsen et al., 1975). Continuing efforts to develop tests sensitive to lesions of the CANS led to measures that incorporated binaural interaction tasks (e.g., localization, binaural fusion, masking level differences) and dichotic presentations (Berlin, Lowe-Bell, Jannetta, & Kline, 1972; Katz, 1962; Kimura, 1961a, 1961b; Matzker, 1959; Musiek, 1983a; Olsen, Noffsinger, & Carhart, 1976; Sanchez-Longo, Forster, & Auth, 1957; Speaks et al., 1975). Temporal ordering and sequencing tasks were incorporated in the mid-1960s (Efron, Yund, Nichols, & Crandall, 1985; Lackner & Teuber, 1973; Milner, 1962; Milner, Kimura, & Taylor, 1965; Musiek & Pinheiro, 1987; Pinheiro & Ptacek, 1971; Ptacek & Pinheiro, 1971).

More recent approaches to assessment of the CANS have involved electrophysiologic measures, although the first reports suggesting their potential for assessment of the CANS were published in the early 1930s (Adrian, 1930; Saul & Davis, 1932; Wever & Bray, 1930). Extensive investigation of auditory evoked responses since that time has demonstrated the value of these reponses for neuroaudiologic evaluation of patients with known or suspected lesions of the CANS (Musiek, Baran, & Pinheiro, 1994). Although the auditory brainstem response (ABR) is a highly efficient measure of the integrity of the eighth cranial nerve and the brainstem (Schwartz, 1987), late latency responses and event-related responses (P300, mismatch negativity [MNN]) may hold more promise for revealing the electrophysiological correlates of deficits observed in central auditory processes (Kraus, McGee, Ferre et al., 1993; Musiek et al., 1992).

Children

In contrast to the rather extensive history of central auditory testing of adults with neurologic impairments (Baran & Musiek, 1991), central auditory evaluative procedures for pediatric populations have gained momentum only in recent years as efforts to understand and remediate learning disabilities and attention deficit disorders often associated with CAPD have intensified (Chermak, 1996). It is well known that young children's central auditory processing is less efficient than adults' (Allen, Wightman, Kistler, & Dolan, 1989; Elliott, 1986; Elliott & Hammer, 1988; Hall & Grose, 1990, 1991; Maxon & Hochberg, 1982; Musiek, Baran, & Pinheiro, 1990; Musiek, Verkest, & Gollegly, 1988; Sussman, 1991; Werner, 1992; Willeford, 1977). Children's reduced efficiency is probably related to maturational differences in neural and linguistic development and response strategies, as well as peripheral processing differences (Chermak, 1996). Despite these differences, early pediatric evaluative efforts relied on central auditory tests developed for adults, with norms adjusted to account for normal developmental differences (Keith & Jerger, 1991). However, given the multiplicity of factors underlying performance differences between children and adults, it is unlikely that simply renorming tests designed for adults ensures adequate assessment of central auditory function in children (Chermak, 1996).

Responding to the need for more appropriate assessment tools, pediatric central auditory tests have been developed incorporating stimuli and procedures that minimize linguistic-cognitive demands while emphasizing auditory-perceptual demands (Cherry, 1980; Jerger & Jerger, 1984; Keith, 1986). Reflecting perhaps a watershed development in pediatric evaluation of central auditory processing, current interest in electrophysiological indices of central auditory function includes children as subjects (Jerger et al., 1988; Jirsa & Clontz, 1990; Kraus, McGee, Micco et al., 1993). The reader is referred to Baran and Musiek (1991), Hall (1992), Keith and Jerger (1991), and Musiek and Baran (1987) for more comprehensive historical reviews of central auditory testing.

Management

As in the history of central auditory assessment, the development of treatment approaches for children and adults with central auditory dysfunction has differed markedly. Management of central auditory dysfunction in adults has included both medical and behavioral therapies. In contrast, given the unremarkable neurologic findings in most cases of pediatric CAPD, behavioral therapies have been employed almost exclusively to manage CAPD in children (Musiek et al., 1985).

Although some surgical procedures have been effective in reducing the auditory sequelae of intracranial lesions in adults, other surgical procedures used to treat disease (e.g., epilepsy) may compromise auditory structures (e.g., temporal lobe, corpus callosum), thereby exacerbating central auditory processing deficits (Cranford, Kennalley, Svoboda, & Hipp, 1996; Kinney, Hughes, & Hardy, 1985; Musiek et al., 1994). Pharmacologic therapies are not available to treat central auditory processing deficits associated with neurodegenerative diseases (e.g., Alzheimer's disease, multiple sclerosis, Parkinson's disease). (See Chapter 10 for pharmacologic treatments under investigation.) Behavioral therapies have focused on the personal hearing aid and FM systems and other assistive listening technologies to improve speech understanding in noise, the most common sequela of central auditory dysfunction in adults (Stach, 1990; Stach, Loiselle, & Jerger, 1991; Stach, Loiselle, Jerger, Mintz, & Taylor, 1987).

Behavioral management programs for children with CAPD were designed to address skill deficits and, more recently, focused on use of FM technology (Blake, Field, Foster, Platt, & Wertz, 1991; Chermak, 1981; Chermak & Musiek, 1992; Lasky & Cox, 1983; Ray, Sarff, & Glassford, 1984; Stach, Loiselle, & Jerger, 1987b; Willeford & Burleigh, 1985). Traditionally, intervention was directed toward enhancing discrete auditory-language skills (e.g., auditory attention, auditory discrimination, auditory analysis and synthesis, auditory sequential memory) that had been identified as areas of deficiency (Barr, 1976; Butler, 1983; Chermak, 1981; Heasley, 1980; Lasky & Cox, 1983; Rampp, 1980; Willeford & Burleigh, 1985). Unfortunately, these approaches have not been particularly effective in reducing the functional deficits associated with CAPD, perhaps because their focus is too narrow or because the deficits targeted are resistant to modification (Chermak, 1981; Chermak & Musiek, 1992; Schneider, 1992; Willeford & Billger, 1978). The management plan described in this book is more comprehensive in scope, espousing a metacognitive approach coupled with auditory and metalinguistic skills development and acoustic signal enhancement. The intervention approach is grounded in theory and supported by data demonstrating the efficacy of several of the component management strategies (see Chapter 7).

SPECTRUM OF COMORBID CONDITIONS

As discussed previously, CAPD has been observed in diverse clinical populations, including those where central nervous system (CNS) pathology or neuromorphological disorder is suspected (e.g., developmental language disorder, dyslexia, learning disabilities, attention deficit disorder) and those where evidence of CNS pathology is clear (e.g., aphasia, multiple sclerosis, epilepsy, traumatic brain injury, tumor, and Alzheimer's disease). Moreover, these conditions are not mutually exclusive and may be characterized as comorbid: An individual may suffer from CAPD, attention deficits, and learning disabilities (Katz, 1992; Keith, 1986; Keller, 1992; Newhoff, Cohen, Hynd, Gonzalez, & Riccio, 1992; Pillsbury et al., 1995; Riccio, Hynd, Cohen, & Gonzalez, 1993; Riccio, Hynd, Cohen, & Molt, 1996). The primacy of any one of these disorders as causal to another, however, remains unclear.

Individuals with diagnoses of CAPD, attention deficit hyperactivity disorder (ADHD), and learning disabilities commonly experience some degree of spoken language processing deficit (Gravel & Wallace, 1992; Westby & Cutler, 1994; Wiig & Semel, 1984). In fact, the most recent definition of learning disabilities establishes language deficits as fundamental ("significant difficulties in the acquisition and use of listening, speaking, reading, writing . . . abilities," National Joint Committee on Learning Disabilities, 1991, p. 19) and has led to terms such as language-learning disabilities and language-related learning disabilities to denote this disability (Gerber, 1993c). Individuals diagnosed with ADHD, learning disabilities, and language impairment frequently experience some deficit in central auditory processing (Chermak et al., 1989; Keith & Engineer, 1991; Keith & Novak, 1984; Keith et al., 1989; Sloan, 1980b, 1986, 1992; Watson & Rastatter, 1985). Indeed, the frequently observed co-occurrence of CAPD and learning disability (Breedin et al., 1989; Chermak et al., 1989; Elliott & Hammer, 1988; Ferre & Wilber, 1986; Jerger et al., 1987) has led to speculation that at least some portion of learning disabilities is due to central auditory deficits (Katz & Illmer,

1972; Keith, 1981a; Knox & Roeser, 1980; Sloan, 1980a). Similarly, the co-occurrence of language impairment and CAPD has led to suggestions that these two deficits may be causally related (Lubert, 1981; Sloan, 1980a; Tallal, 1980; Tallal & Piercy, 1973a; Tallal, Stark, & Mellits, 1985; Tallal et al., 1996).

Also eliciting suggestions of linkage, the association observed between attention deficits and performance on central auditory tests (Campbell & McNeil, 1985; Cook et al., 1993; Gascon et al., 1986) has led to questions about whether CAPD may be a manifestation of impaired attention (Burd & Fisher, 1986; DeMarco, Harbour, Hume, & Givens, 1989; Robin, Tomblin, Kearney, & Hug, 1989) and whether CAPD and ADHD reflect a single developmental disorder (Cook et al., 1993; Gascon et al., 1986). Alternatively, central auditory performance deficits among children with ADHD may indicate the co-occurrence of CAPD, rather than the ADHD itself. This interpretation is supported by Riccio et al. (1996) who reported little correlation between performance on the *Staggered Spondaic Word* (SSW) *Test* and behaviors characteristic of ADHD (i.e., inattention, hyperactivity, and impulsivity). That central auditory performance deficits among children with ADHD reflect the presence of CAPD rather than the ADHD per se is supported further by the frequently reported history of chronic otitis media in children with ADHD (Adesman, Altshuler, Lipkin, & Walco, 1990; Feagans, Sanyal, Henderson, Collier, & Appelbaum, 1987; Pillsbury et al., 1995; Roberts et al., 1989; Silva, Kirkland, Simpson, Stewart, & Williams, 1982) and the association between chronic otitis media and CAPD (Adesman et al., 1990; Brown, 1994; Gravel & Wallace, 1992; Hall & Grose, 1993, 1994; Hall et al., 1994, 1995; Hutchings, Meyer, & Mooore, 1992; S. Jerger et al., 1983; Moore et al., 1991; Pillsbury, Grose, & Hall, 1991; Silva et al., 1986).

Clearly, the validity of these diagnostic labels as clinically distinct entities is questionable. Similar performance deficit profiles, which include inattention, poor listening skills, distractibility, inappropriate social behaviors, and poor academic achievement (APA, 1994; Chermak & Musiek, 1992; Keller, 1992; National Joint Committee on Learning Disabilities, 1991; Seikel, Somers, & Chermak, 1996; Willeford & Burleigh, 1985) render differential diagnosis of CAPD, learning disabilities, and attention deficit disorder especially challenging. Although the relationships among CAPD, ADHD, and learning disabilities are complex and not completely understood, new perspectives and new data may lead to some reconciliation.

Differentiating Attention Deficits and Central Auditory Processing Disorders

Although some evidence suggests that CAPD and ADHD reflect a single developmental disorder (Cook et al., 1993; Gascon et al., 1986), other data and perspectives illuminating the differences between CAPD and ADHD support the clinical utility of these diagnoses. The attention deficits of ADHD typically are pervasive and supramodal, impacting more than one sensory modality (Keller, 1992). In contrast, individuals with CAPD experience attention deficits that may be restricted to the auditory modality. Moreover, the multimodality attention deficits associated with ADHD seem to be restricted to sustained attention (Hooks, Milich, & Lorch, 1994; Seidel & Joschko, 1990), in contrast to the selective (focused) and divided auditory attention deficits that characterize CAPD (Cherry, 1980; Jerger & Jerger, 1984; Katz & Illmer, 1972; Keith, 1986; Lasky & Tobin, 1973). Indeed, the commonly observed left ear deficit on dichotic speech tests seen in individuals with CAPD, as well as their depressed auditory performance under conditions of either contralateral or ipsilateral competition as a function of the level of brain dysfunction, argues against a pervasive attention deficit in CAPD and further distinguishes CAPD from ADHD (Jerger et al., 1988; Musiek, Kibbe, & Baran, 1984; Musiek et al., 1994). Inclusion of a recently released test of sustained auditory attention (vigilance) in the central auditory test battery (Keith, 1994b) should prove helpful in substantiating this distinction.

Differences between CAPD and ADHD are demarcated further by the recent shift in conceptualization of ADHD as a disorder of behavioral regulation rather than attention (Barkley, 1990). Consistent with this reconceptualization, the symptoms of impulsivity and behavioral disinhibition result from neurologically based, "developmental deficiencies in the regulation and maintenance of behavior by rules and consequences" (Barkley, 1990, p. 71). Deficits in rule-governed behavior, resulting from either elevated arousal thresholds (Zentall, 1985) or elevated reinforcement thresholds (Haenlein & Caul, 1987), lead to problems initiating, inhibiting, or sustaining responses to tasks or stimuli (Barkley, 1990). These deficits lead to problems in executive functioning and self-regulation (Barkley, 1990). ADHD is seen, essentially, as a motivational deficit, rather than an attention deficit (Barkley, 1990). In addition to clarifying the nature of ADHD, this reconceptualization centered on poor rule-governed behavior may explain the self-control problems, social skill deficits, and language disorders so frequently observed in ADHD (Augustine & Damico, 1995).

The shifting conceptualization of attention deficit disorders is reflected in the diagnostic subtypes specified in the current *Diagnostic and Statistical Manual of Mental Disorders* (DSM-IV) (APA, 1994). Based on factor analytic studies justifying subgrouping symptoms (Lahey, Schaughency, Hynd, Carlson, & Nieves, 1987; Schaughency & Hynd, 1989; Shaywitz, Fletcher, & Shaywitz, 1994a), the DSM-IV identifies diagnostic criteria for three attention deficit subtypes (APA, 1994). The Combined Type represents attention deficit characterized by hyperactivity-impulsivity and inattention. The Predominantly Inattentive Type presents primary symptoms of inattention. The Predominantly Hyperactive-Impulsive Type presents a primary behavioral regulation disorder and has no precedent in the DSM system. More precise diagnosis of attention deficit using the DSM-IV subtypes may further elucidate distinctions between CAPD and ADHD.

Notwithstanding overlapping symptomatology, clinicians seem able to distinguish behavioral profiles for CAPD and ADHD. In fact, a recent study showed that pediatricians and audiologists view the predominant symptoms of ADHD and CAPD as being rather distinct, with the only strongly shared overlap between groups being inattention and distractibility (Seikel et al., 1996). CAPD was characterized by a selective attention deficit and associated language processing and academic difficulties; ADHD was characterized by inappropriate motor activity, restlessness, and socially inappropriate interaction patterns (Seikel et al., 1996). Other investigators have reported that behavior problems, such as difficulty waiting one's turn and playing quietly and excessive talking, more often characterize children with ADHD than CAPD (Newhoff et al., 1992). Similarly, severe socioemotional sequelae (i.e., conduct disorders, juvenile delinquency) are more common among children with ADHD (Newhoff et al., 1992).

Reconciling the Comorbidity of Attention Deficits and Central Auditory Processing Disorders

By definition, CAPD, ADHD, and learning disabilities are heterogeneous conditions. Clearly, the heterogeneity of the clinical groups identified under these diagnostic labels could render an impression of comorbidity across these disorders, given the range and overlap of performance profiles and etiologies covered by these labels (ASHA, 1996; Goodyear & Hynd, 1992; Hynd et al., 1990; National Joint Committee on Learning Disabilities, 1991). Assuming that these conditions reflect distinct developmental disabilities, however, other factors could both underlie their comorbidity and suggest the clinical distinctiveness of these developmental disorders.

There is no question that, insofar as attention is essential to higher level processing, poor attention can compromise listening. The inability to focus sufficient attention on auditory stimuli might cause auditory processing deficits. Conversely, deficient auditory processing might impair attention. Whether auditory processing deficit causes some attention deficit or a more global attention deficit impedes auditory processing is pivotal to understanding the relationship between the attention deficits of ADHD and CAPD.

Conceptualizing the relationship between attention and auditory processing within the top-down and bottom-up processing models provides a theoretical framework that clarifies the nature of the relationship between ADHD and CAPD (Musiek & Chermak, 1995). According to a bottom-up model, attention is driven by incoming sensory stimulation and garnered by properly integrated and processed sensory stimuli (Musiek & Chermak, 1995). If the acoustic stimuli are not properly processed, as occurs in CAPD, then optimal attention cannot be focused on these stimuli in a timely manner (Phillips, 1990). Consistent with a bottom-up model, therefore, attention deficits are secondary to auditory perceptual processing deficits. In contrast, a top-down model posits CAPD as a manifestation of a global attention deficit. While recognizing that bidirectional interactions between central auditory processing and attention are probably necessary for optimal listening comprehension, the limited evidence available from basic science supports a bottom-up view of attention deficits whereby deficiencies in auditory perceptual processes trigger attention deficits (Musiek & Chermak, 1995). Consistent with this perspective, listening difficulties seen in CAPD result from specific auditory perceptual deficencies rather than global attention deficits (Phillips, 1990, 1995; Tallal et al., 1996).

In essence, the observed comorbidity of CAPD and ADHD may result from attention deficits at different levels of sensory and global dysfunction. Although information processing models may provide some insight regarding the relationship between the attention deficits of ADHD and CAPD, results of neuroimaging studies (e.g., magnetic resonance imaging, electroencephalography) and postmortem studies implicate a neurological basis for the often observed co-occurrence of CAPD, auditory attention deficits, hyperactivity/impulsivity, and learning disabilities.

Postmortem studies have documented brain abnormalities involving auditory regions of the brain in children with learning disabilities (Galaburda & Eidelberg, 1982; Galaburda & Kemper, 1978). Brain imaging studies have revealed morphologic and structural differences in the auditory/language and motor regulation/behavioral inhibition areas of the brains of children with ADHD, as compared with the brains of normal children (Hynd & Semrud-Clikeman, 1989; Hynd et al., 1990; Lou et al., 1989; Mann et al., 1992; Voeller, 1991; Zametkin et al., 1990).

In particular, the planum temporale, insula, and auditory area of the corpus callosum were reported to be significantly smaller on the left or both sides of the brain in children with ADHD, as compared with the control group of children. Hynd (personal communication, 1992) indicated that the morphology of Heschl's gyrus may also differ in children with ADHD, as compared with normal controls. Hynd et al. (1990) reported decreased right frontal lobe width in children with ADHD relative to the control group of children. Lou et al. (1989) reported decreased metabolism in the caudate nucleus associated with ADHD. Mann et al. (1992) found increased slow wave activity in the frontal regions and decreased beta activity in the temporal regions in boys with ADHD, compared to normal control subjects. Morphological differences and possible dysfunction in areas of the brain associated with motor regulation and self-control (e.g., frontal region, caudate nucleus, insula) and auditory/language functions (e.g., temporal region, auditory area of the corpus callosum) offer a neurobiological basis for co-occurring central auditory deficits and behavioral regulation problems in ADHD.

In summary, we have attempted to explain both the distinctiveness and co-occurrence of CAPD and ADHD. At the most basic level, broad definitions may contribute to the apparent comorbidity of these disorders. More important, however, the distributed nature of information processing and underlying brain activation explains overlapping behavioral deficits. We have seen, however, that overlapping behavioral profiles do not necessarily implicate common antecedents. The sustained attention problems observed in ADHD probably result from a supramodal, cognitive deficit. (Alternatively, as discussed above, inattention in ADHD may reflect deficiencies in behavioral regulation rather than attention per se.) In contrast, the selective auditory attention deficits of CAPD result from deficient auditory perceptual processing. Similarly, difficulty following directions is commonly observed among individuals with ADHD and CAPD; however, deficiencies in rule-governed behavior may underlie these difficulties in ADHD, whereas deficient central auditory processing of auditory signals may underlie the same performance deficit in CAPD. Executive dysfunction, as discussed below, may also underlie the resemblance in clinical profiles seen across CAPD, ADHD, and learning disabilities.

Implications for Assessment and Intervention

Additional research is needed to resolve questions surrounding comorbidity. Although extant information processing models and results of neuroimaging studies seem to support both the comorbidity and distinctiveness of the spectrum of disorders we have discussed, additional research is needed to determine conclusively the neurological mechanisms and associated behavioral criteria consistent with a particular diagnostic category. Such information will improve differential diagnosis across the comorbid conditions as well as within the category of ADHD, where a unidimensional perspective on diagnosis has been shown to be inadequate in explaining behavior (Goodyear & Hynd, 1992; Schaughency & Hynd, 1989). Moreover, more definitive diagnostic information should lead to more effective intervention.

Perhaps we will find that these disorders are not truly distinct, but rather reflect differences in expression of a single developmental disorder. We may even see the dissolution of ADHD as a diagnostic category as researchers document problems with the ADHD construct and challenge its validity as a psychiatric disorder (Prior & Sanson, 1986; Reid, Maag, & Vasa, 1993; Rutter & Tuma, 1988). There are actually no empirical markers that identify children with ADHD (Gordon, 1991; Reid et al., 1993; E. Taylor, 1986). The defining characteristics of ADHD are subjective, poorly defined, frequently changing, and disconnected from any theoretical construct or empirical base (Goodman & Poillion, 1992; Maag & Reid, 1994; Reid et al., 1993). Perhaps the basic developmental disorder often labeled as ADHD, particularly the predominantly inattentive type, may in fact be CAPD, which can be identified and quantified using objective criteria.

These circumstances underscore the importance of thorough evaluations using sensitive measures to discern more subtle variations in performance. Given the current uncertainty regarding diagnostic validity of ADHD and the comorbidity across the spectrum of disorders discussed in this chapter, clinicians must accept the challenge to evaluate the integrity of underlying perceptual, linguistic, and cognitive systems to determine the predominant and primary deficits, as well as secondary problems (McFarland & Cacace, 1995). Such an approach requires the interdisciplinary efforts of audiologists, speech-language pathologists, teachers, psychologists, and physicians for assessment and most likely for intervention.

EXECUTIVE FUNCTION

Executive functioning, a component of metacognition, refers to a set of general control processes which ensure that an individual's behavior is adaptive, consistent with some goal, and beneficial to the individual (Borkowski, Milstead, & Hale, 1988; Brown, Bransford, Ferrara, & Campione, 1983; Denckla, 1996; Sternberg, 1985; Torgesen, 1996). Executive functions underlie problem solving and learning (Borkowski & Burke, 1996; Welsh & Pennington, 1988). They are the control processes that coordinate knowledge (i.e., cognition) and metacognitive knowledge, transforming such knowledge into behavioral strategies based on task analyses, planning, and reflective decision making (Barkley, 1996; Butterfield & Albertson, 1995). Executive functions are crucial to learning and problem solving, psychosocial function including self-image, and goal-directed behaviors, including listening (Borkowski & Burke, 1996; Grattan, Bloomer, Archambault, & Eslinger, 1994; Grattan & Eslinger, 1992). Implementing executive functions places significant demands on attention and memory, requiring both sustained and selective attention to enable sensory and perceptual processing of events, both those internal and external to the individual, as well as memory to register, store, and make knowledge and experience available to the individual (Barkley, 1996; Butterfield & Albertson, 1995; Pennington, Bennetto, McAleer, & Roberts, 1996).

Synchronized activation across multiple cortical and subcortical regions, including the frontal lobe, temporal lobe, parietal lobe, basal ganglia, and thalamus, subserves executive functioning (Eslinger & Grattan, 1993; Goldenberg, Oder, Spatt, & Podreka, 1992). Many of the neural networks thought to underlie executive function follow a prolonged course of postnatal development, extending into adolescence and perhaps continuing into adulthood (St. James-Roberts, 1979; Thatcher, 1991; Yakelov & Lecours, 1967); therefore, the system is highly vulnerable to disruption from a variety of causes, including neurobiological stressors, as well as environmental deprivation (Barkley, 1996).

Given the pervasive role served by executive functions, the wide variety of cognitive processes and domain-specific competencies involved in its operation, and its dependence on a large and highly vulnerable neural network, it is not surprising that executive function deficits have been described in a wide variety of clinical populations (Denckla, 1996). Indeed, executive functions have been characterized as the “final common pathway that can be altered by a wide variety of factors” (Eslinger, 1996, p. 386).

Several related disorders, and even some fairly diverse disorders with different symptomatology and different neurobiological etiologies, may manifest executive function deficits. Such deficits are frequently observed in association with brain disease or injury and may underlie childhood neurological disorders, in particular the academic problems experienced by children with learning disabilities or ADHD (Denckla, 1996; Fletcher, Taylor, Levin, & Satz, 1995; Graham & Harris, 1996; Pennington, 1991; Stanovich, 1986; Torgesen, 1994). Moreover, executive function deficits have been identified in children who do not meet eligibility criteria for learning disabilities or ADHD but experience significant difficulties in school (Denckla, 1989). The prevalence of CAPD in the latter group of children has not been determined.

Executive functioning provides a construct useful in understanding a wide range of symptoms observed across a spectrum of overlapping disorders (Pennington et al., 1996). Given the linkage between executive function, rule-governed behavior, and self-control (Hayes, Gifford, & Ruckstuhl, 1996), some have proposed executive dysfunction as the source of the behavioral regulation and inattention problems manifested in ADHD (Barkley, 1994; Denckla & Reader, 1993; Smith, Gould, Marsh, & Nichols, 1995). Similarly, as asserted by Westby and Cutler (1994), the pragmatic and metacognitive behaviors associated with communication are both language-based and rule-governed. Hence, executive dysfunction may explain language deficits in ADHD (Heyer, 1995).

Although executive dysfunction in CAPD has not been examined, it is reasonable to expect that auditory perceptual deficits impede operation of executive functions. The behaviors associated with CAPD (e.g., difficulty in organizing, monitoring, and understanding acoustic signals) suggest limited use of executive function. In contrast to the proposed causal role of executive dysfunction in ADHD (Barkley, 1994; Denckla & Reader, 1993; Smith et al., 1995), executive dysfunction in CAPD would be considered a secondary feature, not a primary cause, of listening difficulties. Such secondary deficits could, nonetheless, compound auditory processing deficits, impede generalization of strategic listening behaviors across settings, and thereby jeopardize treatment efficacy (Borkowski & Burke, 1996).

As a component of information processing theory, executive function is integral to the theoretical foundation of our comprehensive management approach, as discussed in Chapter 7.

Secondary Metacognitive Deficits in CAPD

Individuals with CAPD have deficient experience processing the auditory signal. This experiential deficit can lead to metacognitive deficits since metacognition develops through experience in a skill-based context, such as spoken language processing (Wong, 1991). Although much of the evidence documenting metacognitive strategy deficits has been collected from subjects who were described as learning disabled, subject selection criteria and histories reveal the likelihood that these subjects also presented central auditory processing deficits (Bos & Filip, 1982; Gerber, 1993c; Hallahan & Kneedler, 1979; Kotsonis & Patterson, 1980; Paris & Myers, 1981; Pressley & Levin, 1987; Suiter & Potter, 1978; Swanson, 1989, 1993; Torgesen, 1979; Torgesen & Houck, 1980; Wiens, 1983; Wong, 1987; Wong & Jones, 1982). These data coupled with clincial experience indicate that individuals with CAPD do not seem to exert executive control in deploying strategies to aid in organizing, monitoring, and understanding the acoustic signal, strategies that might facilitate information processing and enable them to compensate to some extent for the deficient central auditory processes that characterize the disorder (Chermak & Musiek, 1992; Gerber, 1993; Pressley & Levin, 1987; Suiter & Potter, 1978; Torgesen & Houck, 1980; Wong, 1987). As passive or inactive listeners, they fail to attend selectively, organize input, deploy listening comprehension strategies, maintain on-task behavior, or employ task-approach skills, including the ability to focus on relevant task information. The data reveal that these individuals present a passive and inefficient approach to problem solving (Swanson, 1989; Torgesen, 1979), a lack of metacognitive awareness (Brown et al., 1983; Hallahan & Kneedler, 1979; Paris & Myers, 1981; Swanson, 1993; Wiens, 1983), and difficulty monitoring comprehension (Bos & Filip, 1982; Kotsonis & Patterson, 1980; Wong & Jones, 1982). They tend not to deploy strategies spontaneously, often requiring external prompting to mobilize a strategy, and have difficulty choosing appropriate problem-solving devices. Less likely to activate schematic knowledge, they do not elaborate and construct information that guides comprehension (Gerber, 1993c).

Passivity and Metacognitive Deficits

Passivity and inactivity can be traced to a compromised self-system, a system that comprises self-efficacy, self-esteem, and attributions. Academic failure frequently seen in CAPD erodes motivation to learn, fosters beliefs of the futility of effortful learning, and results in low self-concept (Wong, 1991). Dysfunctional attributional patterns in which success is attributed to external factors (e.g., luck, a *nice* teacher) develop concurrently, while failure is attributed to internal factors such as inability (Pearl, 1982). These faulty beliefs and attributions engender low self-esteem and self-efficacy. Not unexpectedly, these individuals will avoid the challenging task of listening, particularly in competing backgrounds or when the message is otherwise degraded or difficult to sort. Moreover, they will fatigue and give up prematurely under these circumstances, failing to invoke listening strategies to meet task demands and achieve success. Because deployment of self-regulatory behavior depends on motivation, this sequence of events leads to deficits in executive functions and a passive approach to listening.

Implications for Intervention

Metacognitive deficits in individuals with CAPD are secondary deficits resulting from repeated failure and lack of task persistence, limited use of executive function, inadequate experience with successful listening strategies, and low motivation. Fortunately, metacognitive deficits are responsive to intervention directed toward informed strategy use (Borkowski, Weyhing, & Carr, 1988; Brown et al., 1983; Fabricus & Hagen, 1984; Kendall & Braswell, 1982; Moynahan, 1978; Paris, Newman, & McVey, 1982; Reid & Borkowski, 1987. If left untreated, metacognitive deficits can exacerbate the impact of CAPD for spoken language understanding; with treatment, individuals with CAPD can become skilled listeners who actively engage in discovering what speakers are communicating. To achieve this goal they must be trained to use their metacognitive knowledge and strategies (i.e., executive function) to regulate and guide their listening and extraction of information from the spoken message (Chermak & Musiek, 1992).

Comprehensive treatment of CAPD demands attention to both first-order problems of deficient central auditory processes and second-order metacognitive deficits. Limited success in directly altering deficient central auditory processes has led to increased emphasis on metacognitive interventions (Chermak & Musiek, 1992). The use of metacognitive strategies and instruction for CAPD remediation is detailed in Chapter 8. Additional discussion of future research needs in this area is presented in Chapter 10.

PREVALENCE OF CAPD

Prevalence data for CAPD are lacking. Although numerous reports have appeared consistently in the literature describing auditory perceptual and auditory processing deficits associated with a variety of conditions, no authoritative estimates of the prevalence of CAPD are currently available, with the exception of two studies of older adults.

CAPD was seen in 70% of clinical patients over age 60 years (Stach et al., 1990). In contrast, prevalence of CAPD in older adults was estimated at 10 to 20% based on a stratified random sample of the U.S. population (Cooper & Gates, 1991).

A large number of children, adults, and older adults present symptoms/complaints suggestive of CAPD and are referred for central auditory testing. Confirmation of CAPD is made in a substantial number of these cases. As noted previously, CAPD is frequently reported in association with a history of chronic otitis media (Brown, 1994; Gravel & Wallace, 1992; Hall & Grose, 1993, 1994; Hall et al., 1994, 1995; Jerger et al., 1983; Moore et al., 1991; Pillsbury et al., 1991; Silva et al., 1986), learning disabilities (Breedin et al., 1989; Elliott & Hammer, 1988; Ferre & Wilber, 1986; Jerger et al., 1987; Willeford, 1980, 1985), language impairment (Keith et al., 1989; Tallal et al., 1993; Tallal & Piercy, 1974; Tallal, Stark, & Curtiss, 1976), and attention deficit disorders (Cook et al., 1993; Gascon et al., 1986; Musiek et al., 1984; Pillsbury et al., 1995). CAPD also has been reported in association with voice disorders, autism, stuttering, aphasia, Alzheimer's disease, multiple sclerosis, traumatic brain injury, and psychiatric disorders (Bruder, 1983; Chedru et al., 1978; Divenyi & Robinson, 1989; Efron, 1963; Grimes et al., 1985; Meyers, Hughes, & Schoeny, 1989; Mohr et al., 1990; Robin et al., 1990; Saniga & Carlin, 1991; Strouse, Hall, & Burger, 1995). Given the diverse clinical populations in which CAPD is observed, and in particular, the suggested linkage between CAPD and the rather prevalent otitis media, learning disabilities, and attention deficit disorders, one might expect a fairly significant prevalence rate for CAPD among children and adolescents.

In the absence of specific prevalence data, it may be useful to estimate the frequency of occurrence of CAPD by examining prevalence data for comorbid disorders. Second only to the common cold, otitis media with effusion is the most prevalent illness of early childhood (Teele, Klein, & Roesner, 1989). By 3 years of age, 70% of children will have experienced one or more episodes of otitis media, with over 30% experiencing three or more bouts (Teele et al., 1989). Children with histories of early otitis media demonstrate auditory processing deficits, in particular processing auditory information in background competition, as well as behavioral, attentional, and learning deficits in the classroom (Feagans, Sanyal, Henderson, Collier, & Appelbaum, 1987; Gravel & Wallace, 1992, 1995; Roberts et al., 1989).

The prevalence of learning disabilities in school-age children ranges from 5 to 10% (Interagency Committee on Learning Disabilities, 1987). In fact, nearly half of the children enrolled in federally supported special education programs receive services for learning disabilities (U.S. Department of Education, 1990). Language disorders are quite prevalent (70 to 80%) among youngsters diagnosed with learning disabilities (Wiig, & Semel, 1994), as is CAPD (Breedin et al., 1989; Chermak et al., 1989; Elliott & Hammer, 1988; Ferre & Wilber, 1986; Jerger et al., 1987; Musiek, Gollegly, Lamb, & Lamb, 1990).

ADHD is cited as the most commmon neurobehavioral disorder of childhood, affecting some 3 to 5% of children aged 2 to 8 years (APA, 1994) and as many as 10 to 20% of the school-age population (Shaywitz & Shaywitz, 1988; Szatmari, Boyle, & Offord, 1989). Moreover, estimates of the comorbidity of ADHD and language disorders and/or learning disabilities indicate that between 50% and 70% of children with ADHD also present significant language problems (Goldstein & Goldstein, 1990). Seventeen to 38% of children diagnosed with language disorders also present ADHD (Bleitchman, Hood, & Inglis, 1990; Cantwell & Baker, 1985; Cantwell, Baker, & Mattison, 1979). It is also estimated that between 25 to 50% of children with ADHD present learning disabilities (August & Garfinkel, 1990; Barkley, 1990). Estimates of ADHD among individuals with learning disabilities range between 25% (Holborow & Berry, 1986) to as high as 80% (Safer & Allen, 1976).

Recognizing that learning disabilities and attention deficits persist throughout an individual's life (Adelman & Vogel, 1991; Barkley, 1990; Bashir & Scavuzzo, 1992; National Joint Committee on Learning Disabilities, 1991), it is reasonable to speculate that CAPD identified in youngsters may persist throughout life. On the other hand, there is no reason to expect that older adults with CAPD presented these deficits as youngsters. Hence, we are left with scant data on which to project the prevalence of CAPD. Nonetheless, based on clinical reports, prevalence data available for comorbid conditions, and the authors' clinical experience, we estimate the prevalence of CAPD in children as between 2 to 3%.

SUMMARY

CAPD refers to an observed deficit in one or more of the central auditory processes responsible for generating auditory evoked potentials and the following behaviors: sound localization or lateralization; auditory discrimination; auditory pattern recognition; temporal aspects of audition including, temporal resolution, temporal masking, temporal integration, and temporal ordering; auditory performance with competing acoustic signals; auditory performance with degraded acoustic signals (ASHA, 1996). Although only minimal prevalence data for CAPD are available, CAPD is observed in diverse clinical populations, including those with known lesions or pathology of the central nervous system (e.g., aphasia, Alzheimer's disease, traumatic brain injury) and those where underlying central nervous system pathology or neuromorphological disorder is suspected but unconfirmed (e.g., developmental language disorder, dyslexia, learning disabilities, and attention deficit disorder). The majority of pediatric CAPD probably results from neuromorphological disorder (Musiek et al., 1985; Musiek & Gollegly, 1988; Musiek et al., 1990). Maturational delay and neurologic disorders probably account for a smaller percentage of CAPD (Musiek et al., 1985).

The apparent linkages among the comorbid conditions of CAPD, ADHD, language impairment, and learning disabilities have led to questions concerning causality and the validity of these diagnoses (Campbell & McNeil, 1985; Cook et al., 1993; Gascon et al., 1986; Lubert, 1981; Rees, 1973, 1981; Tallal et al., 1996). Although the primacy of any one of these complex disorders as causal to another remains unclear, consideration of recent data from brain imaging studies, as well as new perspectives on primary and secondary sources of attention, behavioral regulation, and auditory processing deficits, should advance our understanding and improve differential diagnosis and intervention programming. In particular, the possibility that executive dysfunction may be a common link associated with or underlying deficits presented across these comorbid disorders merits further study.

The current model of central auditory processing, whereby a listener actively controls processing and essentially constructs the message, requires reciprocity between bottom-up (i.e., data driven) and top-down (i.e., contextual) processes. This model and the implication of both first-order central auditory processing deficits, as well as second-order metacognitive deficits, in CAPD necessitate comprehensive intervention programming targeting development of both basic auditory and metalinguistic skills and metacognitive strategies.

SUGGESTED READINGS

Baran, J.A., & Musiek, F.E. (1991). Behavioral assessment of the central auditory nervous system. In W.F. Rintelmann (Ed.), *Hearing Assessment* (pp. 549–602). Austin: Pro-Ed.

Berrick, J.M., Shubow, G.F., Schultz, M.C., Freed, H., Fournier, S.R., & Hughes, J.P. (1984). Auditory processing tests for children: Normative and clinical results on the SSW Test. *Journal of Speech and Hearing Disorders, 49*, 318–325.

Carmon, A., & Nachshon, I. (1971). Effect of unilateral brain damage on perception of temporal order. *Cortex, 7*, 410–418.

Galaburda, A.M., Sherman, G. F., Rosen, G.D., Aboitz, F., & Geshwind, N. (1985). Developmental dyslexia: Four consecutive patients with cortical anomalies. *Annals of Neurology, 18*, 222–233.

Hall, J.W. III (1992). *Handbook of auditory evoked responses.* Boston: Allyn and Bacon.

Hughes, L.F., Tobey, E.A., & Miller, C.J. (1983). Temporal aspects of dichotic listening in brain-damaged subjects. *Ear and Hearing, 4*(6), 306–310.

Hynd, G.W., Semrud-Clikeman, M., & Lyytinen, H. (1991). Brain imaging in learning disabilities. In J.E. Obrzut, & G.W. Hynd (Eds.), *Neuropsychological foundations of learning disabilities* (pp. 475–511). San Diego: Academic Press.

Jacobson, J.T., Deppe, U., & Murray, T.J. (1983). Dichotic paradigms in multiple sclerosis. *Ear and Hearing, 4*(6), 311–317.

Jerger, S., Jerger, J., Alford, B.R., & Abrams, S. (1983). Development of speech intelligibility in children with recurrent otitis media. *Ear and Hearing, 4*, 138–145.

Kass, C., & Myklebust, H. (1969). Learning disability: An educational definition. *Journal of Learning Disabilities, 2*, 38–40.

Katz, J. (1983). Phonemic synthesis. In E.Z. Lasky & J. Katz (Eds.), *Central auditory processing disorders: Problems of speech, language and learning* (pp. 269–296). Baltimore: University Park Press.

Keith, R. W., & Jerger, S. (1991). Central auditory disorders. In J.T. Jacobson, & J. L. Northern (Eds.), *Diagnostic audiology* (pp. 235–250). Austin, TX: Pro-ed.

Lou, H.C., Henriksen, L., & Bruhn, P. (1984). Focal cerebral hypoperfusion in children with dysphasia and/or attention deficit disorder. *Archives of Neurology, 41*, 825–829.

Lynn, G.E., & Gilroy, J. (1977). Evaluation of central auditory dysfunction in patients with neurological disorders. In R.W. Keith (Ed.), *Central auditory dysfunction* (pp. 177–221). New York: Grune & Stratton.

Lynn, G.E., Gilroy, J., Taylor, P.C., & Leiser, R.P. (1981). Binaural masking-level differences in neurological disorders. *Archives of Otolaryngology, 107*, 357–362.

Musiek, F.E. (1983). The evaluation of brainstem disorders using ABR and central auditory test. *Monographs in Contemporary Audiology, 4,* 1–24.

Musiek, F.E., & Baran, J.A. (1987). Central auditory assessment: Thirty years of challenge and change. *Ear and Hearing, 8*(Suppl. 4), 22–35.

Musiek, F.E., Gollegly, K., & Baran, J. (1984). Myelination of the corpus callosum and auditory processing problems in children: Theoretical and clinical correlates. *Seminars in Hearing, 5*, 231–242.

Pillsbury, H.C., Grose, J.H., & Hall, J.W. (1991). Otitis media with effusion in children: Binaural hearing before and after corrective surgery. *Archives of Otolaryngology—Head and Neck Surgery, 117,* 718–723.

Pinheiro, M. (1977). Tests of central auditory function in children with learning disabilities. In R. Keith (Ed.), *Central auditory dysfunction* (pp. 223–256). New York: Grune & Stratton.

Sanchez-Longo, L.P., & Forster, F.M. (1958). Clinical significance of impairment of sound localization. *Neurology, 8,* 119–125.

Smith, B.B., & Resnick, D.M. (1972). An auditory test for assessing brain stem integrity: Preliminary report. *Laryngoscope, 82,* 414–424.

Sparks, R., Goodglass, H., & Nichel, B. (1970). Ipsilateral versus contralateral extinction in dichotic listening resulting from hemisphere lesions. *Cortex, 6,* 249–260.

Stubblefield, J.H., & Young, C.E. (1975). Central auditory dysfunction in learning disabled children. *Journal of Learning Disabilities, 8,* 32–37.

Swisher, L.P., & Hirsh, I.J. (1972). Brain damage and the ordering of two temporally successive stimuli. *Neuropsychologia, 10,* 137–152.

Tallal, P., & Piercy, M. (1975). Developmental aphasia: The perception of brief vowels and extended consonants. *Neuropsychologia, 13,* 69–74.

Tallal, P., Stark, R., & Curtiss, B. (1976). The relation between speech perception impairment and speech production impairment in children with developmental dysphasia. *Brain and Language, 3,* 305–317.

Toscher, M.M., & Rupp, R. R. (1978). A study of the central auditory processes in stutterers using the synthetic sentence identification (SSI) test battery. *Journal of Speech and Hearing Research, 21,* 779–792.

Wetherby, A.M., Koegel, R.L., & Mendel, M. (1981). Central nervous system dysfunction in echolaic autistic individuals. *Journal of Speech and Hearing Research, 24,* 420–429.

Yozawitz, A., Bruder, G., Sutton, S., Sharpe, L., Gurland, B., Fleiss, J., & Costa, L. (1979) Dichotic perception: Evidence for right hemisphere dysfunction in affective psychosis. *British Journal of Psychiatry, 135,* 224–237.

CHAPTER 2

NEUROBIOLOGY OF THE CENTRAL AUDITORY NERVOUS SYSTEM RELEVANT TO CENTRAL AUDITORY PROCESSING

Neurochemistry/pharmacology, anatomy and physiology are all important in discussing the central auditory system. This chapter is divided into two main segments: one relevant to assessment, the second to rehabilitation. We have translated basic science concepts and data into a clinical language, and draw practical and theoretical correlates between basic and clinical information. This important but difficult task aids in overall understanding, hopefully without compromising factual data.

Neuroanatomy, neurophysiology and neurochemistry underlie clinical aspects of central auditory assessment and management. A clinician's diagnostic skills in this area of audiology depend on how well he or she understands the neurobiology of the central auditory nervous system (CANS). Audiologists and speech-language pathologists are challenged by the clinical aspects of central auditory processing disorders (CAPD), which require an understanding of the intricacies of hearing and the brain. Clinicians have access to more information than ever in the area of neuroscience as it relates to communication and its disorders. Unfortunately, many audiologists and speech-language pathologists do not or cannot take advantage of the new information on brain structure and function. As a result, patients with CAPD may not receive the best possible treatment. The clinician's recognition of the critical importance of knowledge of CANS structure and function is the first step in improving the ability to manage people with CAPD.

THE BRAINSTEM

The Afferent Brainstem Auditory Pathway: The Cochlear Nucleus

The auditory nerve, which is composed of type-I and type-II fibers, enters the brainstem on the lateral posterior aspect of the pontomedullary junction and projects to the cochlear nuclear complex. The type-I fibers are myelinated and connect to inner hair cells, while the type II-fibers are unmyelinated and connect to outer hair cells. Type-I fibers make up 95% of all the auditory nerve fibers in the auditory nerve trunk. The cochlear nucleus (CN) is divided into three main segments: the anterior ventral cochlear nucleus (AVCN), the posterior ventral cochlear nucleus (PVCN), and the dorsal cochlear nucleus. Fibers of the auditory nerve enter this complex at the junction of the AVCN and PVCN, with each fiber dividing to send branches to the three individual nuclei (Schuknecht, 1974) (Figure 2–1).

The CN is composed of multiple cell types, including pyramidal, fusiform, octopus, stellate, and spherical cells (Pfeiffer, 1966). These cells are grouped into certain areas of the CN. These cells can modify incoming neural impulses in a characteristic fashion, thus providing the foundation for coding information by the type of neural activity within the CN. Each poststimulatory histogram shows the average response of a given neural unit over time to a series of short tones presented at the unit's characteristic frequency (Rhode, 1985). The major response patterns include the following: primary-like, which is an initial spike followed by a steady response until the stimulus stops; the chopper post-stimulatory histogram, which is an extremely fast oscillatory neural response to the stimulus; the onset response, which is a single initial spike to the stimulus onset; and the pauser response, which is similar to the primary-like response, although it ceases soon after the initial spike and resumes a graded response (Kiang, 1975). There is also the "build-up" response, which is

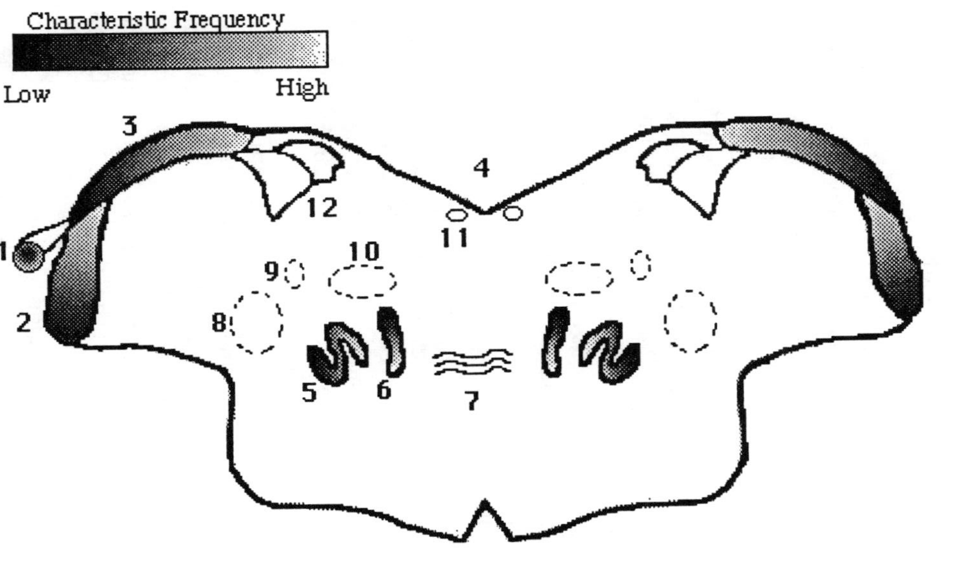

Figure 2–1. A cross section of the brainstem at the level of the ponto-medullary junction at the caudal-most pons.

a gradual increase in cell firing during the presentation of a stimulus (Kiang, 1975; Rhode, 1985). Agreement has been found between the type of cell and the pattern of response, suggesting important relationships between the anatomy (structure) and physiology (function) of cells within the CN. These poststimulatory histograms from the CN provide insight about the complex processing of auditory information at the CN such as the precise timing needed in localizing and identifying interaural time differences (see Rhode, 1991).

Fibers of the auditory nerve entering the CN are arrayed in systematic fashion in each division of the CN, thus maintaining the frequency arrangement relayed from the cochlea (Sando, 1965; Webster, 1971). This tonotopic organization is seen in all three divisions of the CN, with low frequencies represented ventrolaterally and high frequencies represented dorsomedially within each nucleus (Sando, 1965; Webster, 1971). Some tuning curves derived from AVCN units using tone bursts are similar in shape to those of the auditory nerve (Rose, Galambos, & Hughes, 1959). Because some CN fibers yield wider tuning curves than those of auditory nerve fibers (Moller, 1985), one might conclude that CN units may preserve but not necessarily enhance frequency resolution of acoustic information coming from the auditory nerve.

The CN lies in the area of the cerebellopontine angle, which is a lateral recess formed at the juncture of the pons, medulla, and cerebellum. Tumors in this area often affect the CN and may cause central auditory deficits. However, the cerebellopontine angle is sufficiently large to accommodate lesions of sizable mass without compromising neural function (Musiek & Gollegly, 1985; Musiek, Kibbe-Michael, Geurkink, Josey, & Glasscock, 1986).

The CN is unique among brainstem auditory structures because the only afferent input is ipsilateral, and comes from the cochlea via the auditory nerve. Damage to the CN can result in ipsilateral pure tone deficits (Dublin, 1976, 1985; Matkin & Carhart, 1966), and may mimic auditory nerve dysfunction (Jerger & Jerger, 1974). Because the CN is on the posterolateral surface of the brainstem, it often is affected directly by extra-axial tumors, such as acoustic neuromas (Dublin, 1976; Musiek & Kibbe-Michael, 1986; Nodar & Kinney, 1980).

Within the CN a fiber pathway called the tuberculo-ventral tract connects the dorsal CN and ventral CN. This tract is thought to be primarily inhibitory in nature (Ortel, personal communication, 1990). Three primary neural tracts project from the CN complex to the superior olivary complex (SOC) and higher levels of the CANS (Figure 2–2).

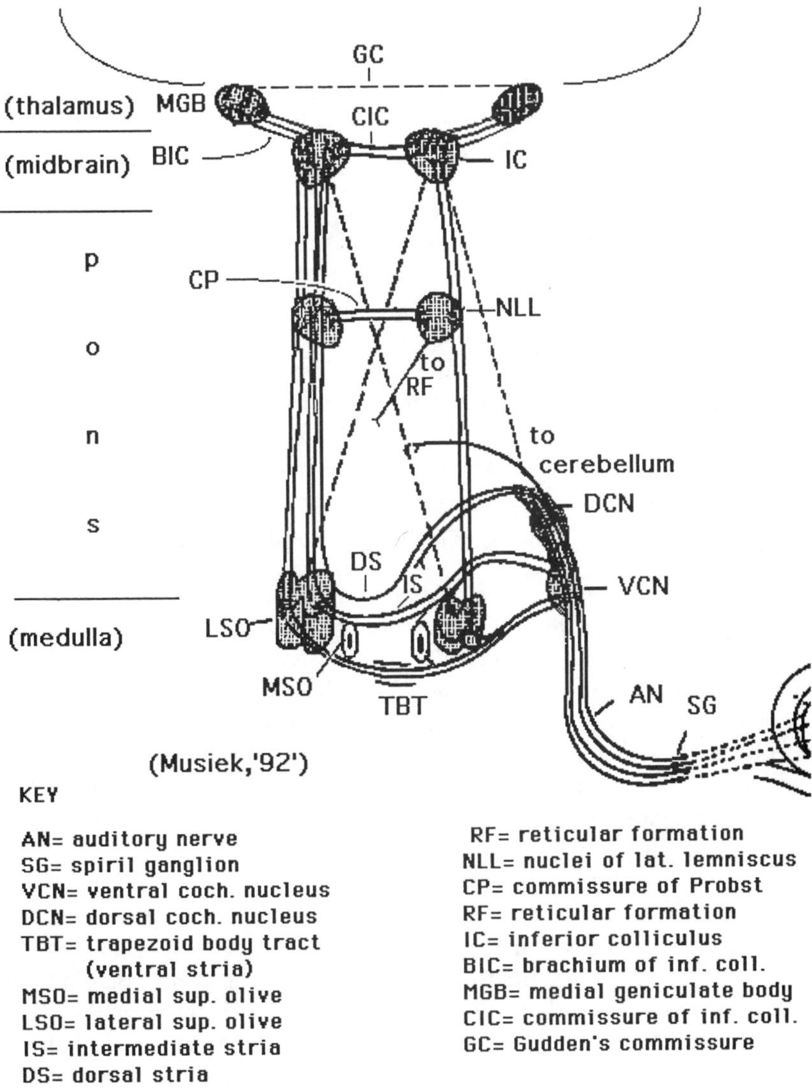

Figure 2–2. The main auditory pathways in the brainstem.

The dorsal acoustic stria is a large fiber tract that originates in the dorsal CN and projects contralaterally to the SOC, lateral lemniscus (Whitfield, 1967), and inferior colliculus (IC) (Kiang, 1975). The intermediate acoustic stria arises from the PVCN and communicates with the contralateral lateral lemniscus (ventral nucleus) and the central nucleus of the contralateral IC (Kiang, 1975). The largest tract, the ventral acoustic stria, emanates from the AVCN and melds with the trapezoid body as it approaches the midline of the brainstem (Whitfield, 1967). The ventral stria projects contralaterally to the SOC and other nuclear groups along the lateral lemniscus. Although these three tracts constitute the primary afferent pathways from the CN, other fibers project ipsilaterally from each division of the CN. Some of these synapse at the SOC and nuclei of the lateral lemniscus within the pons. Others bypass the SOC and the nuclei of the lateral lemniscus, and synapse at the IC only. The dorsal CN also sends a tract of fibers directly to the cerebellum (Whitfield, 1967). Although a variety of neural tracts project from the CN to both the ipsilateral and contralateral sides, the contralateral pathways carry the greatest number of fibers (Noback, 1985).

Superior Olivary Complex

The SOC is located in the caudal portion of the pons, ventral and medial to the CN (Noback, 1985). Although numerous groups of nuclei exist within the SOC (Figure 2–1), only five will be discussed here: the lateral superior olivary nucleus (LSO), the medial superior olivary nucleus (MSO), the nucleus of the trapezoid body, and the lateral and the medial preolivary nuclei. In some animal species the largest and most distinct nucleus is the s-shaped LSO (Moore, 1987). However, evidence suggests that in humans the MSO is the largest of these nuclei (Brugge & Geisler, 1978).

The LSO is innervated bilaterally (Strominger & Hurwitz, 1976) with ipsilateral input from the AVCN, and contralateral innervation from both the AVCN and PVCN (Warr, 1966). The MSO also receives both ipsilateral and contralateral input from the AVCN (Strominger & Strominger, 1971). Although afferent input to the trapezoid body is not understood fully, a major contribution appears to come from the contralateral CN (Strominger & Hurwitz, 1976). Innervation of the lateral and the medial preolivary nuclei is unclear and apparently differs among species, but may come primarily from the ipsilateral AVCN (Strominger & Hurwitz, 1976).

The SOC is a complex relay station in the auditory pathway, and the first (but not only) place where a variety of ipsilateral and contralateral input provides the system with the anatomical basis for unique functions in binaural listening (Willeford & Burleigh, 1985). Interaural time (Masterson, Thompson, Bechtold, & Robards, 1975) and intensity (Boudreau & Tsuchitani, 1970) differences reflected in inputs to the SOC are primary determinants of sound localization. Further, the convergence of neural information from each ear assigns the SOC a critical role in listening tasks that require the integration and interpretation of binaurally presented signals. For example, audiologic tests, such as rapidly alternating speech perception and the binaural fusion test, depend on binaural integration and the interaction of information by the SOC (Tobin, 1985). These tests often yield abnormal results in cases of SOC pathology or degradation of the signal prior to its reaching the SOC (Matzker, 1959). The measurement of masking level differences (MLDs), a sensitive index of brainstem integrity, also requires binaural interaction (Lynn, Gilroy, Taylow, & Leiser, 1981). Temporal cueing at the SOC is critical in MLDs because changing the phase of the stimulus (tones or speech) in the presence of noise results in a change in the ability to detect the signal. Several studies show that low-brainstem lesions affect MLDs, although lesions in the upper brainstem or auditory cortex do not (Cullen & Thompson, 1974; Lynn et al., 1981), which further underscores the role of the SOC in measurement of MLDs and the fusion of binaural signals.

The SOC also appears to be an important relay station in the reflex arc of the acoustic stapedius muscle reflex (Borg, 1973). Although the neurophysiology of the acoustic reflex is still not understood completely (Hall, 1985), it is believed that the reflex involves both direct and indirect neural pathways (Musiek & Baran, 1986). The direct reflex arc appears to consist of a three- or four-neuron chain that is activated when one or both ears are stimulated with sufficiently intense sound. Neural impulses are conducted to the AVCN via the auditory nerve and from there to the ipsilateral MSO and/or facial nerve nucleus. Crossed input appears to come from the AVCN to the contralateral MSO via the trapezoid body. Neurons arising in and around the MSO terminate in the region of the motor nucleus of the facial nerve, from which motor fibers descend to innervate the stapedius muscle. Hence, acoustic stimulation in one ear results in bilateral stapedius muscle contractions (Borg, 1973).

The existence of an indirect pathway for the acoustic reflex has been postulated. Borg (1973) speculated that the indirect reflex arc is a slower polysynaptic pathway which may include the extrapyramidal system of the reticular formation. Despite the lack of complete specification of the neural pathways involved in the reflex arc, considerable clinical acoustic reflex data indicate that this neural pathway exists (Hall, 1985).

As with the CN, tonotopic organization appears to be maintained in all groups of nuclei in the SOC, although the LSO and MSO have been studied most extensively. The LSO has a unique tonotopic arrangement, with lower frequencies represented laterally and higher frequencies medially, following the s-shaped structural contour of the nucleus (Tsuchitani & Boudreau, 1966). The LSO responds to a broader range of frequencies than does the MSO, which has primarily low-frequency representation (Noback, 1985).

The SOC neurons have tuning curves similar to those of the CN (Moller, 1983). Some SOC tuning curves are wide while others are quite narrow. The discharge patterns seen in poststimulus time histograms of SOC neurons are varied but are classified primarily as chopper patterns (Keidel, Kallert, Korth, & Humes, 1983).

Lateral Lemniscus

The lateral lemniscus (LL) is the primary auditory pathway in the brainstem and comprises both ascending and descending fibers. The ascending portion extends bilaterally from the CN to the IC in the midbrain and contains both crossed and uncrossed fibers of the CN and SOC (Goldberg & Moore, 1967) (Figure 2–2).

Within the LL are two main cell groups, the ventral and dorsal nuclei of the lateral lemniscus (NLL), as well as a minor cell group called the intermediate nucleus of the lateral lemniscus. These nuclei are located posterolaterally in the upper portion of the pons, near the lateral surface of the brainstem (Ferraro & Minckler, 1977). Afferent input to the NLL arises from the dorsal CN on the contralateral side, and from the ventral CN from both sides of the brainstem (Jungert, 1958). Both the ipsilateral and contralateral SOC also provide input to the NLL (Noback, 1985). The dorsal NLL from either side of the brainstem are interconnected by a fiber tract called the commissure of Probst (Kudo, 1981). Lemniscal fibers may also cross from one side to the other through the pontine reticular formation (Ferraro & Minckler, 1977). Most of the neurons of the dorsal segment of the LL can be activated binaurally. However, a majority of neurons from the ventral segment can be activated only by contralateral stimulation (Keidel et al., 1983). As with the CN and the SOC, definite tonotopic organization has been demonstrated for both the dorsal and the ventral NLL (Brugge & Geisler, 1978).

Inferior Colliculus

The IC is one of the largest and most identifiable auditory structures of the brainstem (Oliver & Morest, 1984). The IC is located on the dorsal surface of the midbrain, approximately 3 to 3.5 cm rostral to the ponto-medullary junction (Figures 2–2 and 2–3).

From the dorsal aspect of the midbrain, the IC is clearly visible as two spherical mounds (Musiek & Baran, 1986). Two other rounded projections, the superior colliculi, can be seen on the dorsal surface of

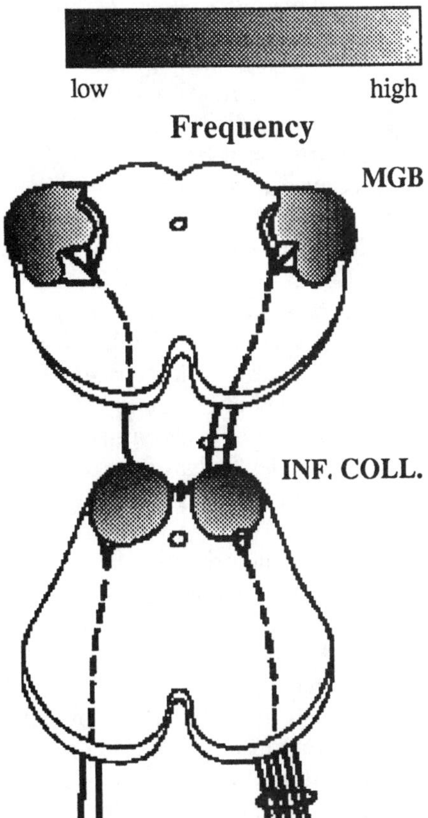

Figure 2–3. The inferior colliculus (mid brain level) and medial geniculate body (MGB) (inferior thalamus).

the midbrain, slightly rostral and lateral to the IC (Musiek & Baran, 1986) (Figures 2–2 and 2–3).

Two major divisions exist within the IC: the central nucleus, or core, which is composed of purely auditory fibers, and the pericentral nucleus, or belt, which surrounds the central nucleus and consists primarily of somatosensory and auditory fibers (Keidel et al., 1983).

The majority of auditory fibers from the LL and the lower auditory centers synapse directly or indirectly at the IC (Barnes, Magoon, & Ranson, 1943). Van Noort (1969) found that the IC receives input from the dorsal and ventral CN, lateral and medial superior olivary nuclei, dorsal and ventral nuclei of the LL, and contralateral IC. Other reports (Keidel et al., 1983; Pickles, 1988; Whitfield, 1967) suggest that the lower nuclei provide both contralateral and ipsilateral input to the IC. Many interneurons appear to exist in the IC, suggesting the presence of strong neuronal interconnections (Oliver & Morest, 1984). The superior colliculi, generally associated with the visual system, also receives input from the auditory system, which is integrated into the reflexes involving the position of the head and eyes (Gordon, 1972).

Although the different functions of the IC have not been defined fully, many of its functional properties have been described. As with other brainstem auditory structures, the IC has a high degree of tonotopic organization (Merzenich & Reid, 1974). Moreover, it contains a large number of fibers that yield extremely sharp tuning curves, suggesting a high level of frequency resolution (Aitken, Webster, Veale, & Crosby, 1975). The IC contains many time- and spatial-sensitive neurons (Pickles, 1988; Knudson & Konishi, 1978, 1980) and neurons sensitive to binaural stimulation (Benerento & Coleman, 1970). This suggests a role in sound localization (Musiek & Baran, 1986). Finally, in considering its neural connections and its position astride the auditory pathways, the IC has been referred to as the obligatory relay nuclear complex in transmitting auditory information to higher levels (Noback, 1985).

Like the LL, the IC has a commissure that permits neural communication between the left and right IC (Whitfield, 1967). A unique feature of the IC is its brachium, a large fiber tract that lies on the dorsolateral surface of the midbrain. This tract projects fibers ipsilaterally to the medial geniculate body, which is the principal auditory nucleus of the thalamus.

Medial Geniculate Body

The medial geniculate body (MGB) is located on the inferior, dorsolateral surface of the thalamus, just anterior, lateral, and slightly rostral to the IC (Figures 2–2 and 2–3). Although the MGB sits in the thalamus and the IC in the midbrain, these structures are located only approximately 1 cm apart. The MGB contains ventral, dorsal and medial divisions (Morest, 1964). Cells in the ventral division respond primarily to acoustic stimuli, while the other divisions contain neurons that respond to both somatosensory and acoustic stimulation (Keidel et al., 1983; Pickles, 1988). The ventral division appears to be the portion of the MGB that transmits specific discrimination (speech) information to the cerebral cortex (Winer, 1984, 1985). The dorsal division projects axons to association areas of the auditory cortex. This division may maintain and direct auditory attention (Winer, 1984). The medial division may function as a multisensory arousal system (Winer, 1984).

Afferent inputs to the MGB are primarily uncrossed, arriving from the IC via the branchium. It is possible, however, that some input may come from the contralateral IC and that some lower nuclei may input directly on the MGB (Pickles, 1988). In the cat, crossed inputs from the IC connect to the medial division of the MGB (Morest, 1964; Winer, 1984).

Tonotopic organization has been reported in the ventral segment of the MGB, with low frequencies represented laterally and high frequencies represented medially (Aikin & Webster, 1972). Tuning curves range from broad to sharp, but MGB fibers in general are not as sharply tuned as those of the IC (Aitkin & Webster, 1972). As with the IC, the MGB has many neurons sensitive to binaural stimulation and interaural intensity differences (Aitkin & Webster, 1972; Pickles, 1988). Based on long response latencies and after-effects of MGB responses to frequency modulation, Keidel et al. (1983) hypothesized that the MGB plays a major role in the processing of natural speech stimuli.

Reticular Formation

The auditory system, like other sensory and motor systems, is intricately connected to the reticular formation (RF). The RF can be viewed as having two subsystems: the sensory or ascending reticular activating system (ARAS) and the motor activating system. Our remarks pertain to the ARAS.

The RF, which forms the central core of the brainstem, is a diffusely organized area with intricately connected nuclei and tracts (Mosenthal, personal communication, 1991). The RF is connected to the spinal cord by reticulospinal tracts and to the cerebrum by many (but poorly defined) tracts, such as the medial forebrain bundle, the mamillary peduncle, and the dorsal longitudinal fasciculus. The RF also contains many brainstem nuclei. The RF has both ascending and descending tracts on each side of the brainstem, which extend from the caudal areas of the spinal cord through the medulla, pons, and midbrain, where diffuse tracts are sent throughout the cerebrum. There are also connections to cerebellum.

When the ARAS is stimulated the cortex becomes more alert and aware. This increased alertness has been shown by changes in electroencephalogram patterns (French, 1957). Conversely, when the RF is turned off, sleep or coma ensues (Mosenthal, personal communication, 1991). The ARAS is a general alarm that responds the same way to any sensory input. The ARAS responses prepare the entire brain to act appropriately on the incoming stimulus (Carpenter & Sutin, 1983). Evidence suggests that the ARAS can become sensitive to specific stimuli (French, 1957). For example, this system has a greater reaction to important stimuli than to unimportant stimuli. This may be one of the mechanisms underlying selective attention and could be related to the ability to hear in the presence of noise. General listening skills also may be affected by the state of awareness. The profuse connections of sensory structures to the RF, and their extensive interactions may make it unnatural to try to separate attention from sensory or cognitive processing of information (see Chapter 1 for a behavioral and processing perspective).

Vascular Anatomy of the Brainstem

Many auditory dysfunctions of the brainstem and periphery have a vascular basis. For example, vertebrobasilar disease, mini strokes, vascular spasms, aneurysms, and vascular loops have all been shown to affect the auditory system (Colclasure & Graham, 1981; Moller & Moller, 1985; Musiek & Gollegly, 1985).

The major blood supply of the brainstem is the basilar artery, which originates from the left and right vertebral arteries, 1 to 2 mm below the ponto-medullary junction on the ventral side of the brainstem. At the low to mid pons level, the anterior inferior cerebellar artery branches from the basilar artery to supply blood to the CN. The CN may also receive an indirect vascular supply from the posterior inferior cerebellar artery (Waddington, 1984). In many cases the anterior inferior cerebellar artery will give rise to the internal auditory artery, which supplies the VIIIth nerve, and then branch into three divisions to supply the cochlear and vestibular periphery. The internal auditory artery sometimes branches directly from the basilar artery (Portman, Sterkers, Charachon, & Chouard, 1975).

At the mid-pons level small pontine branches of the basilar artery, perhaps with circumferential arteries, indirectly supply the SOC and possibly the LL (Tsuchitani & Boudreau, 1966). Also, a strong possibility exists that the paramedian branches of the basilar artery supply the SOC and LL. The superior cerebellar arteries are located at the rostral pons or midbrain level. Their branches supply the IC and in some cases the NLL (Carpenter & Sutin, 1983). At the midbrain level, the basilar artery forms the posterior cerebral arteries. Each posterior cerebral artery has circumferential branches that supply the MGB ipsilaterally (Waddington, personal communication, 1985).

Significant variability has been shown in the vasculature of the brainstem (Waddington, 1974, 1984). Because vascular patterns vary among specimens, no one description can encapsulate all vascular patterns. Because most brainstem auditory structures are on the dorsal side of the brainstem, they may receive secondary and tertiary branches of the key arteries mentioned previously.

Intensity Coding

As sound intensity increases, the firing rate of many of the auditory fibers in the brainstem increases. However, this is a general statement with notable exceptions, as discussed later. Because the range between the threshold and saturation point of any given fiber is much smaller than the range of intensities audible to the human ear, large intensity increases cannot be encoded by individual nerve fibers (Moller, 1983). Rather, at high intensities many neurons must interact to achieve accurate coding. The mechanisms of this interaction are poorly understood (Pickles, 1988), and most information on intensity coding is based on the study of individual neurons.

Neurons of various brainstem nuclei respond to stimulus intensity in three principal ways (Pickles, 1988; Whitfield, 1967). One type of response is referred to as monotonic, meaning that as the stimulus intensity increases the firing rate of the neuron(s) increases proportionally. The second type of intensity function is monotonic for low intensities, but as stimulus intensity increases the firing rate levels off. In the third type of intensity function, the neuronal firing rate reaches a plateau at a relatively low intensity and, in certain cases, actually decreases as intensity increases, resulting in a rollover phenomenon. For example, some neurons in the IC reach their maximum firing rate 5 dB above their threshold (Whitfield, 1967). These three types of intensity coding appear to be common throughout the auditory brainstem, although the extent of each type varies among nuclei groups.

One can hypothesize that a high-intensity signal would not be coded appropriately when there is damage to brainstem auditory neurons of the first type (monotonic) but not to the latter two types of neurons. This could result in higher intensities being coded incorrectly, which might result in what is clinically known as the rollover phenomenon (Jerger & Jerger, 1971).

Timing

The latency of brainstem neuronal responses varies depending on the type of auditory stimulus and the neuron or neuron group analyzed (Pickles, 1988; Whitfield, 1967). Some neurons react quickly to stimulation while others have lengthy latency periods. Some neurons respond only upon termination of the stimulus.

Phase locking is another phenomenon related to timing in the auditory system (Keidel et al., 1983; Moller, 1985). Many auditory neurons appear to lock onto the stimulus according to phase and fire only when the stimulus waveform reaches a certain point in its cycle. This is particularly evident with low-frequency sounds. Moreover, at lower frequencies certain neurons fire on every cycle, while at higher frequencies they fire only at every third or fifth cycle. This phase relationship is especially apparent in lower auditory brainstem neurons and may have considerable relevance to the mechanisms underlying masking level differences (Jeffress & McFadden, 1971). Generally, the firing rates of brainstem auditory neurons are higher than those of cortical nerve fibers for steady-state signals. The speed with which a neuron can respond to repeated stimuli depends on its refractory period. The refractory period is the interval between two successive discharges (depolarization) of a nerve cell, and depends on the cell metabolism; dysfunction of metabolic activity will lengthen the refractory period (Tasaki, 1954).

In reviewing timing of the auditory system, it is necessary to discuss the contemporary phrase "temporal processing." As Phillips (1995) conveys, this phrase may mean different things to different people. Clinicians often use temporal processing to indicate performance on an auditory test that requires some type of timing decision about the stimuli presented. Basic scientists look at various types of temporal processing and how they contribute to other auditory functions. Phillips (1995) provides several examples of how timing is the key to certain auditory processes. Localization of a sound source, for example, requires relative timing of acoustic signals arriving at the two ears. The pitch percept of complex sounds depends on the timing (and related coding) of rapidly repeating acoustic events. There is also sequencing of successive stimuli, masking of signals (existing close in time), discrimination of element duration, integration of acoustic energy, as well as pitch changes that all can be considered temporal processing. Even detection, recognition, and discrimination processes take time and hence may be considered as having a temporal element.

Origins of the Auditory Brainstem Response

The exact origins of some elements of the ABR are uncertain, but research (Moller, 1985; Wada & Starr, 1983) has clarified the issue. Moller (1985) indicated that wave I of the ABR is generated from the lateral aspect of the auditory nerve, whereas wave II originates from the medial aspect. Wave III probably has more than one generator, as do other subsequent waves of the ABR, but it appears that the CN is the principal source of wave III (Moller, 1985; Wada & Starr, 1983). Wave IV probably has multiple generator sites as well, but it arises predominantly from the SOC with a contralateral influence that may be stronger than the ipsilateral contribution. According to Moller (1985) and Wada and Starr (1983), wave V is generated from the LL. In a simplified view of the ABR origins, it is plausible that the first five ABR waves may be generated entirely within the auditory nerve and pons.

The typical findings of ABR abnormalities on the ear ipsilateral to a brainstem lesion (Chiappa, 1983; Oh, Kuba, Soyer, Choi, Bonilowski, & Viter, 1981; Musiek & Geurkink, 1982) seem to be inconsistent with known neuroanatomy, which shows a majority of the auditory fibers crossing to the contralateral side at the level of the SOC. What these ABR findings mean in reference to brainstem pathways and associated physiology is difficult to say at this point in time. However, it seems important to consider these clinical findings in the framework of how the brainstem pathways may function in the pathological situation.

Animal studies by Wada and Starr (1983), and our own observations with humans, show that the first five waves of the ABR are not affected by specific lesions of the IC. Unfortunately, the ABR may not be a useful tool in evaluating lesions at or above the IC. Powerful clinical tests such as the ABR, MLDs, and acoustic reflexes appear to be restricted to detection of lesions below the midbrain level. In cases where lesions of the IC or the MGB (midbrain and thalamic levels) are suspected, other procedures are necessary to detect and define the abnormality.

THE CEREBRUM

Auditory Cortical Areas

The ascending auditory system continues from the thalamic area to the cerebral cortex through neurons that originate in the MGB and radiate outward to the auditory areas of the brain.

The cerebral cortex (gray matter covering the surface of the brain) is composed of three primary types of nerve cells: pyramidal, stellate, and fusiform. Six cell layers in the cortex can be distinguished by type, density, and arrangement of the nerve cells (Carpenter & Sutin, 1983). In the cortex, there are auditory cells in each layer except layer one that are responsive to acoustic stimuli (Phillips & Irvine, 1981).

Researchers disagree about which areas constitute the auditory cortex. Most of this variability results from adapting animal models to the human brain, and from discrepancy as to whether "association" areas should be included as part of the auditory cortex (Musiek, 1986b). We include these association areas because they are critical to understanding the system, although they also contain fibers that are not sensitive to auditory stimuli.

Heschl's gyrus, sometimes called the transverse gyrus, is considered to be the primary auditory area of the cortex. This gyrus is located in the Sylvian fissure, approximately two thirds posterior on the upper surface of the temporal lobe (supratemporal plane). It courses in a posterior and medial direction. To observe Heschl's gyrus the temporal lobe must be displaced inferiorly or separated from the brain to expose the supratemporal plane (Figures 2–4 and 2–5).

Campain and Minckler (1976) analyzed many human brains and found that the configuration of Heschl's gyrus differed on the left and right sides. In some brains double gyri were present on each side; in other brains double gyri were present only unilaterally. In a study of 29 human brains, Musiek and Reeves (1990) reported that the number of Heschl's gyri ranged from one to three per hemisphere, although there was no significant left-right asymmetry in the number of Heschl's gyri within individual brains. The mean length of Heschl's gyri, however, was found to be greater in the left hemisphere (Musiek & Reeves, 1990).

The planum temporale is an area on the cortical surface that extends posteriorly from the most posterior aspect of Heschl's gyrus to the end point of the Sylvian fissure (Figure 2–4). Geschwind and Levitsky (1968) showed that the planum temporale in the human brain

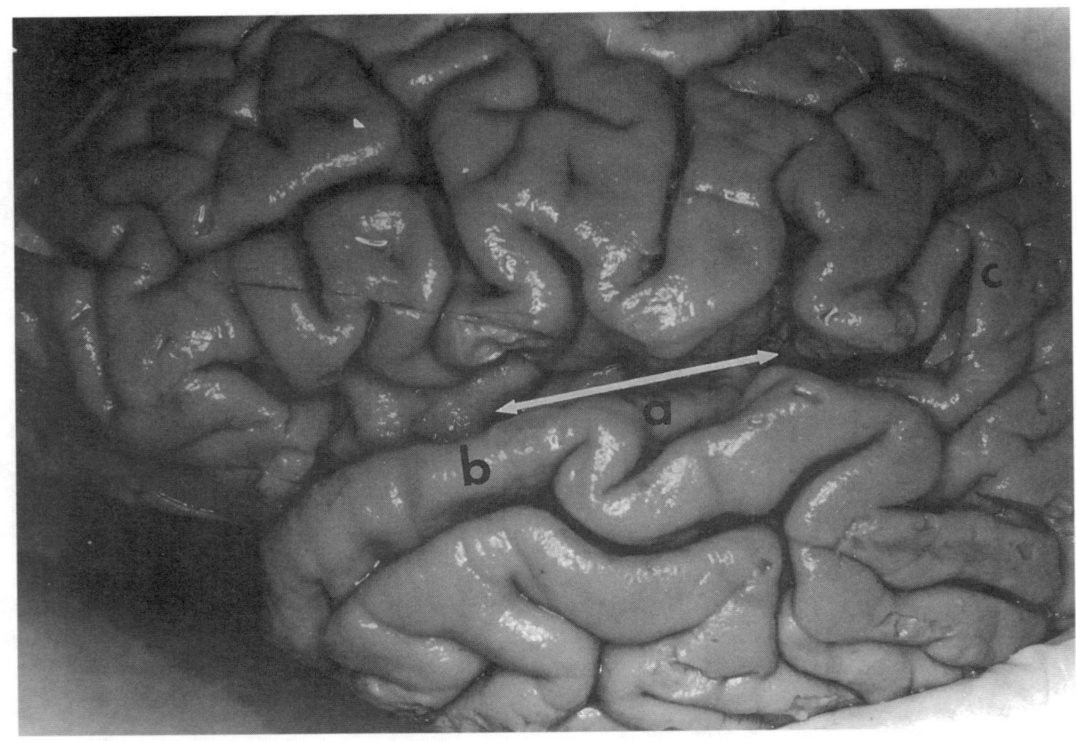

Figure 2–4. The left lateral view of the human brain. The arrow points to the Sylvian fissure. **Key:** a = Heschl's gyrus, b = Superior temporal gyrus, c = Supramarginal gyrus (terminating the Sylvian fissure).

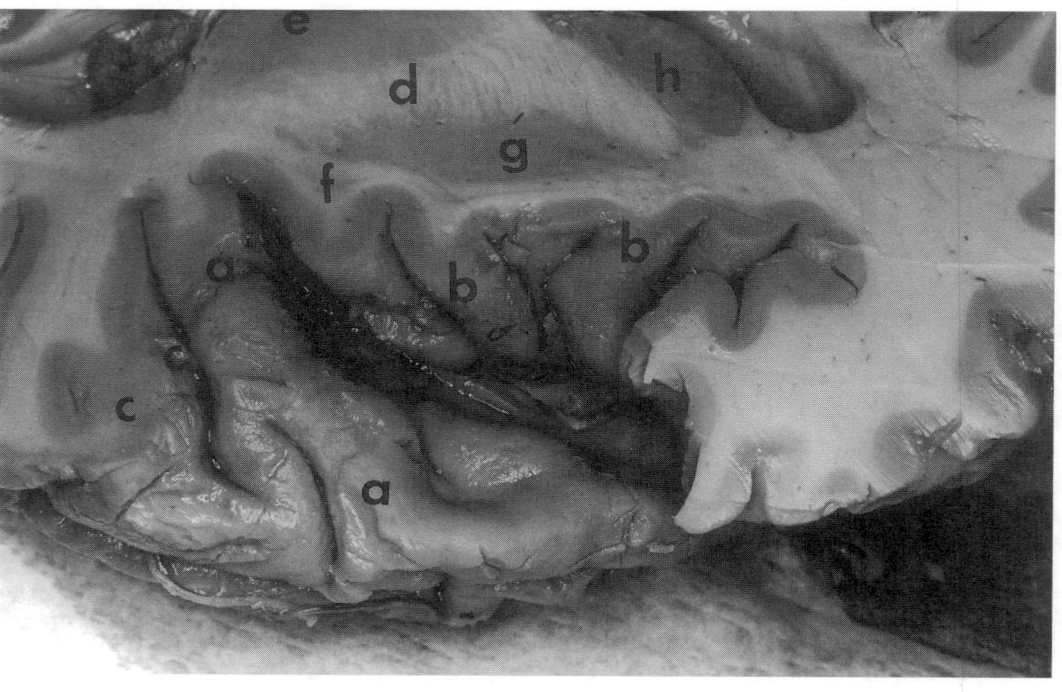

Figure 2–5. The right superior temporal plane of the human brain as seen from above. **Key:** a = Heschl's gyrus, b = Insula, c = Planum temporal, d = Internal capsule, e = Thalamus, f = External capsule, g = Putamen & globus padillus.

is significantly larger on the left side (3.6 cm) than on the right (2.7 cm). Because the left hemisphere is dominant for speech and the planum temporale is located in the approximate region of Wernicke's area, these investigators reasoned that the planum temporale may be an anatomical correlate to (receptive) language in man. Musiek and Reeves (1990) support these earlier findings (Geschwind & Levitsky, 1968) regarding the differences in the length of the left and right planum temporale. They suggest, however, that asymmetries in higher auditory and language function may be due to anatomic differences of the planum temporale, as well as Heschl's gyrus.

The supramarginal gyrus curves around the end of the Sylvian fissure. This area is responsive to acoustic stimulation (Celesia, 1976) and is located in the approximate region of Wernicke's area, as is the angular gyrus, which is located immediately posterior to the supramarginal gyrus (Geschwind & Levitsky, 1968). These are part of a complex association area that appears to integrate auditory, visual, and somesthetic information and is therefore vital in the visual and somesthetic aspects of language, such as reading and writing.

The Sylvian fissure contains the primary auditory area and parts of the language area in humans. Rubens (1986) reviewed early anatomical work on the Sylvian fissure which showed the left Sylvian fissure to be larger than the right. This finding has been confirmed by others, including Musiek and Reeves (1990), who found that asymmetry of the Sylvian fissure was correlated with the greater length of the planum temporale on the left side.

The inferior portion of the parietal lobe and the inferior aspect of the frontal lobe also are responsive to acoustical stimulation (Celesia, 1976; Galaburda & Sanides, 1980). Still another acoustically responsive area is the insula, a portion of the cortex that lies deep within the Sylvian fissure, medial to the middle segment of the superior temporal gyrus (Figure 2–5). The insular cortex can be observed only if the temporal lobe is removed or displaced inferiorly. It appears that the most posterior aspect of the insula is contiguous with Heschl's gyrus.

Within the insula are nerve fibers that are responsive to somatic, visual, and gustatory stimulation. The greatest neural activity, however, results from acoustic stimulation (Sudakov, MacLean, Reeves, & Marino, 1971). It appears that the posterior aspect of the insula, the portion closest to Heschl's gyrus, has the most acoustically sensitive fibers (Sudakov et al., 1971). Located just medial to the insula is a narrow strip of gray matter called the claustrum. Little is known about the function of the claustrum, although it seems to be highly responsive to acoustic stimulation (Noback, 1985; Sudakow et al., 1971).

Anatomical irregularities have been reported in the brains of people with dyslexia (Galaburda, Sherman, Rosen, Aboitz, & Geschwind, 1985; Kaufman & Galaburda, 1989). The planum temporale, normally significantly longer in the left hemisphere, was found to be bilaterally symmetrical in the brains of patients with dyslexia. Moreover, the brains of dyslexic patients contained an unusually high number of cellular abnormalities, referred to as cerebrocortical microdysgenesias. These are defined as nests of ectopic neurons and glia in layer one of the cortex. These ectopic areas are often associated with dysplasia of adjacent cortical layers (including focal microgyria), and sometimes with superficial growths known as brain warts. Although these focal anomalies may exist in up to 26% of normal brains, they are usually found in small numbers and in the right hemisphere. In patients with developmental dyslexia the anomalies occur in greater numbers, often in the left hemisphere in the area of the perisylvian cortex (Kaufman & Galaburda, 1989). These findings are interesting in several ways. One is that these areas of symmetry versus asymmetry and microdysgenesis seem to involve areas that in humans are considered (for the most part) auditory regions of the cerebrum. Also, why is there such a high incidence of cortical dysplasias in individuals with learning disorders? Could one speculate that these morphological abnormalities have functional, or perhaps we should say dysfunctional, correlates? Obviously, more studies are needed to relate these findings to behavioral consequences.

Thalamocortical Connections

Ascending auditory fiber tracts originating in the MGB follow various routes to the cortex and other areas of the brain. One group of fibers provides input to the basal ganglia (the large subcortical gray matter structures composed of the caudate nucleus, putamen, and globus pallidus) (Figure 2–5). The lenticular process, or nucleus, consists of the putamen and globus pallidus and lies between the internal and external capsules (white matter neural pathways) (Figure 2–5). Animal studies (LeDoux, Sakaguchi, & Reis, 1983) have shown that the MGB sends out fibers that connect to the putamen, the caudate nucleus, and the amygdaloid body (a small almond-shaped expansion located at the tail of the caudate nucleus).

In addition to these connections to the basal ganglia, two major pathways run from the MGB to the cortex. The first pathway, consisting of all auditory fibers that originate in the ventral MGB, takes a sublenticular course through the internal capsule to the Heschl's gyrus. The second pathway, consisting of auditory, somatic, and possibly visual fibers, proceeds from the MGB through the inferior aspect of the internal capsule and ultimately under the putamen to the external capsule. From the external capsule, fibers connect to the insula (Streitfeld, 1980). Other connections run from the MGB to the auditory cortex and probably overlap the two mentioned here. The pathways described here typify the multiple and complex connections of the thalamocortical auditory anatomy.

Intrahemispheric Connections of the Auditory Cortex

The primary auditory cortex has both intrahemispheric and interhemispheric connections. Lesions of the primary auditory area in primates have resulted in degeneration of the caudal (posterior) aspect of the superior temporal gyrus and the upper bank of the adjacent superior temporal sulcus (Seltzer & Pandya, 1978). This degeneration pattern suggests the presence of a multisynaptic pathway in the middle and posterior areas of the superior temporal gyrus (Jones & Powell, 1970). The superior temporal gyrus also has fibers that connect to the insula and frontal operculum.

There are few connections between the auditory area and the temporal pole (i.e., the anterior-most aspect of the temporal lobe) (Noback, 1985). By testing patients whose temporal poles had been removed, some audiological studies have examined the validity of various central auditory tests. Given the anatomy of this region, these patients would not be expected to show central auditory deficits.

Auditory cortical areas and other areas of the temporal lobe are connected to areas in the frontal lobe by way of the arcuate fasciculus, one of the "long" association pathways. This large fiber tract travels from the temporal lobe, up and around the top of the Sylvian fissure, and extends anteriorly to the frontal lobe (Streitfeld, 1980). The arcuate fasciculus is combined with a larger tract called the longitudinal fasciculus, which courses in the same direction through similar anatomic regions. Two of the important regions connected through the arcuate fasciculus are Wernicke's area in the temporal lobe and Broca's area in the frontal lobe (Carpenter & Sutin, 1983).

Interhemispheric Connections

The main connection between the left and right hemispheres is the corpus callosum (CC) (Figure 2–6), which is located at the base of the longitudinal fissure.

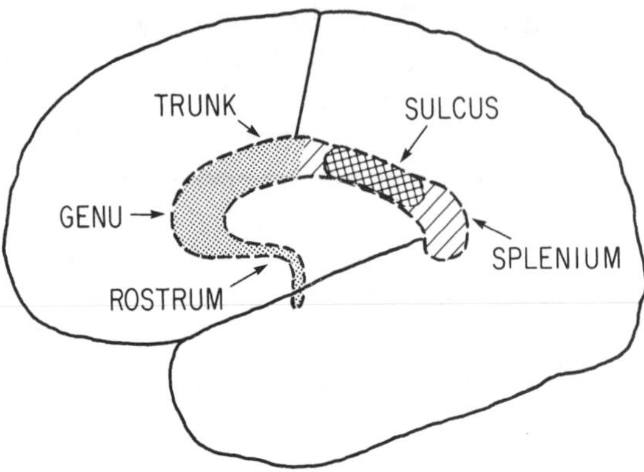

Figure 2–6. The regions of the corpus callosum. Cross-hatched area indicates the auditory region.

The CC is the largest fiber tract in the primate brain. It is covered by the cingulate gyri and forms most of the roof of the lateral ventricles (Selnes, 1974). In the adult, the CC is approximately 6.5 cm long from the anterior genu to the posterior splenium and is approximately 0.5 to 1 cm thick (Musiek, 1986b). The CC has great morphological variability but seems to be larger in left-handed than in right-handed people (Witelson, 1986).

The CC is composed of long, heavily myelinated axons. The CC is not only a midline structure (Musiek, 1986b), as it essentially connects the two cortices and therefore must be considered to span much of the intercortical space above the basal ganglia and lateral ventricles. It is likely that in many "cortical" lesions some region of the CC is involved because it encompasses such a large portion of the cerebrum.

The fibers of the CC are primarily homolateral (connecting to the same locus in each hemisphere), although some fibers are heterolateral (connecting to different loci on each hemisphere) (Mountcastle, 1962). The heterolateral fibers may require a longer transfer time than their homolateral counterparts. One reason for this difference is that the heterolateral fibers often have a longer and less direct route to the opposite side. The transcallosal transfer time (TCTT) is the latency of an evoked potential recorded from one point on the cortex after stimulation of the homolateral point on the other hemisphere. In humans, the TCTT decreases with age, reaching minimum values during the teenage years (Gazzaniga & Sperry, 1962). This is consistent with increased myelination of the CC axons (Yakovlev &

LeCours, 1967). In primates and humans the TCTT varies greatly, from 3 to 6 msec, to over 100 msec (Bremer, Brihaye, & Andre-Balisaux, 1956; Chang, 1953; Salamy, 1978). This variability may support the concept of inhibitory and excitatory neurons in the CC.

The neural connections of the CC correspond to various parts of the cortex, and the anatomy of the CC subserves various regions of the cortex. The most posterior aspect of the CC is the splenium, which contains mainly visual fibers that connect with the occipital cortex (Pandya & Seltzer, 1986). The trunk makes up the middle portion of the CC. The posterior half of the trunk is thinner; this thin area is called the sulcus. Most auditory fibers from the temporal lobe and insula are found in this region. The frontal and parietal lobes also are represented in the trunk region of the CC. The anterior part of the CC, termed the genu, contains olfactory fibers and fibers from the anterior insula (Pandya & Seltzer, 1986).

The auditory area of the CC at midline is just anterior to the splenium in the posterior half of the CC. This information comes from primate research (Pandya & Seltzer, 1986), but data on humans help localize the auditory areas of the CC. Baran, Musiek, and Reeves (1986) have shown that there is little or no change in dichotic listening or pattern perception (tasks requiring interhemispheric transfer) performance after the sectioning of the anterior half of the CC. However, patients with a complete section of the CC demonstrate markedly poor performance on these auditory tasks (Musiek, Kibbe, & Baran, 1984).

Although we have considerable information about the anatomy of the CC at midline, we know little about the course of the transcallosal auditory pathway (TCAP). Information about the TCAP comes from anatomic and clinical studies (Damasio & Damasio, 1979). The TCAP begins at the auditory cortex, courses posteriorly, runs superiorly around the lateral ventricles, crosses a periventricular area known as the trigone, and courses medially and inferiorly into the CC proper. Any lesions along the TCAP can result in degraded interhemispheric transfer.

A recent study demonstrates size differences in the CC for children with attention deficits, as compared to control subjects. The CC of the experimental group were smaller in the auditory area and in the genu, as compared to the control group (Hynd, Semrud-Clikeman, Lorys, Novey, Eliopulos, & Lyytinen, 1991).

The vascular anatomy of the CC is rather simple. The posterior fifth (splenium) is supplied by branches of the posterior cerebral artery (Carpenter & Sutin, 1983). The remaining segment of the CC is supplied by the pericallosal artery, which is a branch of the anterior cerebral artery (Carpenter & Sutin, 1983).

Tonotopic Organization

As in the brainstem, distinct tonotopic organization exists in the auditory cortex. Tonotopic organization exists in the primary auditory cortex of the primate, with low frequencies represented rostrolaterally and high frequencies represented caudomedially (Merzenich & Brugge, 1973). Using position emission tomography to measure changes in cerebral blood flow, Lauter, Herscovitch, Formby, and Raichle (1985) demonstrated a similar pattern in the human brain. Tones of 500 Hz evoked increased activity in the lateral part of Heschl's gyrus, while tones of 4000 Hz resulted in increased activity in the medial position. Most tonotopic information on the insular cortex has been obtained from studies in the cat (Woolsey, 1960). In the cat insula, the high-frequency neurons appear to be located in the superior portion, while the low-frequency neurons are located in the inferior segment (Woolsey, 1960).

In the primary auditory area where cells are sharply tuned, highly definable tonotopic organization and isofrequency strips (contours) can be found (Pickles, 1985). There appear to be "columns" within the cortex which have similar characteristic frequencies (Phillips & Irvine, 1981). There also does seem to be a spatial component to frequency representation in the auditory cortex; approximately 2 mm are required to encompass the frequency range of one octave. For extremely high frequencies, less space is needed to represent an octave range (Mountcastle, 1968).

Some types of tuning curves obtained from the auditory cortex are unique. Broad and sharp as well as multipeaked tuning curves have been recorded from cortical neurons (Pickles, 1985). The multipeaked tuning curves may be observed primarily from cortical recordings. Neurons in the primary auditory cortex appear to receive a narrow frequency-tuned excitatory input from the contralateral ear. This frequency-intensity response area may be flanked by inhibitory inputs that originate from adjacent cochlear sites (Phillips, 1990). Cortical neurons may respond briskly to brief acoustic events but show poorer spike discharge rates to maintained, steady-state acoustic signals (Musiek, 1986a).

Intensity Coding

The discharge or firing rate of cortical neurons in primates varies as a function of intensity and takes two forms: monotonic and nonmonotonic (Pfingst & O'Conner, 1981). Most neurons in the primary auditory cortex display rate-intensity functions similar to the auditory nerve (i.e., the firing rate is monotonic for increments of approximately 10 to 40 dB). Intensities above 40 dB do not result in increased firing rates. Many of the neurons in the auditory cortex are sharply nonmonotonic. In some cases, the firing rate may be reduced to a spontaneous level with a 10-dB increase above the optimum intensity (Pickles, 1988).

Phillips (1990) reported similar results with cats, identifying both monotonic and nonmonotonic profiles. For some nonmonotonic neurons, firing rates decreased precipitously, often to zero, at stimulus levels slightly above threshold. Phillips (1990) also found that the introduction of wide-band noise raised the threshold level of the cortical neurons. However, once threshold sensitivity was achieved in noise, the firing rate increased in a manner similar to the nonmasked condition, with the intensity profile remaining basically unchanged. With successive increments in the level of the masking noise, the tonal intensity profile is displaced toward progressively higher SPLs.

Animal studies show some cortical neurons to be intensity selective. Certain cells respond only within a given intensity range, but collectively the neurons cover a wide range of intensities. For example, cortical cells may respond maximally, minimally, or not at all at a given intensity. When the intensity is changed, different cells may respond at a maximum level, and the previous neurons may respond minimally or not at all (Merzenich & Brugge, 1973).

Timing

Like the brainstem, the auditory cortex responds in various ways to the onset, presence, and offset of acoustic stimuli. Abeles and Goldstein (1972) found four types of responses of cortical neurons to a 100-msec tone. One type of neuron sustained a response for the duration of the stimulus, although the firing rate was considerably less at the offset of the tone. "On" neurons responded only to the onset, and "off" neurons responded only after the tone was terminated. The fourth type responded to both the onset and the offset of the tone, but did not sustain a response during the tone.

Additional information on timing or temporal processing in the auditory cortex can be found in the work of Goldstein, DeRibaupierre, and Yeni-Komshian (1971). These investigators studied cells in the primary auditory area (A1) of rats and found four categories of response to clicks presented at different rates. Approximately 40% of the A1 cells responded to each click at rates of 10 to 1000 per second, while 25% of the A1 cells did not respond at all. The third classification of A1 cells showed varying response patterns as the click rate changed, and the fourth group of cells responded only to low click rates. In a review of the literature, Eggermont (1991) noted that a number of studies found click-following rates of auditory cortex neurons to be in the 50–100 (per second) range or less. Eggermont also pointed out that recording methodology may influence the quantification of the response rates of these neurons. However, it seems apparent that cortical neurons have difficulty following high rate periodic events.

Timing within the auditory cortex plays a critical role in localization abilities. Many neurons in the primary auditory cortex are sensitive to the interaural phase and to intensity differences (Benson & Teas, 1976). In a sound field, more cortical units fire to sound stimuli from a contralateral source than from an ipsilateral source (Eisenmann, 1974; Evans, 1968). This finding provided the basis for the initial clinical work on sound localization.

As early as 1958, Sanchez-Longo and Forster (1958) reported that patients with temporal lobe damage had difficulty locating sound sources in the sound field contralateral to the damaged hemisphere. Recently, Moore, Cranford, and Rahn (1990) studied the abilities of both normal and brain-damaged subjects to track a fused auditory image as it moved through auditory space. The perceived location of the auditory image, which varies according to the temporal relationship of paired clicks presented (one each, from matched speakers), is referred to as the precedence effect.

Although the normal subjects were able to accurately track the fused auditory image, two subjects with unilateral temporal lobe lesions (one in the right hemisphere and one in the left) exhibited auditory field deficits opposite the damaged hemispheres. Results of these investigations (Baran et al., 1986; Musiek et al., 1984) are consistent with other localization and lateralization studies which show contralateral ear effects (Liden & Rosenthal, 1981; Pinheiro & Tobin, 1969).

Electrical Stimulation of the Auditory Cortex

Penfield and associates (Penfield & Rasmussen, 1950; Penfield & Roberts, 1959) conducted several auditory stimulation experiments during neurosurgical procedures done on humans. These investigators electrically stimulated areas along the margin of the Sylvian fissure while the patient, under local anesthesia, reported what he or she heard. Many of Penfield's patients did not report any auditory experience or sensation during electrical stimulation. However, some patients reported hearing buzzing, ringing, chirping, knocking, humming, and rushing sounds during stimulation of the superior gyrus of the temporal lobe. These sounds were mainly referred to the contralateral ear and, to a lesser extent, to both ears.

During electrical stimulation of the auditory areas of the brain, patients often reported the impression of hearing loss, yet they heard and understood spoken words. Patients also claimed that the voice of the surgeon changed in pitch and loudness during electrical stimulation. In 1963, Penfield and Perot reported cases in which electrical stimulation of the left posterior-superior temporal gyrus and Heschl's gyrus resulted in patients hearing voices shouting and other similar acoustic phenomena. When the right auditory cortex was stimulated, most patients who responded heard music and singing.

Lateralization of Function in the Auditory Cortex

One key principle in central auditory assessment using behavioral tests is related to lateralization of the deficit. It is well known that behavioral tests often result in deficiencies in the ear contralateral to the damaged hemisphere. This contralateral ear deficit may relate to the fact that each ear provides more contralateral than ipsilateral input to the cortex. This view has strong physiological support. Mountcastle (1968) reported that the threshold for activation of cortical neurons by contralateral stimulation is generally 5 to 20 dB lower than for ipsilateral stimulation. Celesia (1976) has shown that near-field evoked potentials recorded from the auditory cortex in humans during neurosurgery are of greater amplitude for contralateral than ipsilateral ear stimulation.

Similar findings showing a stronger contralateral representation have also been reported in cats (Donchin, Kutas, & McCarthy, 1976). Late auditory evoked potentials recorded with electrodes over the temporal/parietal areas of the human scalp also have revealed differences between contralateral and ipsilateral stimulation. Generally, the auditory evoked potentials recorded from contralateral stimulation are earlier and of greater amplitude than those recorded ipsilaterally (Butler, Keidel, & Spreng, 1969). However, this is not always the case, and controversy surrounds these findings for far-field evoked potentials (Donchin et al., 1976).

Behavioral Ablation Studies

Ablation experiments have served as the basis for the development of several auditory tests. By monitoring auditory behavior in animals, the effects of partial or total ablation of the auditory cortex have been measured and have been valuable in the localization of function. Kryter and Ades (1943), in one of the first studies involving ablation of the cat auditory cortex, found little or no effect on absolute thresholds or differential thresholds for intensity. These findings are consistent with data subsequently obtained from humans with brain damage or surgically removed auditory cortices (Berlin, Lowe-Bell, Janetta, & Kline, 1972; Hodgson, 1967).

However, several other investigators (Heffner & Heffner, 1986; Heffner, Heffner, & Porter, 1985; Phillips, 1990) report that bilateral ablations of the primate auditory cortex result in severe hearing loss for pure tones. Bilaterally ablated animals demonstrated gradual recovery, but many retained some permanent pure-tone sensitivity loss, especially in the middle frequencies (Heffner & Heffner, 1986). Unilateral cortical ablations resulted in hearing loss in the ear contralateral to the lesion with normal hearing in the ipsilateral ear (Heffner et al., 1985). Permanent residual hearing loss has also been reported in humans with bilateral cortical lesions (Auerbach, Allard, Naeser, Alexander, & Albert, 1982; Jerger, Weikers, Sharbrough, & Jerger, 1969; Yaqub, Gascon, Al-Nosha, & Whitaker, 1988). Differences among animal species are shown in findings with opossums (Ravizza & Masterton, 1972) and ferrets (Kavanagh & Kelly, 1988) in which auditory threshold recovery is almost complete following bilateral lesions of the auditory cortex.

The effects of auditory cortex ablation on frequency discrimination remains unclear, even after many years of research. Some early studies (Allen, 1945; Meyer & Woolsey, 1952) reported that frequency discrimination was lost after ablation of the auditory cortex, but later studies (Cranford, Igarashi, & Stramler, 1976) contradicted these early findings. These discrepancies may be related to the difficulty of the discrimination tasks, as each study employed a different test paradigm to measure pitch perception. The complexity of the tasks, and not the differences in frequency discrimination, is probably responsible for the discrepant findings (Pickles, 1988).

Since ablation of the auditory cortex has little or no effect on absolute or differential thresholds for intensity or frequency, more complex tasks were sought to examine the results of cortical ablation. Diamond and Neff (1957) used patterned acoustic stimuli to examine the ability of cats to detect differences in frequency patterns after various bilateral cortical ablations. After ablation of primary and association auditory cortices, the cats could no longer discriminate different acoustic patterns, and despite extensive retraining, they could not relearn the pattern task. Based on subsequent studies, Neff (1961) reported that auditory cortex ablations primarily affected temporal sequencing and not pattern detection or frequency discrimination of the tones composing the patterns. Colavita (1972, 1974) demonstrated in cats that ablation of only the insular-temporal region resulted in the inability to discriminate temporal patterns. The early research of Diamond and Neff influenced Pinheiro in her development of the frequency (pitch) pattern test, a valuable clinical central auditory test in humans (Musiek, 1985; Musiek & Pinheiro, 1987; Pinheiro & Musiek, 1985). Another pattern perception test, duration patterns, has emerged as a potentially valuable clinical tool (Musiek, Baran, & Pinheiro, 1990). Temporal ordering appears to be a critical part of pattern perception, which is affected by lesions of the auditory cortex.

Other studies show that the temporal dimension of hearing is linked to the integrity of the auditory cortex. Gershuni, Baru, and Karaseva (1967) demonstrated that a unilateral lesion of a dog's auditory cortex resulted in decreased pure tone sensitivity for short but not long tones in the ear contralateral to the lesion.

In contrast, Cranford (1979) showed that cortical lesions had no effect on brief tone thresholds in cats. Cranford (1979) also demonstrated that auditory cortex lesions in cats markedly affected the frequency difference limen for short but not long duration tones presented to the contralateral ear. Following the animal study, Cranford, Stream, Rye, and Slade (1982) examined brief tone frequency difference limens in seven human subjects with unilateral temporal lobe lesions. Findings with human subjects were essentially the same as those with animals. Brief tone thresholds for subjects with temporal lobe lesions were the same as those of a normal control group, but the brief tone frequency difference limen was markedly poorer for subjects with lesions. The frequency difference limen was poorer for the contralateral ear for stimulus duration under 200 msec.

Vascular Anatomy in the Auditory Cortex

The primary artery that supplies blood to the auditory cortex is the middle cerebral artery (MCA) (Waddington, 1974). The MCA branches directly from the internal carotid artery at the base of the brain. Although its route varies considerably among specimens, it courses primarily within the Sylvian fissure in an anterior-to-posterior direction (Waddington, 1974). The MCA varies in length, and may be only 2 cm long before its branching becomes diffuse (Geshuni et al., 1967). However, in some cases it may run almost the entire length of the Sylvian fissure before it becomes the angular artery, which courses posteriorly and laterally on the brain surface.

In viewing the anterior aspect of the MCA, the first major branch that supplies an auditory region is the fronto-opercular artery. This artery takes a superior course, supplying the anterior portion of the insula. The central sulcus artery just posterior to the fronto-opercular artery supplies the posterior insula and the anterior parietal lobe. Branching inferiorly from the MCA are three arteries that course over the middle and posterior part of the temporal lobe (Waddington, 1974). These three arteries (anterior, middle, posterior temporal) supply the middle and superior temporal gyri. A combination of the MCA and angular artery probably supplies the primary auditory area as well as the angular gyrus and part of the supramarginal gyrus. The other part of the supramarginal gyrus is supplied by the posterior parietal artery.

Vascular insults involving the MCA can cause considerable tissue damage to gray and white matter in the temporal-parietal regions of the brain. These lesions, among the most common anomalies affecting the auditory cortex, are devastating not only to the morphology of the auditory cortex but also to its function.

The Efferent Auditory System

Although the efferent auditory system likely functions as one unit, the pathways are divided into two sections. The caudal-most part of the system (the olivocochlear bundle) has been studied, but little is known about the more rostral system. The rostral efferent pathway starts at the auditory cortex and descends to the medial geniculate and the midbrain regions, including the IC. A loop system appears to exist between the cortex and these structures, and fibers descend from the cortex to motor neurons in the brainstem. The IC also receives efferents from the medial geniculate (Pickles, 1988). Efferent fibers may give rise to other efferent fibers along the entire length of the pathway. This would provide a complete efferent connection from the cortex to the periphery (Harrison & Howe, 1974). Although there is evidence for this complete pathway, the definitive anatomy is not known.

Electrical stimulation of the cortex results in the excitation or inhibition of single units in the lower auditory system (Ryugo & Weinberger, 1976). Physiologic evidence exists for a descending train of impulses that eventually reaches the cochlea from the cortex (Desmedt, 1975).

The olivocochlear bundle (OCB) is the best known circuitry of the efferent system. The OCB has two main tracts: the lateral and the medial (Warr, 1980). The lateral tract originates from cells near the lateral superior olive and is composed mostly of uncrossed, unmyelinated fibers which terminate on the (ipsilateral) dendrites beneath the inner hair cells. The medial tract of the OCB is composed of myelinated fibers that originate in the area around the medial superior olive. Most fibers cross to the opposite cochlea, where they connect directly to the outer hair cells. The lateral and medial OCB also connect to various divisions of the cochlear nucleus before they course along the vestibular nerves in the internal auditory meatus (Pickles, 1988; Warr, 1980).

Some early physiologic studies show that stimulation of the crossed OCB fibers results in reduced neural response from the cochlea and auditory nerve (Galambos, 1956). However, stimulation of the lateral aspect of the SOC has lowered the threshold of fibers in the CN (Comis & Whitfield, 1968). Hence, it appears that the OCB has the potential to excite or inhibit the activity from the cochlea.

Pickles and Comis (1973) showed that the application of atropine (a cholinergic blocker) in the region of the OCB resulted in poorer hearing in noise. Other studies show that the OCB has an important role for hearing in noise (Dewson, 1968; Nieder & Nieder, 1970). The mechanism underlying this facilitation for hearing in noise may be related to the ability of the medial OCB to trigger outer hair-cell expansion/contraction, thereby enhancing or damping basilar membrane activity. An important part of this OCB function has to do with its neurotransmitters. The OCB is a central mechanism which has some control over the periphery.

AUDITORY NEUROCHEMISTRY

Neurotransmitters are neurochemical agents that carry information across the synapse between nerve cells. Many characteristics of auditory function and processing may be influenced by the type of synapse and the specific neurotransmitters involved. Because many of the known neurotransmitters are associated with the central auditory system, we review neurochemistry as part of a discussion of auditory neuroanatomy and physiology. Much of the research on auditory neurotransmitters has profound clinical implications.

The Anatomy of Neurotransmission

The main structure in neurotransmission is the synapse. The synapse is the connecting link between nerve cells and involves the synaptic button of the axon, which communicates neurochemically with the dendrites (or in some cases the cell body) of another nerve cell. The neurotransmitters are released by vesicles and diffuse across the synaptic region to bind to receptors, which are proteins embedded in the adjacent cell membrane The binding of a neurotransmitter can cause several events to occur. One event is the change in ion flow across the cell membrane, which can cause a change in the receptor potential (postsynaptic cell). After a number of transmitter-receptor interactions have occurred in a restricted time period, the postsynaptic cell will depolarize and fire its own impulse or action potential. This action is associated with an excitatory neurotransmitter (Musiek & Hoffman, 1990).

An inhibitory neurotransmitter can cause hyperpolarization of the postsynaptic cell membrane, which makes the cell difficult to excite (i.e., fire an impulse) (Musiek & Hoffman, 1990). Other biochemical actions of the cell can influence the nature of the synapse but are beyond the scope of this review.

Presently, many therapeutic drugs are used to affect the synaptic activity. An agonist may mimic natural neurotransmitters by binding to and activating the postsynaptic receptor. An antagonists causes an opposite effect—it can bind to the receptor but not activate it. By binding to the receptor it also blocks the natural neurotransmitter function.

Auditory Neurotransmission (Afferent)

If neurotransmitters can control synaptic activity, it may be possible to control the functions that are based on these synaptic interactions. The neurotransmitters must first be identified and localized. Strict criteria must be met before a chemical can be considered a neurotransmitter (Musiek & Hoffman, 1990). Once these neurotransmitters are identified, treatments with agonists and antagonists may provide new information on function and dysfunction of a system.

The neurotransmitter that operates between the cochlear hair cells and the fibers of the auditory nerve is not known, but glutamate is thought to be a possibility (Bledsoe, Bobbin, & Puel, 1988). Glutamate or aspartate are thought to be involved in auditory nerve-to-CN transmission (Bledsoe et al., 1988; Guth & Melamed, 1982). The CN probably has several excitatory neurotransmitters, including aspartate, glutamate, and acetylcholine (ACh) (Altschuler, Wenthold, Schwartz, Haser, Curthoys, Parakkal, & Fex, 1984; Godfrey, Park, Dunn, & Ross, 1985; Oliver, Potashner, Jones, & Morest, 1983). Gamma amino butyric acid and glycine are inhibitory amino acids found at high levels in the CN (Godfrey, Carter, Berger, Lowry, & Matschinsky, 1977). Both gamma amino butyric acid and glycine are also found in the SOC (Helfert, Altschuler & Wenthold, 1987; Wenthold, Huie, Altschuler, & Reeks, 1987). Excitatory amino acids, such as quisqualate, glutamate and N-methyl-D-aspartate (NMDA), have been localized in the SOC (Otterson & Storm-Mathison, 1984). Glycine and glutamate are likely neurotransmitters in the IC (Adams & Wenthold, 1987). Both NMDA and aspartate have been shown to increase activity at the level of the IC (Faingold, Hoffman, & Caspary, 1989).

There are little data on auditory cortex neurotransmitters. There is some evidence that ACh and some opiate drugs affect auditory cortex activity or evoked potentials; however, more research is necessary to understand the neurochemistry in this brain region (McKenna, Ashe, Hui, & Weinberger, 1988; Velasco, Velasco, Castaneda, & Sanchez, 1984).

Auditory Neurotransmission (Efferent)

More information is available on efferent than afferent neurotransmitters. Specifically, the neurotransmission of the olivocochlear bundle (OCB) has been studied extensively. The OCB system can be viewed as two systems. One system is lateral and originates from the area around the lateral superior olive. The second system is medial and rises from the region of the medial olive. Both systems are cholinergic (Altschuler & Fex, 1986). The lateral system also has enkephalin and dynorphin, which are opioid peptides (Hoffman, 1986). These efferent neurotransmitters can be found in the perilymph of the cochlea. Applying ACh to the OCB mimics effects of electrical stimulation of the OCB (Bobbin & Konishi, 1971).

Auditory Function

Studies have examined neurotransmitter effects on auditory function as measured either electrophysiologically or behaviorally. For example, auditory nerve activity during sound stimulation was reduced when glutamatergic blockers were perfused through the cochleas of guinea pigs (Cousillas, Cole, & Johnstone, 1988). An increase in spontaneous and acoustically stimulated firing rates of CN fibers was noted with the application of aspirate, an excitatory amino acid. This effect was reversed when an antagonist drug was administered. A similar study using agonists (glutamate, aspartate, NMDA) and antagonists at the level of the IC showed similar neural modulating results (Faingold, Hoffman, & Caspary, 1989).

In humans, the late auditory evoked potential (P2) showed an increase in amplitude when naloxone, an opioid antagonist, was administered. In the same study fentanyl, an opioid agonist, reduced the P2 amplitude (Velasco et al., 1984).

Auditory function of the OCB and neurotransmission have been studied. As mentioned, the OCB plays a role in enhancing hearing in noise (Pickles & Comis, 1973; Winslow & Sachs, 1987). This role may be mediated by the chemical interaction of the OCB and the hair cells of the cochlea. The fact that outer hair cells can expand and contract may be intimately related to the OCB because neurotransmitters may control this hair-cell function. This in turn may allow OCB modulation of incoming impulses via the outer hair cells by regulating their motor activity.

Recent studies on chinchillas have shown that the auditory nerve action potential can be enhanced significantly by injecting pentazocine, an opioid agonist (Stahley, Kalish, Musiek, & Hoffman, 1991). This effect, noted only at intensity levels near threshold, clearly involves the OCB system, since opioids are found in the (lateral) OCB system.

Studies on auditory function and neurotransmission eventually may provide a pharmacological way to enhance hearing. Research in this area emphasizes neurochemistry's intimate role in auditory physiology.

IMPLICATIONS FOR (RE)HABILITATION

Habilitative approaches for CAPD should be generated from basic knowledge in the main areas related to function of the CANS, including maturation course, the effects of auditory deprivation, sensory stimulation, and brain plasticity. These areas overlap and should not be considered as mutually exclusive. Rather, these headings are primarily for organizational purposes. We provide an overview of these major areas and relevant examples of experiments that demonstrate underlying mechanisms.

Maturational Course

Different parts of the brain and auditory system develop and mature at different rates. In a general sense, the auditory system matures in a caudal to rostral manner. Maturation of the auditory system evolves around several mechanisms, including cell differentiation and migration, myelination, arborization, and synaptogenesis. We discuss the last three mechanisms.

Myelination

Myelin is white matter of the nervous system which covers and insulates the axons of a nerve fiber (Figure 2–7).

Generally, the amount of myelin on a nerve fiber indicates how fast the impulses are conducted. A heavily myelinated nerve fiber will conduct impulses quickly (some large fibers up to 100 meters/sec), whereas nerve conduction is slow in unmyelinated fibers (< 2 meters/sec) (Mountcastle, 1968). Slow conduction limits the types of processing that take place. Some examples come from the studies on the quaking mouse, a species that, because of a genetic disorder, does not produce myelin. Auditory brainstem response testing on these mice indicates that their interwave latencies are almost twice as long as in control mice (Shah & Salamy, 1980). In another study on myelination, the amount of myelin was measured in rats for 50 days postnatally. The study measured the amount of cerebroside (a lipid in the blood) which increases with the amount of myelin. As the rat pups grew older the amount of myelin increased and the interwave latency of the ABRs decreased (Shah & Salamy, 1980).

Myelination of the brain occurs at different rates for different regions. It appears that the brainstem auditory tracts complete myelination before the subcortical regions of the brain. In humans most of the ABR indices reach adult values at around 2 years of age. However, the middle latency and late auditory evoked potentials do not approach adult characteristics until much later, and the P300 auditory potential does not mature until adolescence or the early teenage years (Musiek & Gollegly, 1988). The development course of these evoked potentials is consistent with the caudal-to-rostral myelination pattern in the brain.

Behavioral auditory tests also have an extended maturational course. Masking level differences (MLDs) are larger in preschoolers than in infants (Nozza, Wagner, & Crandell, 1988). Jensen and Neff (1989) have shown that auditory frequency and duration discrimina-

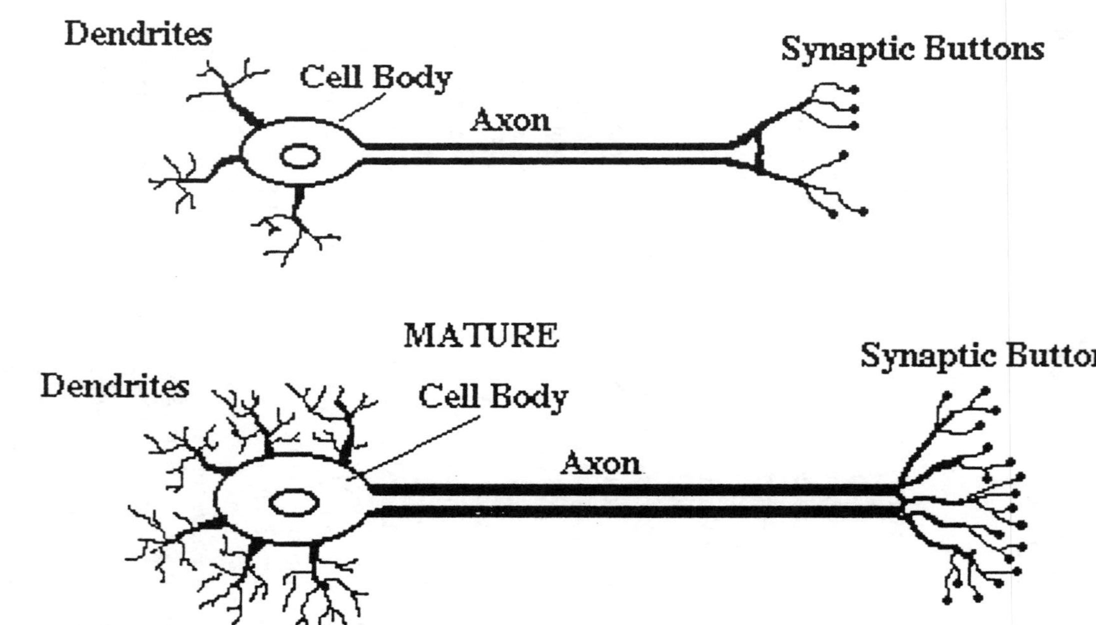

Figure 2–7. An immature and mature nerve cell. Note thicker myelin on the axon and more synaptic buttons and dendrites on the mature cell.

tion is better in 6-year-old children than in 4-year-olds, but not as good as in adults. Dichotic listening and frequency pattern performance do not reach adult values until approximately 10 to 11 years of age. With the possible exception of MLDs these auditory behavioral tasks are mostly associated with cerebral functions, reflecting the long maturational course for the neural substrate related to these functions. Again, this functional developmental timetable is consistent with the myelination time course (Yakovlev & Lecours, 1967).

What is the myelin (maturational) time course to which we refer and what is its foundation? Yakovlev and LeCours (1967) reported on years of study of human brains in regard to myelination at various ages and anatomical regions. Using a Loyez (silver) staining technique they quantified the amount of myelin in a given region of the brain. Their large collection of brains covered a wide range of ages. Yakovlev and LeCours (1967) showed that the optic tracts myelinated before the auditory tracts did. The prethalamic auditory tracts are essentially myelin-complete at 5 to 6 months after birth. However, post-thalamic auditory tracts are not myelin-mature until 5 to 6 years of age. The corpus callosum and certain auditory association areas may not have completed myelinogenesis until 10 to 12 years or older. The somatosensory evoked potentials used to measure interhemispheric transfer time by comparing ipsilateral to contralateral stimulation latencies indicated that corpus callosum maturity ranges from about 10 to 20 years of age (Salamy et al., 1980). This was interpreted also as an index of myelination of the CC.

Another important factor of myelin maturation is the great variability in its rate (Moore, 1983; Yakovlev & LeCours, 1967). If myelination rate varies, the processes it underlies may also vary. Therefore, if a certain amount of maturation is needed to complete a task and that maturation has not been achieved, the task cannot be completed. It is likely that the difference in children's performance on certain auditory tests may be related to differences in the amount of myelination in critical regions of the brain.

Arborization and Synaptogenesis

The term arborization is used to mean axonal or dendritic branching. This is a maturational process of the nerve cell critical to the functioning of groups of neurons. Generally, as the cell matures there is greater arborization; however, increased arborization may also be a result of certain types of continued stimulation after the nerve cell is mature (Figure 2–7).

A nerve cell is composed of three main parts: soma (cell body), axon, and dendrites. The cell body and axons change with maturity. Axonic and dendritic branching is one of the most dynamic maturational actions of the cell. In the very early maturational course, growing axons make their way to specific areas of the immature brain. After reaching its destination, the axon develops branching (i.e., arborization), and each branch has a bulbus terminal. These bulbs in turn make synapses with dendrites (Kalil, 1989). In the first year of life, one cortical neuron may connect with as many as 10,000 other neurons through axonal/dendritic branching (Crelin, 1973). Arborization continues to increase for several years (Crelin, 1973). It is difficult to determine when arborization reaches its maturational peak, because it is influenced by environmental experience (Kalil, 1989). Arborization provides an anatomical basis for more complex interactions among neurons in the brain. Appropriate connections are needed for appropriate function; thus, dendritic branching without connection to other cell bodies or axons is of little value. The course of dendritic maturation appears to show the greatest change in the first few years of life, but the extent of these changes in regard to age is indeterminable.

Recent information about synaptic development suggests an important role of action potentials. When young axons are prevented from generating action potentials, the synaptic structures (i.e., terminal bulbs) do not develop (Kalil, 1989). Therefore, these electrical impulses (most of which come from external stimulation) of the axon are crucial to synaptogenesis.

The synapse is the communication between neurons which involves the transfer of a neurotransmitter. Earlier we discussed this aspect of neurochemistry. Because dendrites are necessary for synapses, their maturity directly influences the overall amount of synaptic development. In studies on kittens an increase in synapses occurs at the inferior colliculus until 14 days of age. Also, the number of synaptic terminals is considerably greater in an 8-day-old kitten than in a 3-day-old kitten (Reynolds, 1975).

Maturation is not the only influence on the synapse that can result in its change. Stimulation can alter the number of synapses and synaptic density after the system is mature. Conversely, a lack of stimulation (deprivation) may reduce the number of synaptic components.

Auditory Deprivation

If a sufficient amount of auditory stimulation is not achieved, structural and function development may not reach its optimal level. Considerable effort has been necessary to establish scientific evidence to support this concept. A number of approaches demonstrate the effect of deprivation on the auditory system. In animals the periphery can be compromised (i.e. suturing the ear canal, ablating the middle ear or cochlea, sectioning the auditory nerve). Another procedure to create deprivation effects is to raise animals in a sound-attenuated environment. In humans, clinical cases of otitis media or sensorineural hearing loss have been used to represent a form of deprivation for study. Many studies on auditory deprivation exist, and a select few are discussed here.

Structural Changes From Auditory Deprivation

The most marked and consistent alteration of auditory brainstem nuclei is a result of ablation (in some form) of the cochlea or sectioning the auditory nerve. Studies show that, after cochlear ablation, the CN neuronal area and synaptic endings are compromised (Jean Baptiste & Morest, 1975; Kane, 1974; Morest, 1982). Partial cochlear hearing loss as a result of oval window puncture also has been shown to affect the mean cell area of auditory brainstem nuclei in chickens (Tucci, Born, & Rubel, 1987).

After intense noise exposure, which damaged major portions of the inner and outer hair cells of the cochlea, degeneration of the cells of the cochlear nucleus and areas of the SOC was observed in cats. Maximal degeneration of the brainstem nuclei occurred 7 to 60 days after noise exposure (Morest, 1982). A similar study in chinchillas revealed degeneration at the CN, SOC, and IC (Morest, 1982). Similar findings have been reported when ototoxic drugs were used to damage the cochlea's cellular structure (Hall, 1976). When one ear's cochlea is damaged the resultant central degeneration generally occurs in the ipsilateral CN and in the contralateral SOC and IC (Morest, 1982). The studies using ablation or induced trauma on the cochlea created a deprivation of sound and resulted in central compromise. However, these types of deprivation may be different than that of a conductive loss or of leaving the ear intact and changing the sound environment.

Conductive hearing loss, as a form of deprivation, has been created in a number of ways (i.e., ligating the ear canals, removing the ossicles). In most cases, this type of hearing loss, when the loss was incurred early in life, has resulted in reduced cell areas in the CN, SOC, and IC (Evans, Webster, & Cullen, 1983; Webster, 1983). Conductive loss induced later in life affects the size of the brainstem nuclei; this effect remains over an extended time period (Webster, 1988).

Webster (1988b) also demonstrated that sound amplification during deprivation (conductive loss) resulted in negating the central effects of hearing loss. However, Tucci, and Rubel (1985) showed no effect on the size of nucleus magnocellularis (avian homologue to CN spherical cells) from either plugging the ear or from ossicle removal. Results using sound isolation to precipitate effects on central structures are mixed. Webster (1983) and Webster & Webster (1977) showed degeneration of caudal pontine auditory structures related to sound isolation, but others have reported no effect (Coleman & O'Connor, 1979; Feng & Rogowski, 1980).

The general trend revealed in the literature is that deprivation of sound stimulation can negatively influence the central structures of the auditory system. It also appears that greater structural changes are noted if deprivation takes place during critical developmental periods (Webster, 1983). This could be interpreted as indicating that acoustic stimulation is necessary during the critical period to ensure normal neuronal development. However, dysfunction can occur without noted changes in structure, and physiological effects of deprivation must be examined.

Electrophysiologic Changes From Auditory Deprivation

As mentioned, various types of auditory deprivation appear to affect CANS function. For example, Clopton and Silverman (1978) showed that deprivation from an induced conductive loss resulted in increased latency of spike discharges at the IC. A similar but smaller effect was noted in older animals undergoing the same type of deprivation. Tucci, Born, and Rubel (1987) measured spontaneous neural activity in the chicken's brainstem after ossicle removal and found essentially no change. However, after an oval window puncture spontaneous activity decreased. Marked changes in spontaneous firing rate at the CN due to cochlea removal have been well documented (Korber, Pfeiffer, Warr, & Kiang, 1966). Interestingly, a study using the auditory brainstem response (ABR) to measure brainstem function showed shorter latencies for mice raised in a sound-isolated environment, as compared with control animals.

As stated, evidence exists for auditory deprivation resulting in physiological compromise of central auditory nuclei in animals. One of the most critical questions is whether fluctuating hearing loss, such as caused by otitis media, can result in some types of central auditory compromise. Electrophysiologic approaches, such as the ABR, can be used with humans to determine the integrity of the brainstem auditory pathway and to examine the effect of otitis media. The ABR has been used to study children with otitis media to monitor brainstem integrity. Essentially all studies have indicated some type of brainstem dysfunction (Gunnarson & Finitzo, 1991; Lenhart, Shaia, & Abedi, 1985; Folsum, Weber, & Thompson, 1983). A study by Gunnarson and Finitzo (1991) measured ABRs in children (ages 5 to 7 years) who were tested at infancy. The children were divided into three groups: infants with normal ABRs up to 2 years of age, infants with fluctuating conductive loss, and a group with abnormal ABRs and more severe conductive loss than those in group 2. Group 1 differed from groups 2 and 3 in the latency of waves III and V as well as interwaves I–III and I–V. The ABR binaural interaction was also measured and was present in eight of nine children in groups 1 and 2, but in only four of nine children in group 3.

Auditory deprivation can take many forms and is a continuum ranging from nearly complete to only mild conditions. Although studies are difficult to perform and can be contradictory, the concept that auditory deprivation may result in central compromise should be strongly considered clinically and experimentally. The effects of deprivation may too subtle to be measured with our current tools. As our technology increases we may be able to better define the subtle dysfunctions related to auditory deprivation. We must examine the following questions: If auditory deprivation is a negative influence is auditory stimulation a positive influence? Can changes in the CANS be brought about by systematic acoustic stimulation?

Auditory Stimulation And Plasticity

Auditory stimulation and plasticity are related and interactive, and we shall discuss them together. Auditory stimulation (experience) is an easily understood term, but plasticity has many different connotations. Neural form and connections take on a predictable pattern (probably genetically determined) often referred to as neural specificity; exceptions to this predictable pattern represent neural plasticity (Lund, 1978). This relates to the common suggestions that changing patterns of neural form and connections are the bases for behavioral change and learning which occur throughout life. Often considered are three basic types of plasticity: developmental, compensatory (after lesions or damage), and learning related (Scheich, 1991). The concepts of auditory stimulation and plasticity are important to habilitation of central auditory processing problems. Knowing whether a neural change can or cannot be brought about by stimulation has critical implications for therapy.

Stimulation or the influence of environmental sounds is key to plasticity. We refer to studies that provide examples of the effect of stimulation on the neurobiology of the hearing system.

Hassmannova, Myslivecek, and Novakova (1981) clearly showed the influence of systematic auditory stimulation in early life. Rat pups (2 weeks old) were stimulated with interrupted tonal stimuli for 30 sessions (each session was 30 minutes) for 2 weeks. Near-field auditory evoked potentials were recorded. The ribonucleic acid (RNA) content of the auditory cortex was measured immediately after the stimulation period for one group of animals, and 4 weeks later for another group of animals. These measurements were compared to those obtained from control animals. Both groups of experimental animals showed significantly decreased latencies for the evoked potentials and greater amounts of RNA in auditory cortex than did control animals. The animals that were tested 4 weeks after the stimulation period showed less of an effect that those tested immediately after the experimental period.

The stimulation of various systems other than the auditory supports the concept that neuronal change is likely. Results from animal studies on the visual and cerebellar systems show that sensory/motor stimulation influences neuronal morphology and function (Bailey & Chen, 1988; Greenough & Bailey, 1988). Recent investigations show a greater number of synapses per neuron in the visual cortex of animals that were reared in complex visual environments, as compared to animals raised in simple visual surroundings (Bailey & Chen, 1988). In another study, four groups of rats were trained on four motor tasks. The first group of rats was trained on a simple motor task, with the next three groups trained on subsequently more complex motor tasks. The group of rats trained on the most complex task showed significantly greater neuronal thickness and synaptic density in the cerebellar neurons than did the other three groups of animals (Greenough & Bailey, 1988).

As mentioned, plasticity appears to be related to maturation. Specifically, the younger the brain the more plastic it is. This concept is supported by behaviorally based studies on sound localization in barn owls. Barn owls have identical head orientation to either visual or auditory localization cues in space. Hence, the difference between visual and auditory localization can be used to measure the degree of error if one system or other is compromised experimentally. In a series of studies by Knudsen (1988), young (< 60 days old) and old barn owls had one ear occluded and their localization ability was measured. As expected, both groups had compromised localization immediately after occlusion. However, the young barn owls' localization performance began to approach normal after 2 to 3 weeks, while the older barn owls' localization showed little improvement. Knudsen (1988) also showed that in young barn owls with one ear occluded auditory neurons changed their "spatial" tuning when the earplug was in place. When the earplug was removed, the neural spatial tuning reverted back to near its original characteristics. The older barn owls did not show this neural change. This physiologically measured change correlated with a critical time period in which the behavioral localization alteration took place.

In another recent study (Recanzone, Schreiner, Hradek, Sutter, Beitel, & Merzenich, 1991), owl monkeys were trained on a frequency discrimination task. After extensive training, the auditory cortex was tonotopically mapped and the area of the trained frequency was two to eight times larger than in the control animals that did not receive the auditory training. In addition, these trained animals improved their frequency discrimination (measured behaviorally) ability after training. This study was the basis for two subsequent studies on children with language learning problems for which auditory training on specific aspects of temporal processing was performed. These children improved their language abilities and auditory processing (Merzenich et al., 1996; Tallal et al., 1996).

Another example of plasticity is related to peripheral (cochlear) hearing loss and the tonotopic reorganization of the auditory cortex. This is a case where the demonstration of plasticity is not related to stimulation but to frequency-specific deprivation. Schwaber, Garraghty, Morel, and Kaas (1994) tonotopically mapped the auditory cortex of adult macaque monkeys before and after (80 to 90 days) experimentally induced cochlear hearing loss. Three months after the incurred hearing loss the auditory cortex was again mapped and showed extensive reorganization. The deprived region of the cortex became responsive to frequencies of an adjacent auditory region (i.e., in this case the cortical area responded to lower frequencies than before). This research highlights important points. First, this plasticity occurred in adult animals, indicating the process to extend past the maturational period. Also, because the cortical tissue assumes new frequency responsiveness it remains viable, possibly a way to avoid degeneration. Clearly, permanent peripheral damage influences the structure and function of the auditory cortex. A major question, however, is whether the cortex can reorganize back to the original tonotopic arrangement if hearing is restored at the damaged frequencies and, if it can, what is the critical time period for this to happen.

Another concept related to brain plasticity is that of long-term potentiation, which can be defined as the condition when the strength of transmission at many synapses increases with repetitive use. The increase in synaptic potentials appears to take place in the amygdala and hippocampal areas of the brain, which are generally linked to memory (Gustafsson & Wigstrom, 1988). Long-term potentiation can be demonstrated months after the initial stimulation regime (Gustafsson & Wigstrom, 1988). Changes in synaptic morphology and chemical neural transmission seem to be the basis for long-term potentiation. More specifically, this stronger transmission seems to be associated with both chemical and anatomic changes at the synaptic level (Gustafsson, 1988; Smith, 1988).

In summarizing, postulates from Aoki and Siekevitz (1988) are appropriate to mention. These authors state that the type of experience (especially, but not exclusively, in early life) will influence the finite structure and function of the brain. Depending on the type of stimulation, certain neural pathways will be reinforced with use, while others fall into disuse. They likened plasticity of the brain to a highway system that evolves with use. Some highly used roads will be broadened and new ones added where necessary, while less used roads will be abandoned. These changes in the brain related to experience seem to be triggered by certain molecular events that are driven by a protein (MAP2), which affects activity at the synaptic region of the cell.

Theoretically, if proper auditory experience at the proper time is not achieved, then proper neural connections may not be established. However, if the proper auditory neural connections do not evolve due to inadequate experience, some degree of plasticity should evolve if adequate and proper stimulation is achieved. How much plasticity takes place with stimulation depends on the concepts such as critical period and maturity.

In conclusion, we have drawn on studies, theories, and clinical interpretations to provide a neurobiologic framework for central auditory assessment and habilitation. We have reported some older but fundamental aspects of structure and function of the neuroauditory system along with new concepts of higher auditory function. We encourage the reader to become well grounded in neurobiologic correlates to central auditory disorders, as it remains the key to understanding and helping our patients.

CHAPTER

3

SPOKEN LANGUAGE PROCESSING

CHIE HIGUCHI CRAIG

The intent of this chapter is to consider spoken language processing as it relates to the assessment and treatment of individuals with central auditory processing disorders (CAPD). Given the dynamic and ephemeral acoustic characteristics of real-world speech signals and the potentially disruptive nature of background noise and reverberation, real-world spoken language processing is the most powerful and probably the most demanding activity to which the central auditory nervous system is directed. It is, therefore, not surprising when individuals with peripheral hearing impairment and/or CAPD report that understanding speech is their greatest everyday challenge.

SPOKEN LANGUAGE PROCESSING: A DEFINITION

The term *spoken language processing* refers to an interactive system of peripheral and central functions used by listeners to recognize and understand real-world transitory utterances as meaningful words or streams of connected meaningful words. In the extant literature, the term *speech perception* frequently accompanies the term spoken language processing and at times the two terms appear almost interchangeable. Albeit highly related, these terms denote important differences in a researcher's scope of study and scholarly emphasis. Speech perception researchers typically consider issues pertaining to the analysis of speech and other complex sound patterns. They study relationships among acoustic, phonetic, and speech production mechanism properties and how these relationships affect speech recognition performance. Although these issues significantly influence the spoken language process, researchers of spoken language processing place less emphasis on the acoustic-phonetic characteristics of the speech waveform and more emphasis on how the auditory percept is processed linguistically.

Due to the anatomical and physiological complexity of the central auditory nervous system and the intricate and interactive functional nature of the central auditory processing system, a transdisciplinary approach to the study of spoken language processing is recommended. Relatively recent research developments in psycholinguistics, automatic speech recognition, computational simulation, and linguistic theory have significantly increased our understanding of spoken language processing and the way sound is transformed into meaning. Although not all of the work of these disciplines is specifically directed to investigate central auditory processing or CAPD issues, it does, nevertheless, present a body of knowledge critical to the development of improved audiologic assessment and aural (re)habilitation strategies for individuals with CAPD (Lubinsky, 1986; Massaro, 1987). Many of the terms employed in this chapter have yet to attain definitional consensus, thus, an attempt has been made to use terminology that is consistent with various disciplines and theoretical frameworks.

Specifically, the chapter's discussion is divided into several sections. First, theoretical and empirical spoken language findings are discussed from a psycholinguistic perspective with special emphasis placed on the process of real-time spoken word recognition and the time-gating paradigm. Next, the literature is discussed from a clinical perspective, and a rationale for real-time speech recognition assessment is proposed. Finally, new approaches to CAPD aural (re)habilitation are discussed.

A PSYCHOLINGUISTIC PERSPECTIVE

In the past, the role of language processing in spoken word recognition was a neglected area of study. Psychological research focused on the written word, and generally it was assumed that processes involved in vision and reading were also involved in the auditory modality. Contemporary emphasis is on the development of psycholinguistic and linguistic computational models that specifically account for behavioral performance data in spoken word recognition (Cole & Jakimik, 1980; Elman & McClelland, 1984; Marslen-Wilson, 1987).

Models of Spoken Language Processing

Models have been developed to describe the function of numerous subprocesses involving the detection of the acoustic speech signal, perceptual analysis by the central auditory mechanism, and the active participation of higher level capabilities (Forster, 1976; Klatt, 1979; Marslen-Wilson, 1987; McClelland & Elman, 1986; Morton, 1969; Pisoni, 1984; Warren, 1981). Such models describe how listeners: (a) perceive the acoustic signal, (b) conduct auditory analysis involving complex pattern recognition, (c) match acoustic patterns to some internal representation(s), (d) extract meaning from strings of lexical representations, and (e) construct a message level interpretation. The six questions and responses that follow provide a brief review of critical issues that have been addressed by researchers involved in the study of spoken word recognition processing.

1. In the spoken word recognition process, what is the size and nature of the auditory percept or processed unit? Many types of auditory processing units have been considered, ranging from phonetic segments (Forster & Bednall, 1976) to whole words (Morton, 1969). Some models permit different sized units to interact. For example, the interactive-activation model recognizes distinctive features and words (Elman & McClelland, 1984). Another model proposed by Warren (1981) employs several different sizes of perceptual units (e.g., phoneme, syllable, or word) that are operational, depending on the type of stimulus, listener, and listening environment.

2. How is lexical access initiated? Lexical access refers to the beginning stage of the lexical searching process in which the auditory percept comes in contact with various aspects of stored mental representations (Forster, 1976; Pisoni, 1984). Many different forms of mental representations have been suggested, including distinctive features (Klatt, 1979), phonemes (Pisoni & Luce, 1987), and syllables (Mehler, 1981). According to some models, lexical access specifically involves matching perceptions of acoustic-phonetic segments to lexical candidates stored in a similarly segmentally structured memory. In the Neighborhood Activation Model (NAM), segmental structure refers to a lexical organization plan or architecture based on the relative acoustic-phonetic similarity between sounds in words (Luce, Pisoni, & Goldinger, 1990). Proposed by Luce (1986), this computer-based model isolates the acoustic-phonetic properties of a target word to determine which word candidates are potential lexical neighbors. A neighborhood is defined as a collection of words that are phonetically similar to the target word. In 1995, Iler Kirk, Pisoni, and Osberger reported that pediatric cochlear implant users are sensitive to acoustic-phonetic similarities among words. They found that their listeners organized words into similarity neighborhoods and employed a NAM-type process to recognize stimuli from the PB-K word list.

3. How much of the speech utterance (e.g., duration from onset) is required to lexically access particular word candidates? Some theorize that immediate lexical contact occurs with perception (Klatt, 1976). Others suggest an initial syllable or 150 ms of a word (Marslen-Wilson & Tyler, 1980). Most assume that there is a discrete stage of lexical access that in some manner restricts the number and nature of potential word candidates drawn from a mental lexicon.

4. How do listeners segment fluently spoken utterances? Co-articulation and other contextual sources of variance and nonlinearity are common in fluent everyday speech (Pichney, Durlach, & Braida, 1985). For spoken word recognition to occur, a listener must be able to construe transitory, rapidly changing acoustic utterances into discrete words. To reduce the risk of inappropriate segmentation that can lead to unpredictable mental representations and/or ineffective lexical access, several acoustic stream segmentation strategies have been developed. Cutler and Norris (1988) proposed the Metrical Segmentation Strategy, which suggests that, in the spoken English language, strongly stressed syllables demarcate units of lexical access. In addition, Bard, Schillcock, and Altmann (1988) suggested that strong syllables access a few highly activated word candidates and that weak syllables access many candidates, but at lower levels of activation. Models that assume no unique point of initial contact for each word candidate avoid some of the strategic pitfalls associated with segmentation. For example, the interactive activation model allows each activated phoneme to evoke a new subset of word candidates (Elman & McClelland, 1984). This approach bypasses some problems caused by inappropriately high levels of sensitivity (e.g., no allowance for misperception), but also tends to set inappropriately low levels of selectivity, resulting in the activation of very large sets or many sets of word candidates.

5. How are particular lexical items activated and eventually selected? Lexical activation refers to some change in status for a subset of lexically accessed word candidates. Some suggest that activation levels vary due to characteristics of the percept, goodness of fit with the contact representation(s), or internal features of word candidates (e.g., frequency of occurrence) (Marslen-Wilson & Welsh, 1978). Most psycholinguists agree that, once a subset of lexical candidates is activated, the ongoing speech signal continues to provide information that eventually results in word selection. In the spoken language literature the term *word recognition* is reserved for the conclusion of the word selection phase when the listener proceeds with some confidence under the assumption that a perceived utterance matches or will match with a particular word candidate.

6. How does information derived from the auditory percept interact with existing linguistic-contextual information? The term *linguistic-contextual information* can be defined as anything that influences the a priori probability of an upcoming utterance or the post hoc, retroactive recognition of a previously unrecognized past utterance. As early as 1951, Miller, Heise, and Lichten (1951) postulated that, as listeners hear words in succession, context constrains the number of probable word candidates, and word intelligibility increases as the number of potential candidates decreases. Some theorists argue that early sensory information is processed autonomously of context and higher level knowledge and that linguistic-context has an effect only after word recognition occurs (Forster, 1981; Klatt, 1979). Others assert that linguistic-contextual factors such as sentence context influence the early sensory analysis of the input signal and that various higher level knowledge sources interact and direct the real-time recognition process (Grosjean, 1980; Salasoo & Pisoni, 1985; Tyler & Wessels, 1983). The spoken utterance can be characterized by its acoustic-phonetic features, but the characteristic of a listener's percept appears to be determined by aspects of the utterance and its context that are selected and depended upon for message interpretation. Recently, Nittrouer (1996) reported that the relative perceptual weighting placed on various acoustic-phonetic parameters differs for children and adults. Given identical speech signals, what one listener hears and what other listeners hear may vary. For example, adults who are acquiring a second language or dialect often report that they do not hear subtle sound segments or prosodic nuances that may be acoustically available and clearly apparent to native language listeners.

A ubiquitous research finding is that context plays a central role in spoken word recognition processing (Blank & Foss, 1978; Cairns & Hsu, 1980; Marslen-Wilson & Tyler, 1980; Salasoo & Pisoni, 1985). In everyday speech, words occur in context, and context generally improves word recognition performance (Cole & Rudnicky, 1983; Miller, Heise, & Lichten, 1951; Schiavetti, Sitler, Metz, & Houde, 1984). Words spoken in isolation are more easily recognized than nonsense syllables, and words having a high frequency of occurrence are more easily recognized than words with a low frequency of occurrence. Moreover, sentential contexts tend to facilitate recognition accuracy (Craig, 1988; Giolas, Cooker, & Duffy, 1970; Hirsh, Reynolds, & Joseph, 1954; Howes, 1952; Kalikow, Stevens, & Elliott, 1977; Owen, 1961; Pollack, Rubenstein, & Decker, 1959; Rosenzweig & Postman, 1957; Savin, 1963; Schultz, 1964). Linguistic-contextual influences arise from listeners' abilities to use information sources beyond those derived from sensory input. These higher information sources include phonotactic, prosodic, syntactic, semantic, lexical, and pragmatic knowledge.

Semantic-contextual effects have been studied by manipulating the level of target *word predictability*. Word predictability refers to the amount of *fill-in-the blank* meaningfulness in a preceding sentence context (Giolas, Cooker, & Duffy, 1970; Howes, 1952). One of the most extensive investigations studying the effects of contrasting levels of target word predictability was conducted by Kalikow, Stevens, and Elliott (1977). Their predictability-high (PH) sentences contained semantic-contextual information in the form of clue words called *pointer words* in phrases preceding each test word. The predictability-low (PL) sentences were developed without pointer words. Their PH and PL sentences formed the basis for the original and revised versions of the *Speech Perception in Noise* (SPIN) Test (Bilger, Neutzel, Rabinowitz, & Rzeczkowski, 1984). An example of a PH sentence is: "A spoiled child is a *brat.*" An example of a PL sentence is: "Bill won't consider the *brat.*"

Recently, Elliott (1995) discussed a fill-in-the blank auditory function termed *verbal auditory closure*. Verbal auditory closure (VAC) refers to a listener's ability to use spoken contextual information to facilitate speech recognition. Elliott described VAC as a mental ability distinct from general intelligence and other types of mental abilities and proposed the *Revised Speech Perception in Noise* (SPIN) Test as an appropriate measure. In one early experiment (Craig, 1988), we compared speech recognition performances in three conditions of target word predictability. Target words were preceded by a predictability-high (PH), predictability-low (PL), and carrier phrase contexts. The results indicated that some PL contexts may confuse listeners and thus lower their PL word recognition performance. The PH and PL findings were consistent with results reported by Kalikow, Stevens, and Elliott (1977) and indicate that even the subtlest of semantic-contextual information can exert considerable influence on spoken word recognition performance.

In perhaps a more perceptual form of VAC, researchers report a subtle unconscious fill-in-the blank perceptual phenomenon called phonemic restoration. Research indicates that listeners use context to perceptually restore interrupted words. Consciously unaware of any acoustic disruption, listeners report that the interrupted speech appears intact, they are unable to locate the position of the interrupting noise within the word or sentence. Early experiments by Miller and Licklider (1950) revealed that periodically interrupted PB word lists seemed continuous when very brief (50 ms) gaps were filled with noise. However, they noted that, although the speech appeared more natural, word intelligibility was not increased by the noise, so the missing segments were not successfully restored.

Other studies involving speech interrupted by noise have shown that phonemes and whole syllables can be restored in keeping with the context provided by sentences and polysyllabic words. Correspondingly, several investigators have demonstrated increased intelligibility when noise is added to gaps in interrupted, isolated monosyllables, as well as when noise is added to gaps in periodically interrupted sentences (Bashford, Reiner, & Warren, 1992; Bashford & Warren, 1987; Warren, 1970, 1984).

Warren (1982) suggested that the perceptual restoration of speech represents a linguistic adaptation of a nonverbal phenomenon referred to as auditory induction. A perceptual synthesis of contextually appropriate sounds occurs when deleted segments of a signal are replaced by a potential masker. Bashford and Warren (1987) reported that the durational limit for multiple phonemic restorations was longest for normal discourse interrupted by noise and was equal to the average word duration in that stimulus (about 300 ms). They proposed that listeners use linguistic-contextual elements of speech to perceptually synthesize missing acoustic-phonetic components from noise and that this phenomenon varies with the extent of the disruption and the linguistic-contextual information. Phonemic restoration is another example of how the acoustic features of a spoken utterance do not necessarily predict the characteristic of a listener's percept. In phonemic restoration, what a listener hears appears to be determined by aspects of the utterance and its context that are selected and depended on for spoken language processing.

Real-time Spoken Word Recognition

As previously discussed, in real-world speech words occur in a rapidly changing ongoing temporal sequence. The term *real-time speech* refers to the transitory, ephemeral nature of an ongoing speech signal. When speech is presented in a real-time manner, listeners must quickly recognize phonemes, syllables, and words based on preceding linguistic-contextual cues and ongoing acoustic-phonetic information.

A particularly compelling early finding in the spoken language processing literature is that listeners generally complete the word recognition process before having heard the entire target word (Grosjean, 1980; Marslen-Wilson, 1987; Marslen-Wilson & Tyler, 1980). Real-time speech recognition performance findings indicate that contextual factors determine the type of word candidates and size of an initial subset of word candidates (Grosjean, 1980). Real-time processing appears qualitatively different when words occur in meaningful sentences than when words occur in isolation or in anomalous sentences (Salasoo & Pisoni, 1985). Real-time words occurring toward the end of a sentence tend to be recognized earlier and reacted to more quickly than words at the beginning of a sentence (Marslen-Wilson & Welsh, 1978). In 1978, Marslen-Wilson and Welsh proposed a model to explain the phenomena of real-time speech recognition processing and the interactivity of acoustic-phonetic and linguistic-contextual information. Based entirely on behavioral performance data, it was named the *Cohort model.*

The Cohort Model

According to the original and revised Cohort model (Marslen-Wilson, 1987; Marslen-Wilson & Welsh, 1978; Slowiaczek, Nusbaum, & Pisoni, 1987):

1. The real-time lexical process involves mapping acoustic-phonetic input onto representations of the phonological word form and accessing its semantic, syntactic, and/or lexical content;
2. Higher-level representations are constructed incrementally as each spoken word is recognized and the lexical content is immediately employed in the development of higher level information;

3. Initial sounds, to a greater extent than middle or ending word sounds, elicit a multiple activation of a cohort of word candidates; and
4. Following initial cohort activation, an interaction of top-down and bottom-up word isolation schema occurs and each cohort member is dynamically assigned and reassigned activation levels until word acceptance is achieved.

Two types of behavioral assessment techniques have been developed to test the Cohort Model and study how listeners recognize words in real-time. The first technique involves a reaction-time type of response task. Listeners are asked to immediately repeat or shadow the pronunciation or mispronunciation of ongoing speech samples (Marslen-Wilson & Welsh, 1978). This type of measure is considered indirect because it requires the addition of a correction factor (50–75 ms) to compensate for an assumed latency period between the listener's internal decision process and expressed response (Marslen-Wilson, 1987). An advantage of this technique is that it presents the listener with a natural stream of ongoing samples of fluent speech; however, disadvantages include the time-pressured nature of the response task and a lack of information regarding appropriate correction factors for various populations (e.g., children and elderly adults).

The second major real-time spoken word recognition assessment technique is commonly referred to as the *time-gating paradigm*. Unlike reaction-time measures, time-gated spoken word recognition measures do not involve time-pressured listener response tasks nor do they require any correction factors. Although some researchers do not consider time-gating an on-line paradigm because it can reflect postlexical access operations, many consider it a direct method of evaluating on-line recognition performance. Tyler (1992) submitted that time-gating is a measure of on-line recognition because listeners' responses to time-gated speech reflect the automatic, unconscious intermediate lexical representations of the spoken utterance. The time-gating paradigm has been applied by many to obtain real-time word recognition performance measures and to study psychological mechanisms underlying spoken language processing and real-time spoken word recognition (Bard, Schillcock, & Altmann, 1988; Salasoo & Pisoni, 1985; Tyler, 1984).

Originally developed by Pickett and Pollack (1963) and subsequently reintroduced and refined by Grosjean (1980), the time-gating paradigm involves the repeated presentation of a gated-in portion of a target word that is incrementally increased in duration. Most time-gating applications employ gated individual or isolated words, but some use gated groups of words (Bard, Schillcock, & Altmann, 1988; Grosjean & Hirt, 1996). Usually, the amount of the gated increment is fixed by a prespecified amount of time ranging from 20 to 100 ms. As in real-time, when gates are increased, more of the target word accumulates until, with the addition of the final gate, the word is presented in its entirety. Listeners are asked to guess the target word being presented and to indicate how confident they feel about their response. As in real-time, in beginning gates, listeners base their word responses only on the preceding context and initial portions of a target word. In subsequent gates, word responses are based on larger and larger fragments of the target word. It is assumed that the nature and precision of a listener's responses reveal the sequence and timing of critical events that occur during the real-time recognition process (Cotton & Grosjean, 1984; Grosjean, 1980; Tyler & Wessels, 1985).

One early event occurring at the gate when the listener initially identifies the target word is referred to as the *isolation point* (IP), with its corresponding *confidence level* (CIP). Unlike conventional measures of word recognition which reflect only accuracy, time-gated measures also reflect how a listener's confidence changes during the recognition process. The IP and CIP measures reflect a listener's performance in an earlier stage in the process.

A later event can be observed at the gate when the listener recognizes the target word with a high level of confidence. This event is referred to as the *total acceptance point* (TAP). Grosjean (1980) demonstrated that the results obtained using measures of IP, CIP, and TAP were consistent with previous real-time results obtained using reaction-time type of response tasks. He further reported that the time-gating measures were significantly influenced by such stimuli-related factors as word frequency, predictability, and length.

A CLINICAL PERSPECTIVE

Evidence of hearing loss or speech perception problems must be identified and addressed in managing individuals with CAPD. As suggested by the previous discussion, conventional speech audiometric measures, even those obtained under challenging listening conditions (e.g., filtered speech, speech-in-noise, competing speech), provide limited information regarding an individual's spoken language understanding. A listener's ability to perceive the speech waveform signal and conduct auditory analysis (e.g., complex pattern recognition) plays a germinal role in spoken language processing. Little is known, however, about how spoken language processing system (dys)functions in the presence of a sensorineural hearing impairment. For example, how do perceptual distortions associated with sensorineural hearing impairment (e.g., dysacusis, tinnitus, and recruitment) affect the performance of the central auditory nervous system? Salvi, Henderson, Boettchner, and Powers (1992) reported that, in adult animals, the tonotopic organization of the auditory cortex undergoes a significant change in arrangement following cochlear insult. Revoile, Kozma-Spytek, Holden-Pitt, Pickett, and Droge (1995) further indicated that listeners with hearing impairment show poorer identification of consonants presented in carrier sentences than when acoustically identical consonants are presented in VCV utterances extracted from the carrier phrase context. Taken together, these results confirm the interdependence of peripheral and central auditory systems, an interdependence that most likely impacts all levels of auditory processing, including spoken language processing. (See Model of Central Auditory Processing in Chapter 1, Auditory Stimulation and Plasticity in Chapter 2, and Customizing Intervention in Chapter 7.)

The Word Recognition Score

Numerous disciplines, including speech-language pathology and audiology, have employed word recognition performance to evaluate a listener's speech perception abilities. In the psycholinguistic literature, the term word recognition refers to an event marking the conclusion of the word selection phase. In speech audiometry, the term word recognition score typically refers to a measure that reflects a listener's ability to perceive and correctly identify a set of speech materials presented at suprathreshold hearing level. The set of speech materials is commonly contained in word lists (e.g., NU-CHIPS, WIPI, PBK-50, PB-50, SSW, W-2, and W-22).

Originally, these types of word lists were developed to assess the long-term spectral efficacy of speech communication equipment, and they primarily reflect acoustic-phonetic considerations (Egan, 1948; Hirsh et al., 1952; Lehiste & Peterson, 1959; Tillman & Carhart, 1966). Suprathreshold speech audiometric procedures produce measures that are highly associated with such acoustical indices as the

Articulation Index (AI) and pure-tone threshold measures (Fletcher, 1929, 1953; Fletcher & Galt, 1950; French & Steinberg, 1947). Researchers observe good agreement between conventional word recognition performance data and AI-based predictions among hearing-impaired listeners (Humes, Dirks, Bell, Ahlstrom, & Cincaid, 1986). Mueller and Killion (1990) proposed an easy AI application for rehabilitation counseling purposes and the determination of appropriate hearing aid fittings. Such clinical applications of speech audiometric word list measures appear very useful for determining a listener's speech perception capabilities and appropriate acoustically based intervention strategies such as hearing aid fittings. Problems arise, however, when clinical predictions regarding spoken language processing or real-world listening behaviors are based solely on these types of word recognition measures which do not individually or in combination provide an adequate reflection of listeners' spoken language processing (dis)abilities (Humes et al., 1994). If our clinical goal is to determine how listeners understand speech under everyday real-time circumstances (e.g., in the evaluation of the efficacy of a particular aural (re)habilitation strategy or in the assessment and treatment of CAPD), then spoken word recognition performance needs to be evaluated in the context of the real-time lexical processing system and not solely within the confines of the acoustic-phonetic or perceptual domain.

Time-Gated Recognition Measures

Although no extant psycholinguistic model specifies the entire range of normal psychoperceptual and psycholinguistic processes, the Cohort Model presents a sufficiently well-developed account of a number of basic properties of real-time spoken language processing. Unlike some of the computational linguistic models, it was developed to reflect observed human behavior, and thus, offers a theoretical framework suitable for the development of central auditory processing assessment and CAPD (re)habilitation procedures.

Time-gated word responses can be quantitatively scored for accuracy and qualitatively evaluated by observing the acoustic-phonetic and/or linguistic-contextual nature of early, intermediate word responses leading up to word recognition. Elliott, Hammer, and Evan (1987), for example, used a time-gating paradigm on words selected from the NU-CHIPS Test (Elliott & Katz, 1980) to study IP and TAP among children, teenagers, and older adults. They reported that the teenagers achieved IPs at lower gates than children or older adults and that the older adults' IP performance was comparable to the children's performance. They concluded that differences in auditory sensitivity did not explain the age-related findings, but that word frequency effects and temporal processing differences were major factors.

Time-gating applications among children have considered: (a) the amount of input required for recognition, (b) the importance of word initial vs. word final information, (c) the number and structure of word candidates prior to isolation point (Walley, 1988), (d) context (Craig, Kim, Rhyner, & Chirillo, 1993), and (e) the effects of language delay and reading problems (Elliott & Busse, 1987). Studies among elderly listeners have considered: (a) the amount of acoustic-phonetic information required (Craig, 1992), (b) effect of preceding and following linguistic-contextual information (Wingfield, Goodglass, & Smith, 1994), and (c) performance comparisons with other age groups (Craig et al., 1993; Elliott, Hammer, & Evan, 1987).

In the past 10 years, our laboratory has studied speech audiometric factors that might influence or contraindicate clinical application of the time-gating paradigm. We obtained time-gated word recognition performance measures at various presentation levels using conventional speech audiometry test materials (e.g., NU-6 and Revised SPIN test). We studied time-gated word recognition performance among a variety of listeners including children, young adults, older adults, native English speakers, non-native English speakers, individuals with normal hearing, and individuals with hearing impairment. In addition, we applied perceptual restoration research techniques.

The link between the time-based features of perceptual phonemic restoration research and time-gating research has important implications for speech perception and spoken language processing research. Both techniques manipulate attributes of temporal sequencing and timed disruptions of the acoustic signal. In time-gating, the timed feature is the prespecified gate duration. In phonemic restoration, the timed feature is the number of interruptions and the duration of the masked or missing portion of the speech stimuli. Both methodologies focus on a listener's ability to use acoustic-phonetic and linguistic-contextual cues for word recognition.

Based on our research findings (Craig, 1992; Craig & Kim, 1990; Craig et al., 1993; Craig, Warren, Bashford, & Chirillo, 1994), we have concluded that:

1. Across a wide age range, listeners with normal hearing and hearing impairment employ various forms of verbal audi-

tory closure to significantly accelerate the real-time spoken word recognition process;

2. Under predictability-high (PH) linguistic-contextual conditions, the activation of word candidates does not depend solely on target word audibility or on acoustic-phonetically segmented lexical access. Semantically related word candidates are activated well in anticipation of target word onset, initial PH word sounds expedite the isolation of a unique word candidate, and listeners require little additional signal to recognized the target words with confidence;
3. All types of listeners are able to complete PH word recognition processing when the recognition processing of words in a predictability-low (PL) context has barely begun. However, many types of listeners are able to recognize PL or isolated monosyllabic words within the first third of the word's presentation;
4. It appears that even among listeners with normal hearing, age-related temporal processing problems place older listeners at some disadvantage when they listen for rapidly changing acoustic-phonetic elements of real-time speech;
5. Older adults, both those with normal hearing and those with hearing impairment, place greater reliance on linguistic-contextual information than ongoing acoustic-phonetic information and, therefore, are at a greater disadvantage when contextual information is less available; however, when contextual information is available they tend to compensate very effectively;
6. Children and young adults with hearing impairment, who have less spoken language experience, can demonstrate effective use of the acoustic-phonetic elements of real-time speech, but appear less able to use linguistic-contextual information to accelerate the real-time word recognition process.
7. The time-gating paradigm is an effective and feasible clinical tool for the assessment of real-time spoken word recognition performance.

CAPD and Real-time Spoken Word Recognition

Real-time spoken word recognition findings indicate that everyday receptive communication problems appear to be exacerbated by temporal processing deficits of central origin (e.g., deficits in temporal discrimination, resolution, integration, and/or ordering), particularly if portions of an ongoing signal become inaudible due to hearing impairment or a degrading listening condition (ASHA, 1996). Under some listening conditions, individuals with CAPD and/or hearing impairment may demonstrate discrete dysfunction(s) in one or more of the spoken language subprocesses: encoding of the percept, matching the percept to internal representation(s), conducting lexical access and/or lexical activation, employing higher level resources, extracting meaning from strings of lexical representations, and/or constructing a message level interpretation. However, in real-time, discrete perceptual and central (dys)functions interact and the spoken language processing consequences are difficult to predict. For example, even with limited spoken language experience/expertise a young child can perceive and temporally process sufficient acoustic-phonetic information to recognize most real-time spoken language in a timely manner. In contrast, a child with CAPD with the same limited spoken language expertise/experience may be unable to compensate and fail to understand the real-time message.

Tallal and Newcombe (1978) proposed that temporal challenges inherent to the perception of rapidly changing speech signals not only influence phoneme perception, but also influence larger units of speech recognition, as well as listeners' abilities to effectively perform speech segmentation. Tallal and Stark (1981) studied children with impaired language and found that auditory processing difficulties were observed for most syllables containing consonants, but not for isolated vowel syllables. They concluded that children with language impairment have difficulty processing acoustic-phonetic cues that are of brief duration and are followed in rapid succession by other acoustic-phonetic cues. Tallal (1980a) submitted that the processing of rapidly changing properties of speech is the major challenge to the effective central auditory processing of speech. When a child with CAPD is also faced with degraded acoustic signals (e.g., speech-in-noise or speech produced very rapidly), barriers to effective real-time spoken language processing are significantly raised. These barriers place children with CAPD at risk for learning disability and/or specific language impairment.

Depending on the communication situation, older adults with age-related hearing impairment may use their wealth of spoken language experience to adequately bypass real-time barriers until age-related temporal processing problems begin to appear or the real-time listening task is further complicated by troublesome real-world listening dilemmas (e.g., noise, reverberation, or rapid, poorly pronounced speech signals). The Committee on Hearing, Bioacoustics, and Biomechanics (CHABA) Working Group on Speech Understanding (1988) published a comprehensive review and tutorial in which numerous sensory and processing factors that influence an elderly listener's ability to understand speech were discussed. In that report, and in further comments (Jerger, Stach, Pruitt, Harper, & Kirby, 1989), it was suggested that central auditory deficits in the older adults significantly contribute to the age-related decline in speech understanding. More research is needed to better understand temporal resolution changes associated with aging, as well as how many older adults successfully compensate when real-time spoken language processing factors and/or backgrounds of competing noise challenge their auditory processing capacity. (See Life Span Considerations in Chapter 7.)

Aging not only causes a deterioration in peripheral hearing sensitivity (Bunch, 1929, 1931; Goetzinger, Proud, & Emery, 1961; Patterson, Nimmo-Smith, Weber, & Milroy, 1982), but also is associated with changes in central neurophysiologic aspects of speech recognition (Jerger, 1973; Marshall, 1981; Nicolas, Obler, Albert, & Goodglass, 1985). Research findings indicate that elderly adults may face significant barriers when they listen for rapidly changing acoustic-phonetic elements of real-time speech. Using simple temporal sequencing, speech identification, and minimal contrasting discrimination tasks, researchers report that, although peripheral hearing impairment accounts for much of their age-related speech identification problems, age-related temporal processing deficits also contribute to reduced performance among older adults (Humes & Christopherson, 1991; Humes & Roberts, 1990; Trainor & Trehub, 1989). It has been shown that, among listeners with good word recognition scores, time-compressed NU-6 test speech samples were less intelligible as a function of age and that older listeners demonstrated steeper rates of accuracy decline as speech rate increased (Konkle, Beasley, & Bess, 1977; Wingfield, Poon, Lombardi, & Lowe, 1985). Fox, Wall, and Gokcen (1992) found that older adults showed a decrement in their ability to temporally process dynamic perceptual cues for vowel identification. Gordon-Salant and Fitzgibbons (1993) studied percent-correct recognition scores based on three forms of time-distorted speech (time-compression, reverberation, and interruption) and reported that age-related factors other than peripheral hearing loss contributed to the diminished speech recognition performance of older listeners.

Research findings indicate that older adults place greater reliance on linguistic-contextual information than ongoing acoustic-phonetic information. Therefore, their lexical searching process may appear less flexible, albeit more efficient (Wingfield & Stine, 1992). Nittrouer and Boothroyd (1990) studied how contextual factors influenced the recognition of phonemes in words and words in sentences among children and older adults. When compared to the performance of young adults, both child and older adult listeners demonstrated poorer recognition abilities and similar context effects, except the children used sentence meaning constraints less effectively than either the young or older adult listeners, and the older adults used lexical constraints to a greater extent than either of the two younger groups.

New Aural (Re)habilitation Approaches

Recent research developments in real-time aspects of aural (re)habilitation and innovations in speech conversion technology afford the development of a new generation of CAPD-related aural (re)habilitation strategies. An effective extant aural (re)habilitation strategy involves the employment of assistive listening devices such as personal FM amplification systems (Stach, Loiselle, & Jerger, 1987a, 1987b, 1991). The overall real-time recognition benefits of this approach are obvious. An FM amplifier treats the spectral acoustic characteristics of the speech signal and circumvents the problem of background noise. By increasing the speech-to-noise ratio of the ongoing signal, a listener with CAPD can process real-time spoken language more effectively and potentially compensate for other types of spoken language processing barriers.

Related to the *improve-the-signal* type of aural (re)habilitative approach, Pichney, Durlach, and Braida (1985, 1986) have studied the spectral elements of *clear speech*. They have attempted to apply their findings to the design and development of new hearing aid technology. Clear speech refers to speech produced by a speaker who has been instructed to speak as clearly as possible, as if trying to communicate in a noisy background. These researchers report substantial differences between the intelligibility of clear and conversational speech for listeners with hearing impairment and attribute these intellibility differences to a variety of factors including speaking rate, consonant power, and occurrence of phonologic phenomena. Recently, their attention has been focused on the role of average speaking rate in the high intelligibility of clear speech.

Based on Tallal's earlier findings that fast speech elements usually present in consonants are major barriers to effective speech perception among children with language-based learning impairments, Merzenich, Jenkins, Johnston, Schreiner, Miller, and Tallal (1996) reported on new adaptive training exercises designed to improve the temporal processing of children with language-based learning impairment. They indicated that, with 8 to 16 hours of training, these children demonstrate improvements in their ability to recognize brief and fast sequences of speech. The benefits of this approach appear especially helpful in offsetting the challenges of temporally processing real-time speech.

Currently, in our laboratory, we are studying the potential aural (re)habilitative benefits of an innovative real-time speech rate conversion device. We believe such real-time devices (Nejime, Arisuka, Imamura, Ifukube, & Matsushima, 1996) may aid in the (re)habilitation of many types of listeners including those experiencing real-time spoken language processing problems associated with CAPD. Developed in Japan, at the NHK (Japan Broadcasting Corporation) Science and Technical Research Laboratories, the Real-Time Speech Rate Conversion System was first announced at the International Conference on Spoken Language Processing (ICSLP '94). It is currently contained in a new down-sized portable device.

Important features of the NHK Real-Time Speech Rate Conversion System include:

1. Manipulation of the presentation rate of real-time speech without significantly disturbing voice pitch, quality, or other important suprasegmental aspects of the ongoing signal;
2. Listener-regulated adjustment of the rate of speech presentation; and
3. Quasi-Lip-Synchronization methods to address potentially problematic dissynchrony between real-time visual and rate-converted auditory signals (Miyaska, Nakamura, Seiyama, Imai, & Takagi, 1994).

In operation under multilingual listening conditions, the NHK device appears to transform rapidly presented speech to speech presented at a slower and more intelligible rate without disturbing the fidelity of the speech signal. We are involved in studying several aural (re)habilitative-related applications of the NHK device to determine if by slowing the rate of real-time speech: (a) speech becomes more intelligible to many types of listeners, (b) age-related temporal processing problems can be overcome, (c) different types of listeners can make more effective use of acoustic-phonetic and/or linguistic-contextual information, and (d) after some training period, some types of listeners can acquire sufficient real-time spoken language experience to naturally accelerate their spoken word recognition process.

SUMMARY AND CONCLUSIONS

The purpose of this chapter was to consider spoken language processing as it relates to the assessment and treatment of individuals with CAPD. The impact of CAPD on real-world spoken language processing varies from listener to listener and situation to situation; therefore, an individualized approach to the design and development of appropriate CAPD assessment and (re)habilitation strategies appears most appropriate. A review of extant spoken language processing research findings and anecdotal reports indicates that if one signal-related barrier (e.g., telephone speech) is present, real-time spoken word recognition performance remains relatively unaffected. However, if that signal-related barrier becomes unduly challenging (e.g., static on the telephone line) or more than one signal-related barrier exists (e.g., noisy background), then it is predictable that real-time speech understanding performance will be seriously disrupted.

Among individuals with CAPD, the challenging effects of any signal-related barriers are seriously compounded if hearing loss, temporal processing deficit, spoken language inexperience, and/or lack of language expertise also are involved. Faced with the dynamic and ephemeral qualities of a real-time speech signal, how can children with CAPD attain the linguistic expertise or spoken language experience needed to accelerate their real-time word recognition process? How can an older adult overcome age-related hearing impairment and/or temporal processing problems and maximize the ameliorative effects of his or her spoken language expertise and experience? Our proposed approach to the development of new aural (re)habilitation strategies for individuals with CAPD is to find effective methods to either accelerate a listener's real-time word recognition process and/or slow down the rate of real-time speech presentation.

Clinicians who assess and treat individuals with CAPD must recognize the significant interactive real-time nature of the spoken language understanding process. Background listening conditions, as well as situational real-time temporal processing demands and listeners' abilities to effectively use linguistic-contextual information, determine everyday receptive communication success or failure. To effectively treat individuals with spoken language processing disabilities, sound must be transformed into meaning in a timely manner. In the real-world, speech intelligibility is important, but it is the listener who is able to recognize words from their earliest onset who demonstrates the most powerful perceptive and processing capabilities (Marslen-Wilson & Tyler, 1980). Clinical insight gained from conventional speech audiometric testing, coupled with applications of real-time word recognition assessment techniques may offer clinicians new and more effective approaches to the treatment of CAPD. Without additional transdisciplinary research and professional education, however, the potential of these new real-time strategies will not be fully realized.

SUGGESTED READINGS

Altmann, G.T.M. (Ed.). (1990). *Cognitive models of speech processing*. Cambridge, MA: ACL-MIT Press Series in Natural Language Processing.

Frauenfelder, U.H., & Tyler, L. (Eds.). (1987). Spoken word recognition. In J. Mehler (Ed.), *Cognition: An International Journal of Cognitive Sciences, 25* (Spec. issue).

Kent, R.D. (1992). Auditory processing of speech. In J. Katz, N.A. Stecker, & D. Henderson (Eds.), *Central auditory processing* (pp. 93–105). St Louis, MO: Mosby Year Book.

Marslen-Wilson, W. (Ed.). (1992). *Lexical representation and process.* Cambridge, MA: MIT Press.

Tyler, L. (1982). *Spoken language comprehension.* Cambridge, MA: MIT Press.

Warren, R.M. (1982). *Auditory perception.* New York: Pergamon Press.

CHAPTER

4

CONSIDERATIONS IN THE ASSESSMENT OF CENTRAL AUDITORY PROCESSING DISORDERS

This chapter, along with the following two chapters, are devoted to current approaches to the assessment of central auditory processing disorders (CAPD). Special emphasis is placed on CAPD as it relates to people with learning problems. This chapter serves as a basis for the following two chapters, as much of the discussion is critical to both behavioral and electrophysiologic test procedures. Chapters 5 and 6 consider differences and similarities in the testing and interpretation of adults and children with CAPD. Although behavioral and electrophysiologic tests are presented in separate chapters, these procedures must be used in combination when appropriate. One of the most important advances in the evaluation of CANS disorders is the understanding of interactions between behavioral and electrophysiologic test procedures.

A number of central auditory tests, either behavioral or electrophysiological, have been used successfully in defining CAPD in children with learning problems (Bornstein & Musiek, 1992; Ferre & Wilbur, 1986; Jerger, Martin, & Jerger, 1987; Jirsa, 1992; Ludlow, Cudahy, Bassich, & Brown, 1983). Therefore, some of the questions surrounding the assessment of CAPD are not whether these tests are valuable, but rather which tests have the best efficiency, validity, and reliability and how certain tests combine with others to yield increased information. Questions about the optimal use of central tests also are pertinent. In this chapter these questions are discussed along with such topics as current test materials and philosophical considerations relevant to assessment of CAPD. An extensive review of the literature regarding central auditory tests is not the aim of this chapter, nor is the assessment of adults with neuroauditory disorders, although reference will be made to these topics to provide information important to the use and understanding of test procedures.

ADVANTAGES AND LIMITATIONS OF THE AUDIOLOGIC APPROACH

The audiologic approach is one method of assessing CAPD. The audiologic approach, for our purposes here, is the assessment of CAPD using audiologic methodology, instrumentation, and acoustic controls. This approach can be contrasted to CAPD evaluation that uses checklists, screening procedures, and language evaluations without the audiologic elements just mentioned. The audiologic approach has clear advantages and limitations in testing for CAPD. Current technology allows excellent control of acoustic stimuli in audiology. This is helpful not only for acoustic calibration, but also for designing and implementing tests that can challenge the processes of the central auditory nervous system. Among these are procedures that test ears individually and in a variety of binaural conditions. The audiologic approach also can provide acoustic environmental control, which is critical in the assessment of validity and reliability.

The control of acoustic stimuli and the test environment provided by the audiologic approach also brings with it additional cost and restrictions on utility. Tests that do not require earphones or a sound room can be administered in more situations than tests that require these audiological necessities. An issue central to the audiologic approach in assessing CAPD is whether the additional cost related to better acoustic control and manipulation of stimuli is offset by improved validity, sensitivity, and specificity. A long history of good acoustic control in the field of audiology would argue that this so. However, there may a place for both CAPD tests that have exquisite manipulation and rigorous acoustics and tests that do not. Given the limitations of certain test environments, such as in most schools, there may be a use for less stringently controlled tests (e.g., the Children's Token test; Wepman discrimination test; Goldman, Fristoe, Woodcock test). These tests must be interpreted carefully due to their limitations and should be viewed not as diagnostic, but rather as screening procedures.

In considering the audiologic approach, the basic audiologic evaluation must precede any assessment of central auditory function. Measurements of pure tone and speech sensitivity and recognition, as well as immittance testing, can provide information on peripheral hearing status. Clearly, peripheral hearing loss can affect central test results and must be considered carefully. Optimal interpretations of central results cannot be made without knowledge of peripheral hearing status.

Considerable damage can be done to the cochlea without significant effects on pure tone thresholds. This is a rare situation, but it does exist. The use of otoacoustic emissions may help to define subtle cochlear damage. This procedure is discussed as an aid in CAPD assessment in Chapter 6.

TEST VALIDITY, RELIABILITY, AND EFFICIENCY

Many factors play a role in the selection of a test or test battery for assessing central auditory function, for example, the length of time necessary to administer, score, and interpret a test. Another factor is whether the test can assess processes linked to central auditory function. Although peripheral and central auditory processes overlap, and certainly the two systems must work together, some tasks are better suited for central than for peripheral assessment. The most critical factors for test selection are test validity, reliability, and efficiency (sensitivity and specificity).

The determination of test validity, reliability, and efficiency in regard to central auditory assessment is an important but not always clearly understood concept. A valid test is one that accurately measures the factors it is designed to measure. In the area of central auditory assessment, it is presumed that the tests used will measure central auditory dysfunction. The best way to determine if a central test is valid is to measure its performance on patients with proven lesions of the CANS. This requires recruiting a clinical population to test the test(s), as well as careful localization of the lesion site by radiographic, surgical, or other nonaudiologic means. Also critical in validation is an anatomical definition of the CANS to ensure that the lesion, or lesions, are in fact present in the CANS. This method of validation clearly has many shortcomings (i.e., a less-than-direct relationship between structure and function; the lack of specific, isolated lesions; the lack of detailed anatomical information on the lesions), but remains invaluable to evaluate the worth of CANS tests (Damasio & Damasio, 1989; Jerger, Johnson, & Loiselle, 1988).

The validation of central auditory tests on children with learning disabilities (LD) is not a feasible approach simply because not all children with LD have central auditory deficits (Hurley, Singer, & Schultz, personal communication). Therefore, there is no gold standard with which to measure test accuracy. Comparisons across several central tests can be made on an LD population to help determine which tests are most sensitive in defining this population; however, this approach is not commensurate with validation of central auditory dysfunction.

Evidence shows that central auditory deficits in children with suspected processing disorders have patterns similar to those with confirmed lesions of the CANS (Jerger, et al., 1988; Musiek, Gollegly, & Baran, 1984). This finding emphasizes that central auditory tests do measure central auditory dysfunction and that this dysfunction may have a common basis. In Chapter 2 we discussed morphological abnormalities in children with LD. This indicates an anatomical deviancy in the auditory regions of the brains of children with LD, as is the case in adults with confirmed lesions. Therefore, tests that are sensitive to confirmed lesions of the CANS are likely to be sensitive to children with LD who have heterotopias or other morphological deviance on the superior temporal plane.

Test-retest reliability is important to all tests. In theory, perfect reliability exists when scores from the original test and the retest are the same. This is predicated on maintaining a perfectly static condition in regard to the elements measured, but this is problematic, especially in patients with CNS lesions. It is well known that the CNS changes when it is compromised by trauma, disease, or in some other manner. For example, in trauma or disease neural tissue may degenerate or reorganize in a different manner at a much later time. These factors, along with changes in alertness, cognitive status, and compensation strategies, can alter test performance. Because of this, information on test-retest reliability (especially moderate or long-term) may be difficult to obtain with clinical populations. Obtaining valid measures of test-retest reliability is problematic with the normal population. Certainly, central auditory tests exist for which test-retest reliability measures are available. For example, the *SCAN* (Keith, 1986), the *Selective Auditory Attention Test* (SAAT) (Chermak & Montgomery, 1992; Cherry, 1980), *Dichotic Digits Test* (Musiek, Gollegly, Kibbe, & Verkest-Lenz, 1991), *Auditory Duration Patterns Test* (Pengilly, 1992), compressed speech testing (Beasley, Forman, & Rintelmann, 1972), and the P300 (Kileny & Gripal, 1987) are central tests with reported information on test-retest reliability. However, these data are not available for many of the central tests commonly used clinically.

Test efficiency is derived from sensitivity and specificity indices (Turner, 1991). Sensitivity is the percentage of test results that indicate an abnormality when a true abnormality exists. Specificity is a percentage of test results that indicate that no abnormality exists. Generally, when sensitivity increases, specificity decreases. This reciprocal relationship is related directly to the criteria used for pass versus fail. One can change criteria to fail more subjects and the sensitivity will improve, but this criteria change will also make the test less specific (i.e., it will fail people who function normally). If there is an increase in sensitivity but an equal decrease in specificity, the efficiency will remain about the same. The pass-fail criteria determine test specificity and sensitivity. The best situation is to have both high sensitivity and specificity, but this is not always possible. However, depending on the demands of the clinical situation, one can bias criteria to enhance sensitivity at the cost of decreased specificity or vice versa. For example, if the clinical consequence was much greater for a false-negative than for a false-positive result, the pass-fail criteria could be adjusted to increase the sensitivity of the test.

When considering a test for clinical use, it is important to obtain information about the test's efficiency. Although sensitivity and specificity information are available for a number of central auditory tests, there are far too many tests for which this information is not available. In the next chapter we present more information on test efficiency.

TESTING A VARIETY OF AUDITORY PROCESSES

Many auditory processes are involved in the appropriate perception of an acoustic event (Handel, 1989). Most of these processes are interdependent. An example of this interdependence is detection and discrimination. Before one can discriminate among acoustic events, they must be detected. Also, nearly all auditory processes involve both the peripheral and central systems. Some processing requires more central than peripheral function; for other processing the inverse is required. Usually, the more complex the acoustic task in listening, the more the central system becomes involved. A speech-in-noise task requires more central auditory function than hearing a pure tone in a quiet room. We use a variety of auditory processes in everyday situations. Some of these processes are known and can be tested; others are not known or are only poorly understood. Many of these processes overlap and interact in complex ways. The brain orchestrates many of the processes to allow us to perceive and gain meaning from many acoustic events.

Similarly constructed auditory tests probably assess similar functions. For example, the *Staggered Spondaic Word* test is similar to other dichotic word tests, and therefore the processes tested are likely to be similar. Given limited time, the clinician often must assess as many auditory processes as possible in an effort to find potential weaknesses. Therefore, there are advantages to selecting tests that are fundamentally different in their construction (Musiek & Chermak, 1994), as this would allow the clinician to test a greater variety of auditory processes.

In many cases, more than the auditory system is involved in CAPD. Other sensory and cognitive systems can also be compromised in CAPD. If a test battery can differentiate among various sensory systems, it can offer a great advantage toward isolating a specific type of problem (Cacace & McFarland, 1995).

Test Battery Considerations

In a test battery the same tests should not be used in every situation (Pinheiro & Musiek, 1985). The clinician should choose from a variety of tests that best fit the patient or test situation. The examiner should understand the strengths and weaknesses of each test and should know the anatomic and physiologic underpinnings of the tests. The clinician also should be aware of trends on the initial tests and select subsequent tests that may verify or disprove these trends.

Again, it is valuable to select tests that assess different processes. Two tests that measure similar processes, even though highly efficient, would better be replaced by less efficient tests that assess different processes. Some tests are influenced greatly by peripheral hearing loss, such as dichotic CVs; other tests, such as duration pattern perception or the P300 (Musiek, Baran, & Pinheiro, 1990; Speaks, Niccum, & Van Tassel, 1985), are less affected.

Why some tests are influenced more than others by peripheral hearing loss is unclear, but we offer factors cogent to the problem. One factor is the acoustic composition of the test(s). The greater the complexity of intensity and frequency interactions, especially over a restricted time period, the greater the peripheral influence. For example, dichotic CVs have some fast intensity and frequency transitions critical to their understanding; therefore, great demands are made on the cochlea. People with cochlear hearing loss have difficulty recognizing CVs even when they are not in the dichotic condition. However, the duration patterns test is composed of steady state pure tones (no change in frequency or duration) of considerable duration with a relatively long interstimulus interval. The integrity of this stimulus can be preserved, even in a mildly damaged end organ. Hence, people with cochlear hearing loss generally perform better on patterns tests than on CV tests. Another factor related to the influence of cochlear loss on central tests is where the majority of the processing must take place. Take again the example of dichotic CVs and duration patterns tests. Although both tests require peripheral and central processing, the CV tests require more peripheral processing than do the patterns tests. The patterns tests require all acoustic elements to be perceived before the many cortical processes are initiated to decode the pattern. The CV test's main central activity is the dichotic segment of the test, while even in a monaural condition people with cochlear loss have trouble recognizing CVs. To view these two factors in another manner, CV tests require more intensity and frequency resolution than do patterns tests, and frequency and intensity discrimination are perhaps more the domain of the periphery than of the brain (although brain disorders can certainly influence intensity and frequency resolution). More complex processing is brain related for patterns, whereas CVs have processing liability both in the periphery (cochlea) and brain.

Hence, for patients with hearing loss, if a central test is chosen, one should choose from tests that are not greatly affected by hearing loss. In addition to sensitivity and specificity, important factors to consider in composing a test battery include test efficiency and the time necessary to administer and score the test. Central auditory tests should require a short time to administer, because long tests are not well tolerated by children or patients with CNS problems. Also, if a test battery is given, each test should be short enough so that the entire test battery is not excessively long. The scoring for tests should be straightforward and require little time. The administration of the test, or tests, should be easy for the clinician and understandable for the patient. Tests that require excessive practice often are not clinically feasible.

Test batteries have several advantages and disadvantages. The complexities and redundancies of the CANS make it necessary to administer several tests in order to obtain an adequate sensitivity for the test battery. Similar trends across tests in a given battery provide the examiner with confidence in the results. These trends also can be helpful in designing rehabilitative strategies for the patient. A potential disadvantage of a test battery is the likelihood of decreased specificity. This may occur because many more opportunities exist for the subject to make errors and many different processes are tested. Using many tests in a test battery is similar to making the criteria for a certain test more stringent. Also, when results across tests are at odds with one another, it is unclear which is accurate. The best guide in this situation is for the clinician to analyze test efficiency data and weigh the tests in regard to their sensitivity/specificity. This assumes that the tests were administered correctly and were appropriate for the patient. Test batteries also require more time to perform than do only one or two tests. Although we do not favor set test batteries, certain categories of tests should be considered when selecting a test battery for children at risk for CAPD.

Test battery interpretation can be most difficult, and there are little published data to direct those interested in this facet of assessment. When making a diagnosis of auditory processing deficit, it is difficult to interpret several tests that show differing results. For example, if five central auditory tests are given and only one is abnormal, is the patient considered to have an auditory processing deficit? Many factors affect the conclusion, such as whether the abnormal test is a dependable and valid test, whether the one test abnormality fits with the patient's history, whether the patient responded well for this particular test, and whether it is reasonable to believe that a very high percentage of patients with auditory processing deficits will fail at least one central test (Musiek, Geurkink, & Keitel, 1982). However, a number of patients without auditory processing deficits may also fail at least one test. Viewing this in another way, if the criteria for diagnosis of CAPD is to fail only one test in the battery, then the sensitivity of this criteria will be high but the specificity will likely be low. A rule of thumb is that for one failed test out of a battery to command the diagnosis of CAPD the scores must be more than three standard deviations below the mean (two standard deviations below the mean usually means failure for a particular test). In most cases, if two or more tests are abnormal, this is usually diagnostic for a central auditory problem. Each individual test must be given its due. If the test is valuable, is administered appropriately, and shows a marked deficit even though other tests do not, it may herald a specific kind of processing deficit. It is helpful to have the corroboration of other tests, but test batteries should be chosen to test different processes; hence, corroboration across the test battery may not always be necessary or possible. In terms of overall interpretation, a deficit on only one test is not as worrisome as are deficits on many tests, and should be discussed with parents, teachers, and doctors in the appropriate perspective. In cases of single-test deficits, a retest at a later time may be appropriate to verify the finding.

In evaluating children, it is rare to administer more than five tests in the battery. Obviously the more tests failed, and the lower the scores on each test, the greater the confidence that a central auditory deficit is present. Also important during interpretation is the relative sensitivity, specificity, and reliability of each test in the battery.

The problem of multiple test interpretation also can be combatted by deriving a composite or total score. Although this approach has obvious advantages, the appropriate weighting of different tests (often needed in deriving composite scores) in the battery can be difficult. Because different tests assess different functions, with some tests more effective than others, weighting test results may be arbitrary. Overall, test battery interpretation is a challenge and is contingent on the examiner's clinical experience, knowledge, and insight.

POPULATIONS FOR CENTRAL AUDITORY ASSESSMENT

Unfortunately, many clinicians believe that children with LD are the only population on which to use central auditory testing. This is a common and appropriate population for central auditory assessment, but far from the only one. In fact, there are many advantages to testing populations other than children with learning disabilities.

Aphasic patients represent a population for which central auditory assessment is underused. An extremely high percentage of aphasic patients have involvement of the central CANS (Divenyi & Robinson, 1989), yet this often goes undetected because it is not assessed. Some tests used in CAPD assessment may not be appropriate for patients with aphasia, but many are—especially the electrophysiological procedures. Many popular speech and language tests for aphasia simply do not provide sufficient insight into the nature and degree of central auditory involvement. Without knowing the full spectrum of communication deficit in the aphasic patient, it is most difficult to design a good rehabilitative scheme.

Most aphasic patients receive therapy that is focused on the expressive mode, while little is done to help remediate the receptive auditory system. It is important for speech-language pathologists and audiologists to combine forces in assessing and managing aphasic patients. However, to make a worthwhile contribution to the team, the audiologist must be well trained in the CANS.

Peripheral hearing as well as CANS function should be assessed in aphasic patients. Because most aphasic patients are older, the chance of their having peripheral hearing loss is quite high. In many cases, aphasic patients with peripheral or central involvement can be helped considerably by high-fidelity assistive listening devices. Hence, knowing the status of hearing in the aphasic patient can be critical to the success of therapy.

Patients who have degenerative neurological diseases that may affect the auditory tracts are another population that deserves central auditory evaluation. In this population, the most common disease entity with an auditory correlate is multiple sclerosis. Abundant evidence indicates that this population of patients can have auditory deficits, primarily when the auditory tracts are involved (Levine et al., 1993). Other neurologic degenerative diseases also have been shown to involve the auditory system, for example, Charcot Marie Tooth disease (Musiek, Weider, & Mueller, 1982), Alzheimer's disease (Grimes, Grady, Foster, Sunderland, & Patronas, 1985), olivopontocerebellar degeneration syndrome (Lynn, Cullis, & Gilroy, 1983), Friedreich's ataxia, Parkinson's disease, and various leukodystrophies (Chiappa, 1983); however, these diseases are not as common as multiple sclerosis, nor have they been studied as much from an auditory perspective.

Patients with seizure disorders with loci at or near the auditory areas of the cerebrum also are candidates for central auditory assessment. This condition can cause dysfunction of the CANS (Collard, 1984). In addition, two primary treatments for intractable epilepsy, corpus callosotomy (split brain) and resection of involved neurological tissue, affect central auditory processing. The split brain procedure and its effect on auditory processing have been well studied (Musiek, Kibbe, & Baran, 1984). Also well studied from an audiological point of view is the effect of temporal lobectomy, which is a common surgical procedure for epilepsy control (Musiek, Baran, & Pinheiro, 1994).

Patients with mass lesions of the CANS also are candidates for central auditory evaluation. Presently, the audiology staff seldom make the diagnosis for these kinds of lesions. However, by using central auditory tests, insight may be gained as to how much the auditory system is compromised and the functional consequences of these lesions. In patients with known lesions of the CANS, it is important to determine whether central auditory function is compromised, as opposed to determining whether a lesion exists in the CNS.

Occasionally, patients with symptoms of mass lesions of the CANS may see an audiologist before a diagnosis is made. In these situations, the audiological assessment must provide insight to the problem and herald a timely referral.

Patients who have received head trauma, especially those with closed head injuries, often have damage to the central and/or peripheral auditory systems. Sometimes central assessment can provide insight into the nature of recovery, or lack of recovery, in these patients. Unfortunately, central auditory evaluations often are not performed on these patients, even though extensive neuropsychological testing often is performed. Within the neuropsychology test battery, subtests are used to evaluate central auditory function. The neuropsychology tests of auditory processes are not as complete, useful, or well controlled as a well-thought-out audiological test battery for peripheral and central auditory function.

Patients who wear, or are candidates for, hearing aids and who do not do well with amplification may require central auditory assessment (Musiek & Baran, 1996). In many cases hearing aids are not effective with these patients because of some central auditory compromise. Often, these patients have some history of CNS involvement, which has affected their central auditory processing. Also, the great majority of hearing aids users are older adults who are at risk for some degree of central auditory involvement. Management of patients who do poorly with amplification can be improved if a central deficit is defined. In some patients, based on their peripheral hearing, both ears may be similar or one ear may be better. However, a central evaluation may indicate an entirely different result in regard to ear symmetry or lack of it. This information may have implications for the management of a patient. Some patients suffer from the binaural interference phenomenon (Jerger, Silman, Lew, & Chmiel, 1993). This is a condition where binaural amplification may be worse than a single hearing aid. This is related to extremely poor speech recognition on one side which contaminates good performance from the other side. This could be caused by either a peripheral or central disorder. Binaural interference is demonstrated by binaural speech recognition scores that are worse than the best monaural score. Although binaural amplification is usually better than monaural, this is not the case when binaural interference is present.

Populations of obscure auditory dysfunction (OAD) also should be evaluated for CAPD (Baran & Musiek, 1994). Patients with OAD are those who complain primarily about difficulty hearing in noise and have normal audiograms. These patients are adults and, at the time of the diagnosis of OAD, do not have any underlying disorder. (Otoacoustic emissions may help with resolving the source of the OAD; see Chapter 6). These patients will often, but not always, demonstrate CAPD. Central function should be measured, and anxiety questionnaires should be administered. Obscure auditory dysfunction represents a relatively large population of patients who, until recently, were dismissed by clinicians as having no hearing problems (Figure 4–1).

TEST MATERIALS AND EQUIPMENT

Central auditory assessment requires test materials for two types of procedures: behavioral and electrophysiological. For many years a common complaint among clinicians was that many of the taped materials were not adequate and were difficult to obtain. This problem has been solved with the development of the compact disc (CD). At least one major CD is readily available for use in central auditory assessment. Compact discs are of high fidelity, allow easy access to many

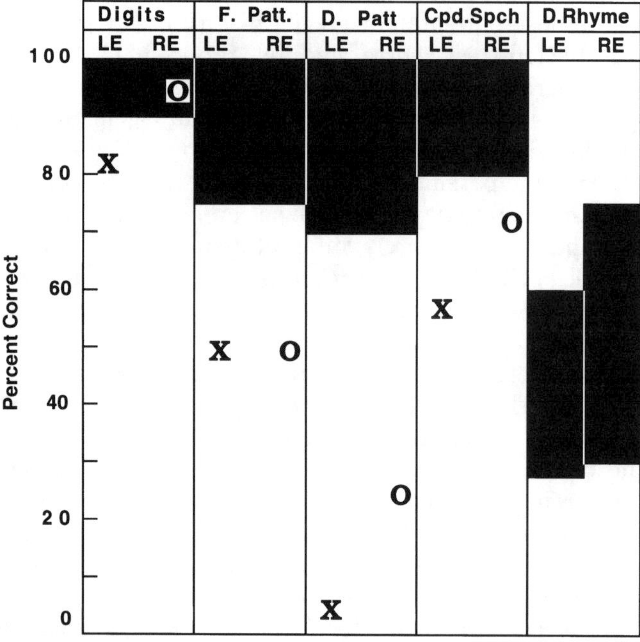

Figure 4–1. Central auditory test results from a 28-year-old woman who had difficulty hearing, especially in background noise, for several years. Her pure tone thresholds and speech recognition ability (at 30 dB SL re: spondee threshold) were normal bilaterally. The central auditory tests show deficits on every test. This patient was eventually given the diagnosis of obscure auditory dysfunction with probable central auditory deficit. **Key:** F. Patt = frequency patterns; D. Patt. = duration patterns; Cpd Spch = compressed speech (45%) with 3% reverberation; D. Rhyme = dichotic rhyme test. Black area indicates normal performance.

tests, and withstand common wear and tear. A number of valuable tests are available only on tape and certainly should be used.

It is important for the clinician to have a number of test materials at his or her disposal. As discussed, there are advantages to customizing the test battery for the patient, which requires an array of test materials. It is an advantage to have CD players that also have cassette tape capabilities. Regardless of how good test materials are, they cannot compensate for shortcomings in instrumentation, such as inappropriate calibration between channels, low-fidelity headphones, or a poor acoustic environment.

Electrophysiologic central tests require physiologic averagers, and several companies make these readily available. Most commercial averagers are excellent for performing auditory brainstem response (ABR) measures. However, those interested in electrophysiologic tests other than ABR should be sure that the averagers have the capability to do such tests as the middle latency response (MLR), late potentials (including the N1, P2, and P300), and the mismatched negativity response (MMN). The P300 and the MMN require special stimulus presentation and special averaging. Therefore, the instrument's capability for these more complex potentials must be demonstrated. To make optimal use of the middle and late potentials, four-channel capacity is important.

SCREENING VS. DIAGNOSTIC TESTS

Both screening and diagnostic test procedures play a role in assessing central auditory dysfunction (Musiek, Gollegly, & Lamb, 1990). This is especially true for children with learning problems. In central auditory evaluation, screening procedures are used primarily to help make an appropriate referral for a complete diagnostic workup. Screening tests are used in lieu of diagnostic tests by clinicians who are uncomfortable with a diagnostic battery or who do not have the resources to conduct a complete central auditory workup. Screening tests should be of short duration and can be conducted in a variety of settings. Some diagnostic tests often used in a battery have been used as screening procedures; however, tests designed for screening probably should not be used as a diagnostic entity. Central auditory test(s) that are short in length (i.e., few items), are used as the sole test, or lack acoustic control, such as would be used for screening, may not be good for in-depth diagnostic testing. The reasons for this are manifold. Screening tests may not have the complexity to test a variety of auditory/language processes, a trait critical to appropriate diagnosis. Tests amenable for screening also may not have the reliability or validity that in-depth batteries or longer tests have; and screening tests may lack flexibility to appropriately test certain patient populations.

The SCAN (Keith, Rudy, Donahue, & Katbamna, 1989) was developed as a screening test for central auditory processing problems in children. The SCAN has three subtests which are purported to evaluate auditory maturation and identify children who may benefit from rehabilitation and further testing. The three subtests include filtered words, figure-ground, and competing words. Details of these subtests are available elsewhere (Keith et al., 1989; Musiek, Gollegly, Lamb, & Lamb, 1990). The SCAN has many favorable features, including ease of use, short duration (requires 20 minutes to complete), availability of norms for a wide age range (3–11 years), and ease of scoring. However, some concerns about the SCAN exist, especially if it is used diagnostically. One concern is the small normative sample for 3- to 4-year-old children, which compromises the interpretation of results for this age group. Also the SCAN has not been validated on subjects with proven CANS lesions. Another concern is that the SCAN does not include a test of temporal processing—a critical process in central auditory function (Pinheiro & Musiek, 1985). It is also important with the SCAN, as with any other tests or test batteries, that language assessments are performed. This is relevant for the SCAN because all the subtests use only words as the stimuli; hence, there is a risk for language problems contaminating the results.

Also available is the SCAN-A, which is an extension of the SCAN and is designed for adolescents and adults (Keith, 1994a). Keith (1994b) also has developed a test that screens for attention-related auditory problems, which is called the Auditory Continuous Performance Test (ACPT).

Other tests can be used for screening, such as *The Token Test* (DiSimoni, 1978), the *Lindamood Auditory Test of Conceptualization* (Lindamood & Lindamood, 1971), the *Flowers-Costello Tests of Central Auditory Abilities* (Flowers, Costello, & Small, 1973), the *Auditory Discrimination Test* (ADT) (Reynolds, 1987), and the *Goldman, Fristoe, Woodcock Auditory Skills Test Battery* (Woodcock, 1976). All these tests have drawbacks, including heavy language dependencies, possible visual cueing, poor acoustics, and lack of any derived laterality information.

BACKGROUND INFORMATION AND PATIENT HISTORY

Acquiring appropriate background knowledge is vital before audiologically testing a child or adult suspected of having CAPD. This background information can be acquired by asking the patient, spouse, teacher, or parents pertinent questions about the medical, communicative, educational, and psychological history of the patient. Some of this information may also come in the form of referral reports.

Medical History

For CAPD assessment, key questions about the patient's medical history relate to neurological or sensory history or symptoms. Diseases, trauma, or symptoms indicative of sensory or neurological involvement are important and include concussions, neurodegenerative problems, epilepsy, vascular symptoms, numbness, coordination problems, vision difficulties, vestibular symptoms, and previous surgeries. For children, the prenatal, perinatal, and postnatal courses should be examined. Any potentially serious problems, such as prematurity, high bilirubin levels, anoxia, cerebral bleeds, hydrocephalus, toxic effects, low Apgar scores, the TORCH complex, birth trauma and otitis media, should be noted. Developmental milestones should be checked. Radiologic, neurologic, or otologic reports should be examined. It also is important to ask about medications the patient is taking. Medications that may cause changes in attention or CNS are important to note, as they may influence test results.

Communication History

A patient's speech, language, and hearing history should be taken. Any speech and language problems should be diagnosed and managed. Children referred for CAPD evaluation should have a complete speech and language assessment. Auditory behavior should be documented (i.e., What is the nature of the hearing difficulty? How long has it been present? In what situations is it most prevalent? How does the patient hear in noise and on the telephone? Does the patient appreciate music? Can he or she follow auditory directions? Has he or she had previous hearing tests? How is the patient's sound localization?). For school-age children, parents and teachers should complete hearing questionnaires, such as the Children's Auditory Processing

Performance Scale (CHAPPS) or Fisher Auditory Problems Checklist (Fisher, 1976). It is important to seek some indication that the patient's auditory behavior is not as it should be. One of the strongest indicators of an auditory processing deficit is a patient who has had many normal audiograms yet continues to seek hearing evaluations because of auditory difficulties.

Psychological and Educational History

Prior to seeing children for CAPD evaluation, we strongly suggest that psychoeducational testing be performed (see Chapter 9). This test information can provide insights into other problems that may influence test administration and results. Psychoeducational test results also can be helpful in designing and implementing management schemes for CAPD.

Overall intelligence quotient and verbal and performance scores should be known. Normal intelligence levels are necessary to understand and perform most tasks of central auditory processing tests. Scholastic achievement results are helpful in locating academic strengths and weaknesses, which will help in tailoring the test approach. Often people with CAPD do better in nonverbally related subjects, such as math, and do poorly in verbally linked subjects, such as reading. Emotional and behavioral problems may alert the clinician to other bases for the difficulties presented, and may also warn of difficulties in reliably testing the patient. Diagnoses of learning disabilities and attention deficit disorder, with or without hyperactivity, are important considerations, because CAPD can coexist with these entities (see Chapter 1). High-school or college students may struggle with learning a foreign language, which sometimes hints at undiagnosed CAPD. For school-age children, one should note how much special educational help the child has received and how often the child is absent from the regular classroom. The last two factors are important in planning the means to integrate programs into the child's daily routine.

Neuropsychological testing can be helpful in adults and children with potential CNS compromise. Educational history from adults and older children may indicate possible learning disabilities that were never diagnosed.

SUMMARY

In this chapter we reviewed the advantages of the audiologic approach to the assessment of CAPD. Control of test stimuli, acoustic environment, and breadth of test paradigms support the use of the audiologic approach to evaluate CAPD. Nonaudiologic central tests can be valuable if used within their limitations. Also, many of these tests are inexpensive and can be administered easily.

This chapter also stresses the importance of test validity, reliability, and efficiency (sensitivity and specificity). This information should guide the clinician in selecting the best tests available. Because many processes contribute to higher order auditory function, a test battery is needed to best evaluate the CANS. A variety of tests that assess various processes should be included in a battery of tests.

Many clinical populations can benefit from central auditory tests. Clinicians can also benefit from testing various populations with central test procedures. Although children with various learning disabilities are a common group on which to apply central tests, other populations, such as those with neurodegenerative disease, older adults, those with OAD, and even hearing-aid candidates can benefit from this type of testing.

Excellent test materials and equipment for administering central auditory tests now exist. Compact discs and physiologic averagers have advanced our abilities to reliably assess central dysfunction. Although these advances will help the clinician, he or she still must depend on good communication with the patient and family and a thorough medical and psycho-educational history.

SUGGESTED READINGS

Jerger, S., Martin, R., & Jerger, J. (1987). Specific auditory perceptual dysfunction in a learning disabled child. *Ear and Hearing, 8*, 78–86.

Jirsa, R. (1992). The clinical utility of the P3 AERP in children with auditory processing disorders. *Journal of Speech and Hearing Research*, *35*, 903–912.

Musiek, F., Gollegly, K., Lamb, L., & Lamb, P. (1990). Selected issues in screening for central auditory processing dysfunction. *Seminars in Hearing, 11*, 372–384.

Turner, R. (1991). Making clinical decisions. In W. Rintelmann (Ed.), *Hearing assessment* (2nd ed., pp. 679–738). Boston: Allyn & Bacon.

CHAPTER

5

BEHAVIORAL CENTRAL AUDITORY TESTS

Behavioral tests remain the mainstay of evaluating the CANS. Although many other aspects of CANS assessment must be considered, behavioral test results are key to the diagnosis of CAPD in adults or children. This chapter discusses salient issues surrounding behavioral tests of central auditory function, but places less emphasis on specific test administration or the history of these tests. Information on specific administration of central auditory tests can be found in articles about the particular test in question.

The types of tests discussed here are placed into categories. The processes represented by these categories are not the only ones that these tests assess or require. The categories represent the main processes and provide a taxonomy that may help in understanding test selection. These processes also can be useful in describing performance on central auditory tests, provide insight into function or dysfunction, and help in planning intervention (see Chapter 7). When developing a test battery, it may be useful to consider one or more tests from each category. Although the central auditory test battery should be tailored to each patient, careful consideration of each category is valuable when choosing tests. We provide a synopsis of processing categories and examples of central auditory tests from each category.

TEMPORAL PROCESSES

Ample evidence shows that temporal processing is an underlying and key component of central auditory function (Bornstein & Musiek, 1984; Pinheiro & Musiek, 1985). The ordering or sequencing of two rapidly presented, successive acoustic stimuli (two consonant-vowels or two complex tones), such as Tallal's tests, is valuable when testing temporal processing abilities in children (Tallal, 1985). Lackner (1982) reported on a similar task using consonant and vowels as the stimuli to sequence. The frequency pattern test also requires (but is not limited to) temporal processing (Musiek & Pinheiro, 1987; Pinheiro, 1977). This test requires the subject to relate the pattern perceived from three brief (150 msec) tones, which are combinations of 880 Hz or 1122 Hz sinusoids with a 200-msec interstimulus interval. The various combinations yield six patterns. Tallal's test has various modifications for administration, while the frequency pattern test does not. Both tests have been used clinically. The duration pattern test (Musiek, Baran, & Pinheiro, 1990) uses the temporal aspect of processing in two ways: ordering of tonal stimuli and duration discrimination. The test is similar to the frequency pattern test, but has as its elements 1000 Hz tones which vary only in duration (either 250 or 500 msec with a 300-msec interstimulus interval).

Other psychoacoustic tasks assess various kinds of temporal processes, but are seldom used clinically. This is unfortunate because a number of temporal paradigms have shown good clinical potential, for example, two-element ordering (Swisher & Hirsh, 1972) and brief tone frequency discrimination (Cranford, 1984). The two-element ordering task by Swisher and Hirsh is similar to Tallal's test. This task requires the sequencing of two dissimilar abrupt acoustic stimuli and is sensitive to cerebral lesions, especially of the left temporal lobe. Cranford's brief tone test establishes a frequency difference limen (DL) for very short tones and for long tones. Difference limens for the long tones are similar for patients with CANS involvement and normal patients. However, for short tones, DLs are much larger for subjects with CANS involvement than for control subjects.

Another temporal facet used is response time to a high-level psychoacoustic task, such as time or frequency discrimination (Thompson & Abel, 1992). Although response-time-oriented tests are different than the previously mentioned temporal tasks, they measure an important time parameter. They also can be applied to almost any behavioral test, which makes them clinically desirable. Thompson and Abel's (1992) work supports the concept that extended processing time translates into extended response time for an auditory task.

The clinician should strongly consider temporal processing tests for inclusion in most central auditory test batteries. Their efficacy is strongly supported by both animal and human studies that show the diagnostic value of temporal processing tasks (Colavita, 1972; Musiek, 1984, 1986; Musiek & Baran, 1987; Neff, 1961).

DICHOTIC LISTENING: BINAURAL INTEGRATION/SEPARATION

Various dichotic speech listening tests are sensitive to CANS dysfunction, and a wide range of tasks are included in this category (Musiek, Baran, & Pinheiro, 1994; Musiek & Pinheiro, 1985). Clinically, two main types of dichotic speech tasks have emerged: binaural separation (also called directed listening) and binaural integration. In binaural separation, the subject is directed to listen to a target stimulus within the dichotic task. While in the binaural integration task, both signals in the dichotic paradigm must be recognized. Two popular binaural separation dichotic tasks are competing sentences and synthetic sentence identification with contralateral competing message (SSI-CCM) (Musiek & Pinheiro, 1985). In the competing sentences test, two simple sentences are presented to each ear, and the subject is asked to repeat the target sentence while ignoring the other sentence. The target sentence is presented at 35 dB sensation level (SL), and the other sentence is presented at 50 dB SL. The SSI-CCM is composed of third-order approximation sentences which are presented to one ear, while meaningful, continuous discourse is presented to the other ear at various message-to-competition ratios. The subject is asked to find the corresponding number of the sentence that is heard (from a closed set visual representation) and relate it to the examiner. The subject is asked to ignore the continuous discourse.

Dichotic digits, staggered spondaic words (SSW), dichotic CVs, and dichotic sentence identification (DSI) are commonly used (binaural integration) dichotic tests (Bellis, 1996; Musiek & Pinheiro, 1985). The digits test requires two digits to be presented to each ear simultaneously while the subject repeats all digits. The same procedure is used with the CVs test, although the CVs are usually displayed (in a closed set) in front of the subject. Often the subjects are asked to write down the CVs they hear. The SSW is a semi-dichotic presentation of overlapping spondees (the second word of the first, and first word of the second spondee). The subject is asked to repeat both spondees. The DSI requires the dichotic presentation of two third-order approximation sentences. Again from a closed set with visual display in front of the subject, the subject reports the two corresponding numbers of the sentences presented.

As with temporal processing tests, other dichotic procedures have been used experimentally and clinically. Some of these procedures, such as the psychoacoustic pattern discrimination test (PPDT) (Blaettner, Scherg, & von Cramen, 1989), use click rather than speech stimuli. The PPDT has regular sequences of noise bursts or click trains that are dichotically presented with random changes. The subject must discriminate the pattern changes. Tests in this category, such as the PPDT, have a temporal facet that plays a role in the task.

Dichotic listening tests are clinically useful. Evidence shows that dichotic tasks in general are sensitive to central auditory dysfunction, and dichotic tests as a category should be strongly considered for inclusion in a central test battery (Musiek & Pinheiro, 1985).

LOW-REDUNDANCY MONAURAL SPEECH TASKS: AUDITORY CLOSURE

Within this group are speech tests in which the speech signals have been degraded or are presented in some type of acoustic competition. Filtered, compressed, expanded, interrupted, and reverberated speech signals have all been used as central tests (Musiek & Baran, 1987; Rintelmann, 1985). In addition, speech signals that are in competition with other speech signals, noise, or are altered in intensity have been used in central assessment. As a group, this category of tests does not have high sensitivity or specificity; however, they do test processes that are different from temporal and dichotic procedures (Musiek, Baran, & Pinheiro, 1994). The reduction in redundancy typical for these tests makes them feasible for assessing auditory closure. The compressed speech task has a temporal element in its design and may provide insight into a temporal processing problem.

Some common low-redundancy monaural speech tasks to consider when developing a test battery include: low pass filtered speech

(LPFS) test (Rintelmann, 1985), the SSI-ICM (Jerger & Jerger, 1974), the compressed speech with reverberation test (Bornstein & Musiek, 1992), and the pediatric speech intelligibility (PSI) test (Jerger, Jerger, & Abrams, 1983). The LPFS test uses PB word lists with the words filtered so that only the low-frequency energy is passed on to the subject. Usually the low band pass cut-off frequencies range between 500 to 1000 Hz, and the subjects simply repeat the words presented. The SSI-ICM is the counterpart of the SSI-CCM, differing only in that both the third-order approximation target sentences and the continuous discourse are presented to the same ear. Again, this type of presentation can be performed at different signal-to-noise ratios. The PSI is adapted for children and has a pointing task for pictured target words and action sentences (placed in front of the child). These words and sentences are set at a selected message-to-competition ratio. Message-to-competition ratio functions can be established for both the PSI and SSI-ICM. The compressed speech tests usually require the speech signal to be passed through instrumentation that compresses the speech, which creates little distortion. Performance is a function of the percentage of compression. Standard speech recognition lists are used in a monaural condition, and the subject simply repeats the words required.

BINAURAL INTERACTION, LATERALIZATION, AND LOCALIZATION TASKS

This category includes a variety of tests. Their commonality is that the two ears (auditory systems) must interact. Speech and tonal masking level differences (MLDs) are binaural interaction tasks that are often used in central auditory assessment (Schoeny & Talbott, 1994). Masking level difference is the difference in binaural threshold for tones or speech in noise that are in or out of phase with the noise, or in or out of phase at the two ears. Specifically, when the signal is out of phase (antiphasic) for the two ears or with the noise there is a release from masking and thresholds improve, as compared to the in-phase condition.

Interaural timing tasks, such as the ones used by Levine et al. (1993), require the subject to make a lateralization judgment (Figure 5–1). Clicks are presented to each ear at varying time differentials. In normal performance, the click that leads in time will result in a sound image that will lateralize to the side of the head to which the lead click is presented. If the two clicks are presented to each ear at

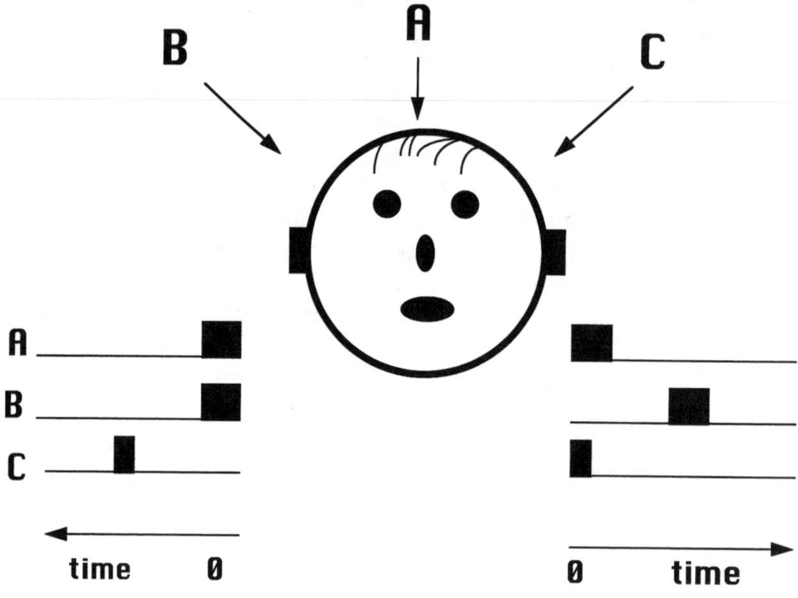

Figure 5–1. Interaural timing task showing that when two clicks are presented at the same time a mid-line image is perceived, as denoted by stimulus combination A. In stimulus combination B, the click to the subject's right side leads in time, which yields an auditory image on the right side of the head. In stimulus combination C, the left stimulus leads in time, resulting in lateralization to the left.

the same time, the image is perceived at mid-line in the head. Similar lateralization behaviors result from intensity differences between the two ears for clicks or tones. That is, the ear presented with the stimulus with the greater intensity results in lateralization to that side, and if the stimuli are of equal intensity, a mid-line image is reported. A number of clinically valuable but seldom used procedures have been developed based on these kinds of lateralization tasks (Groen, 1969; Hausler & Levine, 1980; Levine et al., 1993; Matathias, Sohmer, & Biton, 1985; Pinheiro & Tobin, 1969; Quine, Regan, & Murry, 1983).

Localization of sounds in a sound field has long been used in central auditory assessment (Sanchez-Longo & Forster, 1958). Recently a promising procedure for auditory localization was introduced (Moore, Cranford, & Rahn, 1990). This localization procedure is based on the precedence effect, which can be demonstrated in a soundfield when two stimuli are presented from two speakers located on opposite sides of the room. Interspeaker delays will result in a sound image localized in the field closest to the speaker with the lead stimulus. These time delays can be quantified to provide images at loci anywhere between the two speakers. Moore, Cranford, and Rahn (1990) have devised a useful way to track sound images in a soundfield using a laser pointer and computer.

Binaural fusion tasks were introduced by Matzker (1959) and popularized by Willeford (1977). These tasks require that two signals, one for each ear, are presented often, but not always, dichotically. Each signal is acoustically modified, which makes it difficult to understand by itself, but is easily understood when the signals are fused (supposedly by the CANS). Rapidly alternating speech perception (RASP) (Willeford, 1977) and Segment alternated CVC words tests (Wilson, 1994) require recombination of separate parts of words in order to understand the whole word. That is, word segments are alternated between the two ears at a designated time interval with each ear hearing only part of the word. The brainstem supposedly combines these segments from each ear to provide the perception of the entire word.

SENSITIVITY AND SPECIFICITY OF BEHAVIORAL TESTS OF CENTRAL AUDITORY FUNCTION

As discussed in Chapter 4, key clinical features of a test are its sensitivity and specificity (Figure 5–2). In this chapter, as in Chapter 6, the specificity and sensitivity of individual tests and test combinations will be discussed. True-positive (hit) rates will be used interchangeably with sensitivity, and false-positive rate is the same as 1 minus the specificity (e.g., if specificity is 0.80 or 80%, then the false-positive rate would be 1 – 0.80 = 0.20 or 20%). We provide as much sensitivity and specificity data as possible; however, these data are not always available. In cases where data are not available, we will provide the next best information to give insight into the diagnostic value of the test.

More data are needed on the sensitivity and specificity of central auditory tests. It is difficult to interpret the worth of a test without an indication of its sensitivity and specificity. It also is difficult to compare tests, even with data on true-positive and false-positive

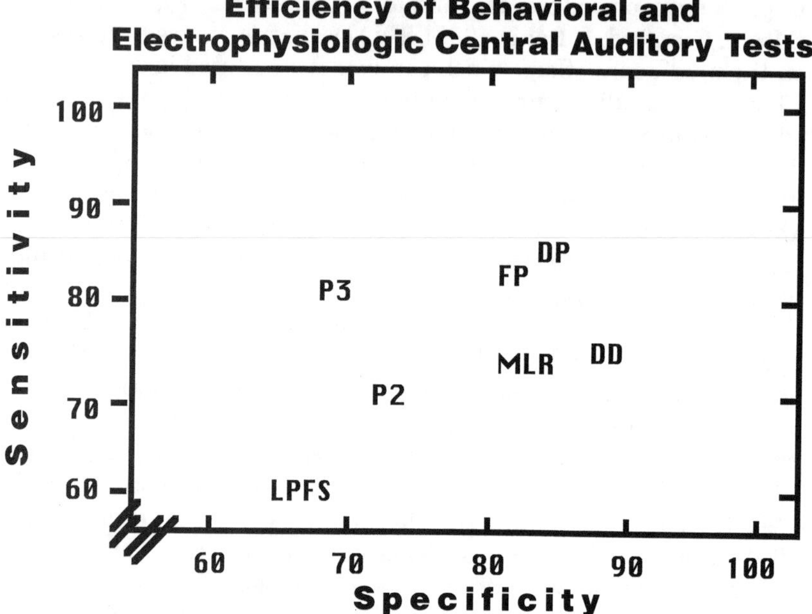

Figure 5–2. One way to view the sensitivity and specificity of central tests is by plotting sensitivity along one ordinate and specificity on the other. These tests are often used in our clinic and sensitivity and specificity data have been established. These results are based on patients with confirmed involvement of the central auditory nervous system. Key: DD = dichotic digits; DP = duration patterns; FP = frequency patterns; P3 = P300; LPFS = low pass filtered speech; P2 = P200; MLR = middle latency response.

rates, unless comparisons have been made on the same populations. The reason for this is that no two groups of subjects with neurological involvement are the same (Damasio & Damasio, 1989). In fact, no two subjects are the same, even if the neurologic lesions are in the same anatomical locus. Therefore, too much emphasis should not be placed on hit and false-positive rates. On the other hand, sensitivity and specificity should serve as a guide to general validity of a given central test; although far from perfect, it is the best indicator we have. In the following paragraphs comments on true-positive and false-positive rates will be offered on some tests for which this information is available. This information has limitations. Most importantly, different pass/fail criteria for different tests influence sensitivity/specificity data. Also, tests may be labeled similarly, but the tasks required of the subjects may differ markedly. The sensitivity/

specificity data suffer from differing pass/fail criteria. Tests termed the same may be different, and their administration may differ. Nonetheless, the following information on sensitivity/specificity is valuable to the clinician as a general guide to the diagnostic value of the more common central auditory tests.

TEMPORAL PROCESSING TESTS

In the temporal processing category, both frequency and duration patterns have true-positive rates of approximately 80% and a false-positive rate under 20% (Musiek, Baran, & Pinheiro, 1990; Musiek & Pinheiro, 1987). These rates were established for subjects with cerebral lesions and for those with mild-to-moderate cochlear hearing losses. Although true-positive and false-positive rates have not been established, other temporal processing tasks appear to have good sensitivity to central auditory dysfunction and may be valuable in the clinical domain. Swisher and Hirsh (1972) showed a marked difference between normal and brain-damaged individuals in the time required to correctly order two acoustic stimuli. For subjects with right-brain damage, the left-ear performance was decreased; for subjects with left-brain damage who were fluent, there was a marked deficit bilaterally. Cranford, Stream, Rye, and Slade (1982) reported on 10 patients with CANS lesions. Cranford used a brief tone frequency discrimination task for which difference limens (DLs) for experimental and control subjects were established. Once the duration of the tones was decreased to less than approximately 50 msec, the DLs for the neurologically involved subjects became larger than the normal range. This was the case in all 10 patients, with the largest DL noted in the ear contralateral to the lesioned hemisphere. Similar findings have been reported by Cranford et al. (1982) in animals with ablations of auditory cortex. Tallal's tasks of sequencing two complex tones, two vowels, or two consonant-vowels have been highly sensitive in separating children with developmental aphasia from normal control subjects (Tallal & Piercy, 1973b). Subsequent studies show the same temporal processing procedure to be valuable in defining children with language learning problems (Tallal, 1985).

DICHOTIC TESTS

Dichotic speech materials have long been recognized as sensitive tools for defining central auditory dysfunction (Musiek & Pinheiro,

1985). True-positive rates have been reported to be a function of the type of dichotic materials used. Unfortunately, few data are available on the false-positive rates of various dichotic speech procedures.

Several validity studies on the dichotic digits have revealed true-positive rates of 75 and 80% and false-positive rates of under 15% (Musiek, 1983a; Musiek et al., 1991). Mueller, Beck, and Sedge (1987) reported sensitivity of 57% and specificity of 75% for veterans with long-standing head injuries of the left temporal lobe. On aphasic patients Niccum, Rubens, and Speaks (1981) reported hit rates of 90 to 100%. Dichotic CVs have been shown to be highly sensitive to lesions of the auditory areas of the cerebrum, but unfortunately are also sensitive to cochlear involvement. Interpreting Olsen's data from a 1977 report, the dichotic CVs showed a true-positive rate of 78% on a group of 40 patients who had undergone temporal lobectomy. Even higher true-positive rates have been reported in other studies. Speaks (1975) reported severely depressed CVs scores for the ear contralateral to the lesion in all 10 of his patients with CNS involvement. Olsen and Kurdziel (1978) demonstrated a 90% true-positive rate for CVs with temporal lobectomy subjects. Mueller et al. (1987) reported 93% sensitivity and 55% specificity for patients with long-standing left temporal lobe trauma. In the same study, Mueller et al. (1987) reported a 66% and 67% sensitivity and specificity for the *Staggered Spondaic Word Test* (SSW). Musiek (1983b) reported a sensitivity of 70% for 30 patients with CANS involvement (18 patients with cortical involvement and 12 patients with brainstem involvement). In examining patients with temporal lobe epilepsy, Collard (1984) found a sensitivity of about 50% for the SSW. Olsen and Kurdziel (1978) found only an 18.2% hit rate for the SSW on 22 temporal lobectomy patients.

Another dichotic test, although not a speech test, is the Psychoacoustic Pattern Discrimination Test (PPDT) (Blaettner et al., 1989). The PPDT has demonstrated a true-positive rate of 86% and a false-positive rate of 7%.

MONAURAL LOW-REDUNDANCY SPEECH TESTS

Sensitivity and specificity data are scarce on monaural low-redundancy speech tests. Our own analysis of the *Low-Pass Filtered Speech* (LPFS) test based on a population of 18 subjects with CANS lesions and 20 subjects with mild-to-moderate cochlear hearing losses was not satisfactory. In this study, the LPFS true-positive rate was barely

60%, and the false-positive rate was approximately 30%. Lynn and Gilroy (1977) used populations of 34 patients with temporal lobe lesions and 27 patients with parietal lobe lesions (presumably outside of the CANS) and showed a sensitivity and specificity of 74%. Karlsson and Rosenhall (1995) reported filtered speech test sensitivity rates of 62%, 49% and 62% on subjects with brainstem lesions (*N* = 27), brainstem vascular lesions (*N* = 15), and temporal lobe lesions (*N* = 31), respectively.

The SSI-ICM was used in a study by Jerger and Jerger (1974) on 11 subjects with brainstem lesions and revealed abnormalities in all 11 patients, resulting in 100% sensitivity. In a study on children with confirmed lesions of the CANS, the PSI-ICM showed abnormalities on six of nine (67%) patients (Jerger, Johnson, & Loiselle, 1989).

Compressed speech has been used in studies on patients with CANS lesions, and some reports provide sensitivity if not specificity data. Baran, Verkest, Gollegly, and Kibbe-Michael (1985) reported a 67% hit rate for 27 subjects with CANS involvement. Karlsson and Rosenhall (1995) related hit rates of 64%, 47%, and 80% for subjects with brainstem, brainstem vascular, and temporal lobe involvement, respectively.

BINAURAL INTERACTION AND LOCALIZATION TESTS

Of the binaural interaction tests, masking level differences (MLDs) is the procedure with perhaps the most clinical and clinical research use. The MLD, whether for speech or tones, is sensitive to lesions of the low brainstem. Lynn, Gilroy, Taylor, and Leiser (1981) reported a 100% sensitivity and specificity for patient populations with pontomedullary lesions, as compared to upper brainstem and cortical lesions. Olsen, Noffsinger, and Carhart (1976) reported a hit rate of 50% for subjects with widespread brainstem involvement. The 50% hit rate is similar to that reported in studies on patients with multiple sclerosis (Jerger, Oliver, Chmiel, & Rivera, 1986; Noffsinger, Olsen, Carhart, Hart, & Sahgal, 1972). A recent study by Karlsson and Rosenhall (1995) revealed a 69% sensitivity result for 27 patients with brainstem involvement.

Interaural timing tests have been administered to patients with multiple sclerosis. Interpreting the results is problematic with this population because not all multiple sclerosis patients have involvement of the CANS. Hausler and Levine (1980) found that 11 of 19 patients with multiple sclerosis and normal audiograms performed abnormally on an interaural timing task. Interestingly, in a later study (Levine et al., 1993), all seven subjects who had multiple sclerosis plaques in the auditory pathway of the brainstem as defined by MRI had abnormal interaural timing performance. Using a different interaural timing task, Quine et al. (1983) showed that 19 of 30 subjects with multiple sclerosis performed abnormally. Without MRI data on all multiple sclerosis subjects, or on patients with lesions clearly located in the auditory brain regions, it is difficult determine the accuracy of the interaural timing tests. However, given the worst scenario (i.e., a group of subjects with multiple sclerosis, some of whom may not have auditory lesions), interaural timing task are still moderately sensitive.

From an historical perspective, early tests for central auditory function involved sound localization. Sanchez-Longo and Forster (1958) used a simple soundfield localization task to assess patients with neurological problems. Their report listed patients with brain lesions at various sites. By interpolating the data from Sanchez-Longo and Forster, we divided the patients into those with auditory lesions and those with nonauditory lesions of the brain. Based on this interpolation, we obtained a sensitivity of 57% and a specificity of 80% from a population of 50 patients. An updated and clinically useful approach to auditory localization in a soundfield was reported by Cranford and colleagues (Cranford, Boose, & Moore, 1990). By interpolating the reported data, 21 of 24 subjects with multiple sclerosis failed this tracking test, for a sensitivity of 88% (Cranford et al., 1990).

TRENDS IN BEHAVIORAL TEST RESULTS

The classic finding on behavioral central tests is a deficit noted in the ear contralateral to the hemisphere with the lesion. The exceptions to this are interesting and informative. In addition, trends differ for patients with brainstem involvement from those with cortical lesions. Findings also can vary depending on the nature of the lesion as well as the test used, which creates a complex situation. In the following sections, we discuss the more common trends for patients with brainstem, cerebral, and interhemispheric lesions.

Brainstem Involvement

Depending on the size and/or location of the lesion(s), the findings on behavioral tests of brainstem function will vary. Although exceptions occur, lesions above the mid-pons often result in depressed scores in the ear contralateral to the lesion. Lesions located in the low-pons often result in ipsilateral deficits. Diffuse lesions or large and invasive lesions of the brainstem may result in bilateral deficits. Tests such as masking level differences and interaural timing tasks will not provide laterality information, but only an abnormal score for brainstem involvement (Jerger & Jerger, 1974; Musiek, Gollegly, Kibbe, & Verkest 1988).

Brainstem lesions generally will not have an effect on pure tone sensitivity or traditional speech recognition ability (Musiek, 1985). However, there are notable exceptions to this trend. If the cochlear nucleus is involved, it is possible that pure tone and speech recognition abilities will be compromised ipsilaterally (Dublin, 1986; Matkin & Carhart, 1966). Also, if a lesion is pervasive enough to markedly affect both brainstem ascending pathways, severe deficits in hearing sensitivity can evolve. In this situation central deafness may well be the diagnosis.

With the exception of MLDs, most behavioral tests will be influenced by lesions above the brainstem. That is, both cortical and brainstem lesions can yield abnormal scores on tests designated primarily for cortical lesions. Although most behavioral tests are not specific to differentiating brainstem and cortical lesions, they are sensitive to both. Also, in general terms, intra-axial brainstem lesions are associated with the higher sensitivity on behavioral tests than extra axial lesions (see Chapter 6 for further discussion).

Cerebral Involvement

The term cerebral is used here to include cortical and subcortical areas of the brain. The classic finding for central behavioral tests of auditory function in patients with unilateral cerebral involvement is deficits for the ear contralateral to the hemisphere involved. This is probably more distinct for dichotic tasks than for low-redundancy speech tasks (Musiek & Pinheiro, 1985).

The "paradoxical left-ear deficit" is a pattern that becomes evident when the corpus callosum fibers in the left hemisphere are affected. In this situation, a lesion in the left hemisphere will result in a left-ear or ipsilateral deficit, but only on dichotic speech tasks. In fact, a left-ear deficit on dichotic speech tasks will result if there is a lesion anyplace along the transcallosal auditory pathway, which extends from the left to right cortex (Musiek, Gollegly, & Baran, 1984). This finding is related to the concept that during dichotic listening the ipsilateral auditory pathway is suppressed in favor of the stronger contralateral pathway (Milner, Taylor, & Sperry, 1968). If a verbal report is required of a subject with corpus callosum involvement, the patient has no difficulty complying because the right-ear pathway has easy access to the speech, or left, hemisphere. Impulses from the left-ear stimuli, however, go to the right hemisphere and must be transferred across the corpus callosum to the left hemisphere for speech coding and a verbal report. When the corpus callosum is involved, this transfer either cannot happen or the integrity of this transfer is degraded and a left-ear deficit results (Musiek, Gollegly, & Baran, 1984).

A patient who has involvement of the corpus callosum and left auditory cortex will show a bilateral deficit on dichotic speech tasks (Musiek & Baran, 1987). This outcome is seen because the classical contralateral deficit results will evolve from the left cortex lesion (right-ear deficit), and due to the callosum involvement a left-ear deficit will also result (Figures 5–3 and 5–4).

Another interesting trend in behavioral tests is presented by the use of the monaurally presented frequency and/or duration pattern perception tests. These tests seem to require interaction of both hemispheres to decode the stimuli for a verbal report. For both hemispheres to interact the corpus callosum must be functional. Therefore, dysfunction in either hemisphere or the corpus callosum results in bilateral ear deficits on pattern perception tasks (Musiek, Gollegly, & Baran, 1984; Musiek, Pinheiro, & Wilson, 1980). It is theorized that the right hemisphere is needed to decode the acoustic contour of the pattern and that the left hemisphere is needed to linguistically label the pattern elements. Although monaural deficits have been noted on pattern perception tests, this finding is not common in patients with lesions of the cortex or subcortex (Musiek, Baran, & Pinheiro, 1990; Musiek, Pinheiro, & Wilson, 1980; Musiek & Pinheiro, 1987).

Because deficits in either hemisphere or the corpus callosum can result in bilateral deficits on pattern tests, these procedures cannot provide laterality information. However, by requiring the subject to hum his or her response, one can check right-hemisphere integrity. If a patient can hum the response but cannot verbally state it correctly, the problem may be in the corpus callosum (transfer) or in the left hemisphere (linguistic labeling). If the result on humming patterns is poor, the right hemisphere may be involved. Therefore, the corpus callosum or left hemisphere cannot be evaluated with pattern tests, and other procedures will be needed (Musiek, 1994; Musiek, Gollegly, & Baran, 1984; Musiek, Pinheiro, & Wilson, 1980).

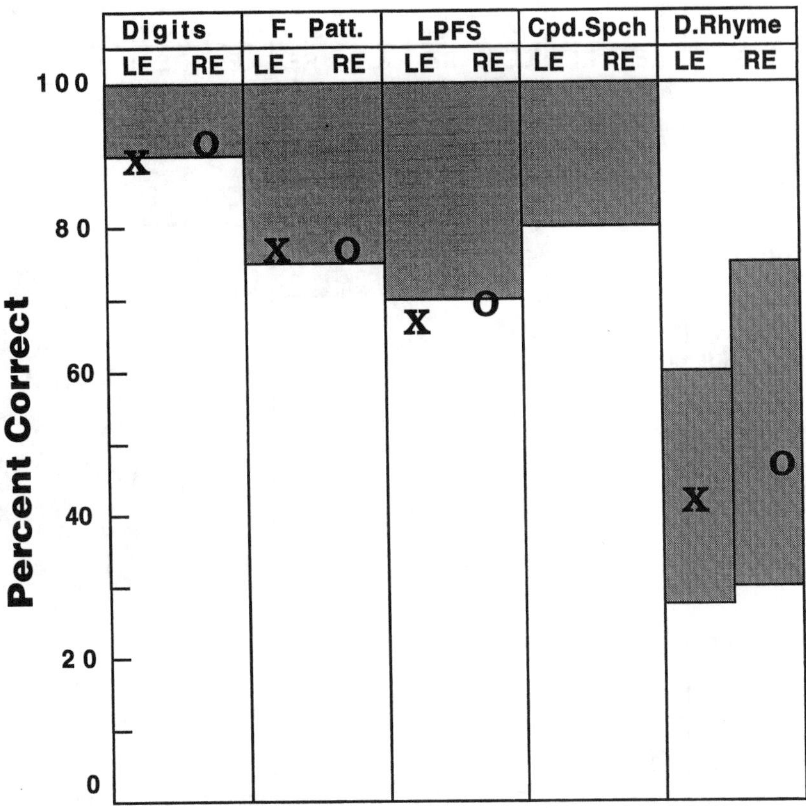

Figure 5–3. Mean composite central auditory test scores for a group of patients (N = 6) precommissurotomy (split brain).

PEDIATRIC CONSIDERATIONS

Many of the tests discussed in the previous synopsis of categories of central tests can be used with both children and adults (Chermak, 1996). Obviously, norms must be established for the various age ranges. Some tests are more amenable for use with children. The PSI and the SCAN may be used with preschoolers (Jerger & Jerger, 1984; Keith, 1986). The language level of the test and its related verbal instructions are a guide to the age for which the test can be used. Many of the tests we use require an age of at least 7 years (second-grade level), as younger children used as controls show considerable variability. The dichotic digits test, SSW test, filtered speech test, and the

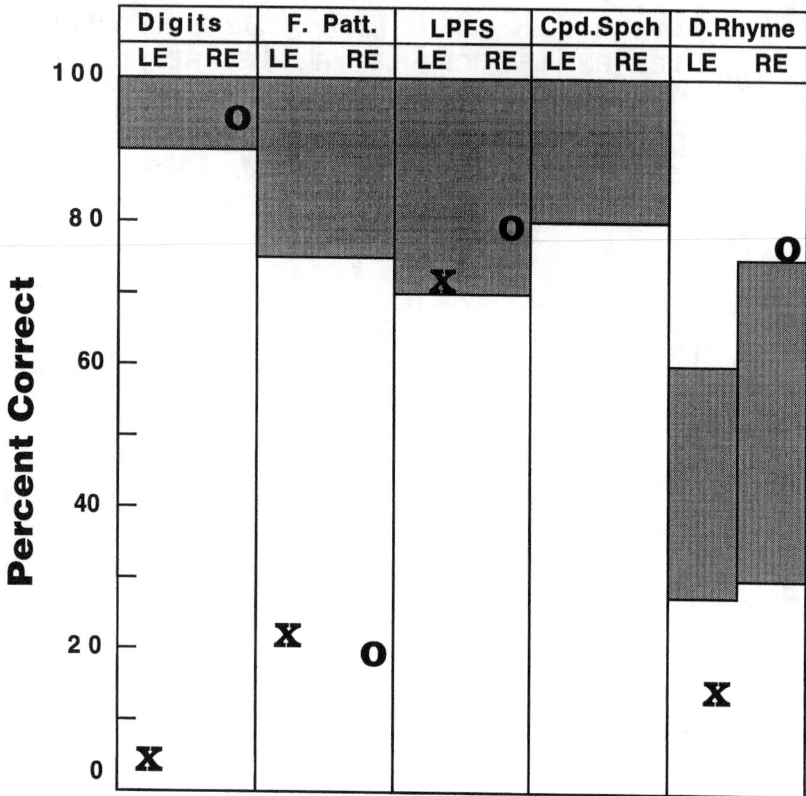

Figure 5–4. Mean composite central auditory test scores for the patients shown in Figure 5–3 postcommissurotomy.

compressed speech test are just some of the tests that can be administered to children between the ages of 6 and 7. Competing sentences and frequency patterns tests seem to provide definitive information for children 8 years and older. Because of its nature, the dichotic rhyme task can be performed by children 4 to 5 years of age. Interestingly, adult values for most of the tasks mentioned are reached at about 10 to 12 years of age (Musiek & Gollegly, 1988). Unfortunately, many of the adult tests for central auditory function have not yet been adapted or normed for children.

Response time is an important index that can be used for both children and adults in central auditory assessment. Regardless of the test, response time measurements can be made (Thompson & Abel,

1992). It is important to make sure that there are no intervening problems, such as motor difficulties, that may affect response time. This can be done by using a reference response time to a simple task, such as a pure tone stimulus. This type of stimulus should not require excessive processing; hence, a clear measure of response time, independent of processing time, can be obtained. Normal values for these reference measures can be obtained. Reaction time also may be employed to assess processing interactions during speech perception. The auditory Stroop task and the auditory Garner paradigm offer two such tasks to study linguistic influences on auditory processing (Jerger, Grimes, Tran, Chean, & Martin, 1996).

Many central auditory tests use speech as a stimulus (or require linguistic labeling). When this is the case, components of spoken word recognition should be considered to influence the outcome (i.e., response of the child) (Jerger & Allen, 1996). Theoretically, in addition to the extraction of auditory information, other components related to spoken word recognition affect the absolute performance on central auditory tests using speech stimuli. Phonetic feature extraction, phoneme identification, word recognition, and the behavioral oral response could, alone or in combination, yield an abnormal behavioral response to a central auditory test item (Jerger & Allen, 1996). Therefore, these components of spoken word recognition and/or the various auditory processes can cause abnormal performance. It is not known to what degree the spoken word components depend on basic auditory processes, or how much each component contributes to a normal or abnormal response, but these are certainly factors in this theoretical construct as it relates to CAPD.

OLDER ADULTS

Many elderly patients have difficulty understanding speech signals and hearing in noise. These common hearing complaints may have different bases. First, nearly all elderly patients have peripheral hearing loss, which can cause these symptoms. Also, problems with speech understanding and hearing in noise may have a central auditory basis, as these symptoms have been linked with CAPD. A third possibility is that both peripheral and central mechanisms are involved in presbyacusis. Considerable debate, data analysis, and theory have evolved to attempt to quantify the degree to which peripheral and central factors cause presbyacusis (Humes & Christopherson, 1991; Stach, Spretnjak, & Jerger, 1990). Although both groups have evidence for their claims, both peripheral and central problems exist in the elderly with great individual variance. Clearly, the elderly perform worse on behavioral central tests, but the contributions of peripheral loss to this decreased performance is difficult to gauge (see Life Span Considerations in Chapter 7). Clinicians must recognize that peripheral hearing loss may be responsible for an adult's spoken language understanding problems, either in part or to the exclusion of central auditory deficits. A comprehensive test battery of peripheral and central tests must be administered to determine the source of difficulty. Moreover, the audiologic results must be interpreted in concert with language and cognitive data. Data should be obtained on the performance of older adults who do not present with CAPD to facilitate interpretation of central auditory test scores. Not only are certain central tests highly influenced by peripheral hearing status, but some central tests (e.g., DSI, SPIN) exhibit uncertain test-retest reliability when administered to older adults (Cokely & Humes, 1992) and therefore may not be useful with this population.

SUMMARY

This chapter focused on behavioral or psychophysical tests of central auditory function. Behavioral tests provide considerable information about central auditory function, and with the increasing use of electrophysiologic tests, their value may increase as new relationships evolve between the physiologic and behavioral measures. It is helpful to categorize the large variety of available tests. The categories of temporal processing, dichotic listening, low redundancy, monaural speech, and binaural interaction tests each represent important parameters of assessment in CAPD. All tests within these categories are not of equal value. In a given patient, some tests may be more effective than others; however, tests from each of these categories should be considered by the clinician because they represent a variety of processes and an approach to assessing these processes in a clinically feasible time frame.

The sensitivity and specificity of behavioral central tests is an important facet of evaluating the worth of a test. Because there is no gold standard with which to compare test results, one must realize the shortcomings of efficiency measures of central auditory tests. Using populations with confirmed, well-circumscribed lesions of the CANS to test the diagnostic value of central auditory tasks has merit and should be considered. The classic result that the ear contralateral to the damaged hemisphere reveals the deficit still proves true. However, we now know that corpus callosum involvement yields left-ear deficits and that certain tests (e.g., pattern tests), because of the way they test the system, may not yield these classic results. The astute combining of different tests can provide insights into underlying mechanisms that are not seen with single tests or tests combined without forethought.

Although many of the commonly known central auditory tests can be used with adults and children, differences between these groups must be realized, especially in regard to maturational trends, language levels, and educational status. There is a need for more tests designed specifically for children, especially tests that do not use speech as a stimulus. And the careful examination of older adults must take language and peripheral hearing status into account. The examiner must use caution in selecting behavioral central tests with speech as a stimulus if spoken word recognition can possibly influence absolute results.

SUGGESTED READINGS

Musiek, F., & Pinheiro, M. (1987). Frequency patterns in cochlear, brainstem and cerebral lesions. *Audiology, 26*, 79–88.

Musiek, F., Baran, J., & Pinheiro, M. (1994). *Neuroaudiology: Case studies* (pp. 115–206). San Diego: Singular Publishing Group.

Swisher, L., & Hirsh, I. (1972). Brain damage and the ordering of two temporally successive stimuli. *Neuropsychologia, 10,* 137–152.

Tallal, P. (1985). Neuropsychological research approaches to the study of central auditory processing. *Human Communication, 9*(Part I), 17–22.

Thompson, M., & Abel, S. (1992). Indices of hearing in patients with central auditory pathology. II: Choice response time. *Scandinavian Audiology, 21*(Suppl. 35), 17–22.

CHAPTER 6

ELECTROPHYSIOLOGIC ASSESSMENT OF CENTRAL AUDITORY PROCESSING DISORDERS

This chapter discusses the electropysiologic assessment of central auditory processing defects (CAPD). However, two of the tests discussed briefly are not electrophysiologic. Acoustic reflex (AR) and otoacoustic emissions (OAEs) testing are not electrophysiologic in nature, but they are discussed in this chapter due to procedural similarities and because they provide a physiological index of auditory function.

The use of electrophysiologic tests for the evaluation of central auditory function reminds us of the breadth of the central auditory nervous system (CANS). The AR, OAEs, and auditory brainstem response (ABR) are tests of brainstem pathways. The middle latency evoked response (MLR), the N1 and P2 responses, the P300, and the mismatched negativity (MMN) reveal function of cortical and subcortical areas of the brain in response to acoustic stimuli.

Evoked potentials (EPs) have not been popular as test for CAPD among audiologists. Recently, however, the use of EPs to assess central auditory function has gained popularity. Although a few speech-language pathologists have experimented with EPs, the use of EPs by this professional group is almost nonexistent. Psychologists (including neuropsychologists), neurologists, and physiologists have the longest history of use of EPs for evaluating the auditory system, both clinically and experimentally. Middle and late potentials tests have existed for many decades, but the advent of the ABR in the 1970s drew much interest and research from audiology, and an increased number of audiologists began to use EPs.

As mentioned in Chapter 4, the use of EPs requires rather expensive equipment, which limits its use. Also, there is concern about whether EPs can enhance diagnostic capabilities relative to detecting dysfunction of the CANS (Musiek, Baran, & Pinheiro, 1994). Again, the best current use of many of these potentials is in combination with good behavioral tests or as additional testing based on behavioral findings.

In this chapter information is presented on each of the EPs mentioned earlier. We will not focus on historical data or on details of the administration of the various EPs, but rather on concepts surrounding EPs as they relate to the CANS and CAPD. Refer to Hall (1992) for more discussion of EP procedures.

THE AUDITORY BRAINSTEM RESPONSE (ABR)

Background

The first diagnostic paper written on the ABR had to do with central auditory function. Starr and Achor (1975) reported on the value of the ABR in defining lesions of the auditory pathways of the brainstem. This report preceded papers on the ABR and acoustic neuromas—probably the most common diagnostic use of the ABR.

The ABR is composed of five waves, which represent a series of synchronous, neural responses generated by the auditory nerve and brainstem (Hall, 1992; Moller, 1985) (Figure 6–1). These neural responses are recorded from electrodes placed on the vertex or high forehead and referenced to the earlobe or mastoid area. The stimulus is usually a click, but can also be a tone pip that can be presented at low (e.g., 15 per second) or high (e.g., 80 per second) rates. By computer averaging thousands of trials and filtering the responses picked up by the electrodes, a readable waveform representing very small voltages can be interpreted.

Waves I and II of the ABR waveform are generated by the peripheral auditory nerve; waves III and the IV–V complex are generated by the brainstem. More specifically, it appears that wave III is related to the cochlear nucleus, while waves IV and V have multiple

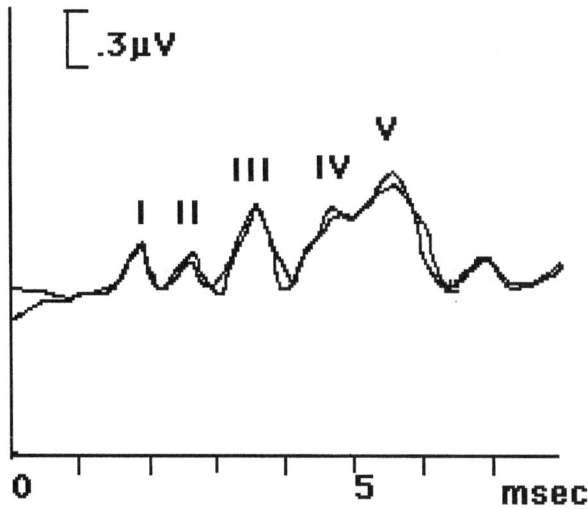

Figure 6–1. A normal auditory brainstem response (ABR) waveform, depicting waves I through V.

generators, with the superior olivary complex and nuclei of the lateral lemniscus playing a major role (Moller, 1985).

The ABR is valuable in the measurement of the integrity of the brainstem auditory pathway. For some populations with CAPD, the ABR is a test of choice; however, the ABR is not often used with children who have learning disabilities (LD). The consensus is that children with LD and no other concomitant problems will have normal ABRs (Marosi, Harmony, & Becker, 1990; Mason & Mellor, 1984; Roush & Tait, 1984). Although rare, it is possible for children with LD to have neurological brainstem involvement and, therefore, require appropriate evaluation. Other clinical populations, such as those with head trauma, neurological disease, auditory deprivation, the elderly, and those suspected of having CAPD, may be well suited to evaluation by ABR.

Sensitivity/Specificity

The history of the sensitivity and specificity of the ABR in detecting acoustic neuromas is well documented (Hall, 1992; Musiek, 1991; Musiek, McCormick, & Hurley, 1996). Reports indicate sensitivity rates of 90% or more and specificity rates of 80% for the detection of tumors of the eighth nerve. However, less information is available on the sensitivity and specificity of the ABR to CANS lesions.

Some early reports on the ABR showed the procedure to be valuable in detecting brainstem abnormality for a variety of lesions (Starr & Achor, 1975; Stockard & Rossiter, 1977). Some later reports, however, indicate that the sensitivity of the ABR to brainstem lesions is not as good as once believed. Chiappa (1983) and Musiek, Gollegly, Kibbe, and Verkest (1988) reported ABR sensitivity rates of just under 80% to a variety of brainstem lesions in adults. Later it was shown that the hit rate for ABR depended on the kind of brainstem involvement (Musiek & Baran, 1991). It appears that the sensitivity of ABR is very high (>90%) for disorders such as intra-axial lesions, but for disorders such as multiple sclerosis the hit rates are lower (60%). Recently, an extensive study provided hit and false-positive rates for the ABR for a variety of confirmed brainstem lesions (Musiek & Lee, 1995). This study demonstrated that, with the use of several indices (i.e., interwave intervals, absolute latencies, amplitude ratio), hit rates were approximately 80% and false-positive rates were approximately 20%. Clearly, the ABR, although valuable, is not as sensitive to brainstem disorders as it is to acoustic neuromas.

Diagnostic Patterns for ABR

Diagnostic indicators for the ABR center around the presence or absence of waves, the absolute latency of waves, interwave latency measurements, and amplitude comparison of waves. Because the brainstem generates waves III, IV, and V, the abnormal latency, amplitude, or absence of these waves should indicate brainstem or central problems (Figure 6–2). An extension of the wave I–III interval could indicate a brainstem lesion or an acoustic neuroma (Musiek, Josey, & Glasscock, 1986; Musiek & Lee, 1995). If there is a wave III–V abnormality, there is a strong likelihood of brainstem involvement, as the generators of these waves would be unaffected by an acoustic neuroma unless it was large (Musiek, Gollegly, Kibbe, & Verkest, 1988; Musiek & Lee, 1995). An extended wave I–V interval is related to the latencies of the wave I–III or III–V interval, and therefore could indicate either an acoustic neuroma or brainstem lesion. The presence of the early waves (I, II, and III) and the absence of the late waves (IV and V) indicate brainstem involvement (Musiek, 1991; Musiek, Gollegly, Kibbe, & Verkest, 1988). The absence of an entire waveform could be related to severe hearing loss, or auditory nerve or brainstem involvement. In brainstem involvement, some hearing loss would probably have to exist to yield this pattern of results.

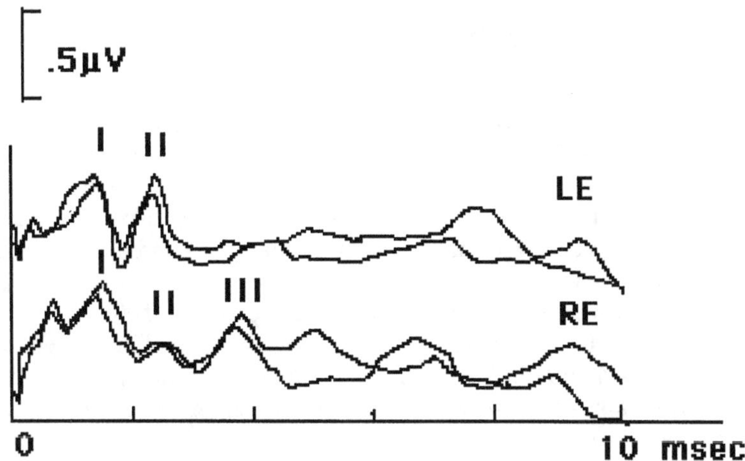

Figure 6–2. Left and right ear ABR waveforms from a 46-year-old patient with multiple sclerosis with brainstem involvement. Normal pure tones thresholds and speech recognition were documented bilaterally.

Amplitude measures for the ABR are not as reliable as latency measures (Hall, 1992). However, the amplitude comparison of waves I to V may have clinical value (Musiek, Kibbe, Rackliffe, & Weider, 1984; Musiek & Lee, 1995).

Adults and Children

Generally, the ABR reaches adult latency values by approximately 2 years of age (Hall, 1992). Thus, children and adults can be evaluated easily with the ABR. Of significance are studies indicating that children who have suffered from otitis media early in life may demonstrate deprivation effects reflected by mild ABR abnormalities (Folsom, Weber, & Thompson, 1983; Gunnerson & Finitzo, 1991). Some elderly patients also may show ABR abnormalities secondary to aging of the CANS (brainstem) (see Willott, 1991, for review). There is great variability in terms of ABR latencies and aging, which is probably related to the difficulties encountered when comparing young and elderly subjects, such as finding young and old with similar hearing sensitivity. Also, aging is physiological, not chronological; a 70-year-old patient may have a physiologically younger auditory pathway than a patient 15 years younger.

THE MIDDLE LATENCY EVOKED RESPONSE

The middle latency evoked response is a synchronous auditory evoked potential that was first described by Geisler, Frishkopf, and Rosenblith in 1958. The potential described by Geisler et al. had a negative wave at approximately 20 msec and a vertex positive peak at approximately 30 msec. Later investigators described several negative and positive waves that have since been included as part of the MLR (Figure 6–3).

The MLR waves occur after the ABR and within 100 msec of the stimulus onset. Geisler et al. (1958) noted that the MLR corresponded closely to the behavioral threshold of hearing. Indeed, since 1958 many articles have been written about the use of the MLR for estimating hearing sensitivity (Musiek & Geurkink, 1981; Thornton, Mendel, & Anderson, 1977; Zerlin & Naunton, 1974). However, despite a promising future in clinical use, interest and research in the MLR slowed due to the notion that the basis of the MLR might be myogenic (Bickford, Jacobson, & Cody, 1964). Although this notion proved false, general interest was curbed (Musiek, Geurkink, Weider, & Donnelly, 1984). Interest in the MLR increased after the advent of the ABR. This revamped interest in the MLR in the 1980s was not directed toward using the MLR for estimating hearing sensitivity and

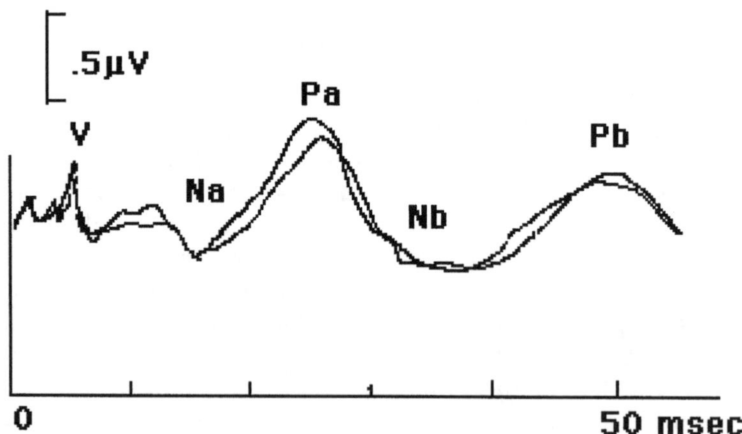

Figure 6–3. A normal middle latency response (MLR) waveform. Both negative and positive waves are denoted as well as the ABR wave V.

diagnosis, but rather for providing information on the integrity of the CANS. Most of our discussion of the MLR will be directed in this area. The MLR is useful in evaluating the CANS and for CAPD due to the location of the generators of this response.

Neural Generators of the MLR

It appears that the MLR has multiple generators, with major contributions from the thalamocortical pathway and, to a lesser degree, from the inferior colliculus and the (mesencephalic) reticular formation (Kraus, Kileny, & McGee, 1994). Studies also show that the auditory reception area of the temporal lobe plays a critical role in the Pa response (Kraus et al., 1994). It is also important to consider that the generators of the MLR in animals could be different from those of humans.

Nonpathological Factors

Many factors can influence the findings of the MLR in assessing the CANS. If the clinician is not aware of these factors, poor, contaminated, or diminished waveforms may lead to misinterpretation of the results.

The influence of sleep is an important consideration when using the MLR in CAPD evaluations. In adults, the amplitude of the MLR waves is attenuated as a function of the stage of sleep (Osterhamel, Shallop, & Terkildsen 1985). In children, sleep also has an effect, but in a different manner (Kraus, McGee, & Comperatore, 1989). In stage-1 sleep and REM sleep, the Pa wave often can be recorded; but in stage-2 and stage-3 sleep, the Pa wave can be recorded only occasionally. In stage-4 sleep, the Pa wave rarely can be recorded.

Although stage of sleep influences the ability to detect the MLR waves in children, the maturation of the CNS also may play a role (Kraus, Smith, Reed, Stein, & Cartee, 1985; Musiek, Geurkink, Weider, & Donnelly, 1984). The MLR waves can be delayed or absent in normal children younger than age 10; hence, maturation must be considered as a factor when using this measure for central assessment. At the same time, in children under age 10, the MLR may possibly be used for monitoring maturation of the CANS.

The filtering of the MLR is another important factor to consider. Analog filtering with narrow band and sharp roll-offs can result in phase shifting or the ringing of filters (Musiek, Geurkink, Wider, & Donnelly, 1984; Sherg, 1982). This in turn may provide a waveform which could be misinterpreted. Wider filtering bands, such as 20 Hz (children) or 30 Hz to 1500 Hz with 6- to 12-db per octave roll-offs, will curb distortions of the waveform. These wider filtering bands, although resulting in noisy waveforms, also allow the simultaneous recording of the ABR. Digital filtering will prevent many of the distortion problems with the MLR waveform.

The rate of stimulus presentation also can influence results. In infants, lower rates of presentation (1 to 2 clicks/sec) have yielded larger waveforms, as compared to 10 clicks/sec (Jerger, Chmiel, Glaze, & Frost, 1987).

Recording the MLR for CANS Assessment

Recording the MLR for central auditory assessment requires multiple electrode placement. A clinically feasible and diagnostically useful electrode array is placement at C3, C4, and Cz. This allows for the comparison of amplitudes and latencies for each hemisphere and mid-line. These comparisons are necessary for measuring the electrode effect, which will be discussed later. The reference electrode can be placed at the earlobe, ipsilateral and or contralateral to the ear stimulated, or at the nose, chin, or nape of the neck (noncephalic). Each of these reference electrode sites have both advantages and shortcomings, but this debate is beyond the scope of this chapter (Hall, 1992; Kraus et al., 1994).

MLR Indices and Interpretation

In central auditory assessment several measurements or indices can be used to determine normality or abnormality of the MLR. Generally, only the Na and Pa waves are used to determine the appropriateness of the response. The other waves of the MLR (Nb, Pb, Nc, Pc) are not reliable enough for clinical use. Both amplitude and latency indices can be used for MLR interpretation; however, the latency measures are not as sensitive as amplitude indices (Kraus, Ozdamar, Hier, & Stein, 1982; Musiek & Lee, in press; Scherg & Von Cramon, 1986).

A key point in the diagnostic use of the MLR is that the intersubject variability for amplitude indices is too great to use clinically (Musiek, Geurkink, Weider, & Donnelly, 1984). However, for older children and adults the MLR should be present; if it is not, there is cause for concern. One of the best indices is the comparison of amplitudes obtained for electrodes placed over each hemisphere. Often the electrode closest to the area of the lesion will be compromised (regardless of which ear is stimulated) in regard to amplitude; hence, there will be a difference when comparing electrodes (Figures 6–4 and 6–5). This difference is called the electrode effect (Musiek, Baran, & Pinheiro, 1994). Studies show the value of comparing MLR amplitudes across electrodes (Kileny, Paccioretti, & Wilson, 1987; Kraus et al., 1982; Scherg & Von Cramon, 1986). Questions remain, however, about how much of an amplitude difference across electrodes is significant. A 50% difference in amplitude has been used to indicate potential dysfunction (Musiek et al., 1994), but recent research indicates that even less of a difference could be diagnostically significant (Kelly, Lee, Charrette, & Musiek, 1996).

Ear effects are another index used in MLR interpretation. This is when one ear, regardless of electrode site, consistently shows reduced amplitudes. Again, a 50% difference in amplitude is considered important; however, this measure appears less valuable diagnostically than electrode measures (Kelly et al., 1996; Shehata-Dieler, Shimizu, Soliman, & Tusa, 1991).

Although Na and Pa latencies can be delayed in CANS disorders, these indices have not proved valuable (Kileny et al., 1987; Shehata-Dieler et al., 1991).

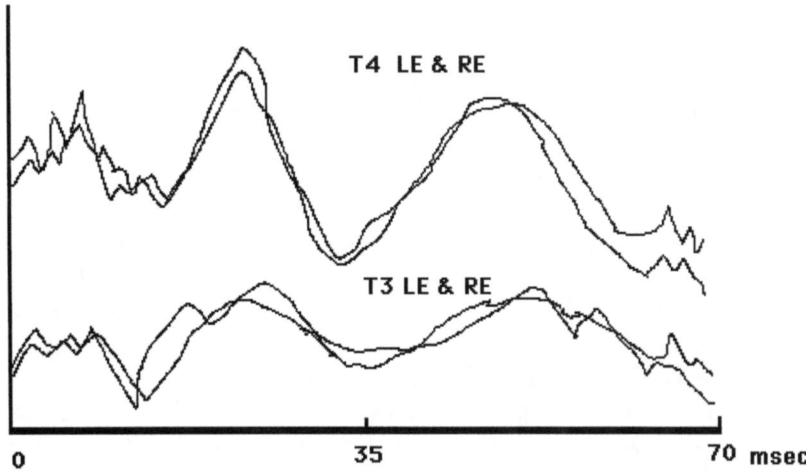

Figure 6–4. Results from a patient with a left temporal lobe tumor. An electrode effect is shown, as the T3 (left) electrode yields a considerably smaller amplitude than does the T4 (right) electrode. The waveforms from each ear are highly similar.

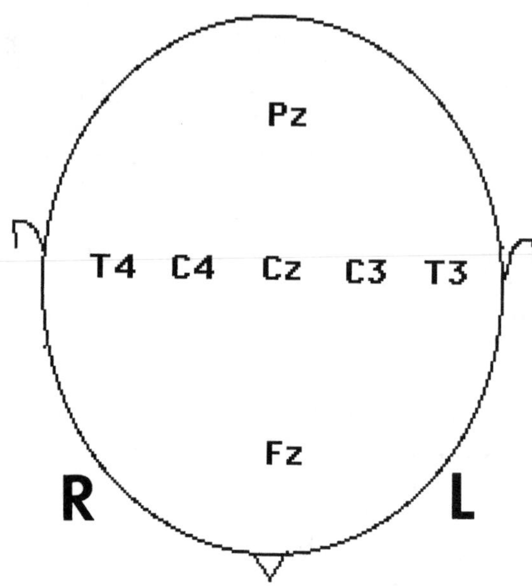

Figure 6–5. Common audiologic scalp electrode sites; view looks down on the top of the head.

The MLR and Central Auditory Lesions

The use of MLRs in subjects with central auditory involvement is a new and partially experimental procedure. There are few sensitivity and specificity data on the MLR, but studies are underway. In the following discussion, studies that have an impact on the MLR's value in CANS involvement are included even when sensitivity and specificity data are not available.

An early study on central lesions and the MLR was conducted by Kraus et al. (1982), who studied 24 patients with central lesions in the auditory areas. Of this group approximately 50% had normal MLRs. Of the patients who had abnormal MLRs, the most telling index was Na-Pa amplitude for the electrode over the involved hemisphere. Kileny et al. (1987) reported similar results. These investigators tested 11 patients with temporal lobe involvement and compared the results to a control group of normal patients and patients with other brain lesions. The MLR demonstrated significantly reduced amplitudes when comparing left and right hemisphere electrode sites. Ibanez, Deiber, and Fischer (1989) found significant electrode effects in 11 of 21 patients (52% sensitivity) who had cortical or subcortical lesions.

Woods, Clayworth, and Knight (1985) tested nine patients with unilateral cortical lesions, and six showed abnormal ear or electrode effects. Also studied were nine patients with subcortical lesions, all of whom showed ear and or electrode effects. Shehata-Dieler, Shimizu, Soliman, & Tusa (1991) showed an electrode effect by reduced amplitude in eight of nine patients tested with the MLR (two patients had large myogenic responses). Statistically, the recordings from the side of the lesions were significantly smaller than those from the intact side. A comparison group of patients with nonauditory lesions of the temporal lobe did not show this trend.

A recent study involving the MLR with 30 patients with multiple sclerosis showed abnormal findings in 22 patients (73.3%). The most common abnormality was absent Na and Pa waves (Celebisoy, Ayogdu, Ekmekci, & Akurekliet, 1996). A recent study on children with LD showed differences in the latencies of the MLR when compared to children with no learning problems (Arehole, Augustine, & Simhadri, 1995). This study revealed extended latencies of the Pa wave in 5 of 11 children with LD; only 1 child of 11 in the control group demonstrated an increased Pa latency. Other case studies on children with LD have shown abnormal MLRs (Jerger & Jerger, 1985; Jerger, Johnson, Jerger, Coker, Pirozzolo, & Gray, 1991). Conversely, Kraus et al. (1985) reported no significant difference in MLRs between children with LD and control patients.

The effect of aging on the MLR has been reviewed by Willot (1991). Willot related that studies show an amplitude and latency increase in the Pa wave with increasing age when a click stimulus is used. As with the ABR, the MLR has great variability across subjects in studies and across studies. The morphology of the MLR also may change with age, influencing amplitude and latency measures (Chambers & Griffiths, 1991).

LATE AUDITORY EVOKED RESPONSES (N1, P2, P3, AND MMN)

In this section, four late auditory evoked responses are discussed. The N1 and P2 complex are the oldest of the late potentials and were reported in 1939 (Davis, 1939). The N1 and P2 also are called both the N100 and P200, corresponding roughly to the time domains they occupy, although in reality the N1 occurs at about 80 to100 msec and the P2 occurs at about 160 to 200 msec (Figure 6–6).

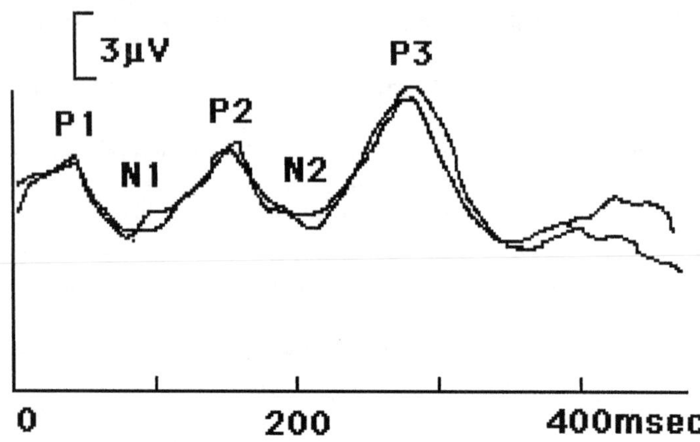

Figure 6–6. Late auditory potentials.

These potentials vary in amplitude from approximately 2 to 6μ volts, and their latencies vary as a function of the type and intensity of the stimulus. These potentials are best recorded from the vertex, but can also be recorded from sites around the vertex (McPherson, 1996). Common filtering for the N1–P2 is 1 to 30 Hz or 1 to 100 Hz.

The P3 or P300, first reported by Sutton, Braren, Zubinand, and John (1965), is larger than the P2 and is a result of the subject focusing on a target stimulus within an oddball paradigm (Figure 6–7). This paradigm has a series of stimuli which are occasionally different. The different stimuli occur approximately 20% of the time, and the subject must identify (usually by counting) when these stimuli occur. When the subject selectively attends to the target stimulus, the P300 results. Two averages exist for the P300: one average is for the electrical response to the target stimuli, which include the N1, P2, and P300, and the second average is for the nontarget stimuli, which yields only an N1 and P2 complex. Subtracting the waveform of the nontarget stimuli from the waveform of the targeted stimuli should provide a waveform of only the P300. The recommended recording montage for the P300 is midline montage of Fz, Cz, and Pz; however, the P300 can also be recorded from lateral areas on the scalp. Optimal filtering for the P300 is controversial, with 0.1 or 1–30 Hz used most often. The amplitude of the P300 is related to the probability of the target stimulus; the greater the probability, the smaller the potential. Clearly, attention plays a major role in the P300.

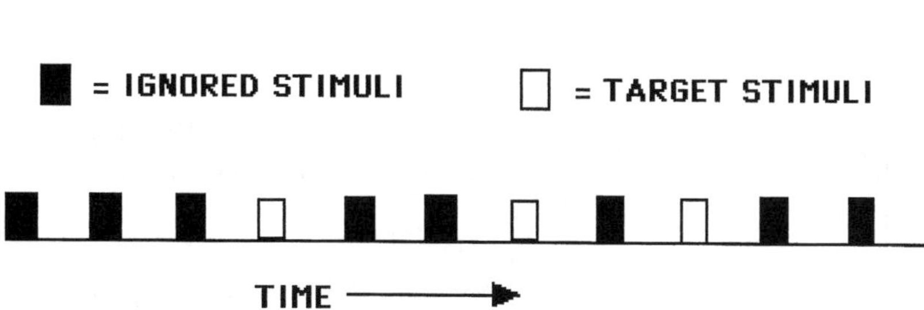

Figure 6–7. A train of stimuli in the oddball paradigm used in event-related potentials, such as the P300 and MMN.

The MMN or mismatched negativity is also elicited passively from an oddball-type paradigm, but unlike with the P300, attention is not required. The subject simply listens to the stimuli. The MMN is an automatic preattention response to stimulus change (Kraus & McGee, 1994). The change in stimulus results in an additional negativity after the N1. Again, two averages are taken, one for the regular or standard stimulus and the second for the deviant stimulus. One average is subtracted from the other and the MMN remains (Figure 6–8). The MMN can demonstrate differences in standard and deviant waveforms for stimuli that vary as little as 8 Hz in frequency and 5 dB in intensity (Naatanen, 1992). Because of its differential sensitivity, the MMN is an ideal procedure for measuring various types of auditory discrimination. This information can then be used diagnostically or for rehabilitative purposes (Kraus & McGee, 1994).

Generators of the Late Potentials

Based on topographic and dipole source analysis and on lesion effects, the N1 and the MMN appear to originate from the primary auditory cortex and association auditory cortex on the superior temporal plane (Knight, Hillyard, Woods, & Neville, 1980; Vaughn & Ritter, 1970).

The P2 response seems to be linked to the temporal lobes and the limbic system. Data are consistent with the auditory cortex as the generator (Hari, Aittonieme, Jarvinen, Katila, & Varpula, 1980; Vaughn & Ritter, 1970). Baumann, Rogers, Papanicolaou, and Saydjari (1990) suggest that the P2 occurs in the primary auditory cortex, along the Sylvian fissure on the side contralateral to stimulation.

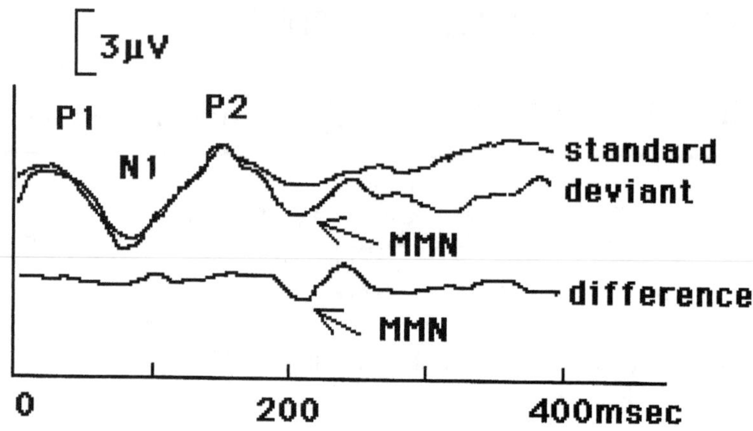

Figure 6–8. A mismatched negativity (MMN) waveform.

The P300 generators are not known; however, some evidence supports the hippocampus and/or the posterior temporal lobe as contributors to this potential (McPherson, 1996). It is reasonable to assume that the area of the brain responsible for memory would play a role in generating this complex potential. Major studies have implicated areas of the auditory cortex as generators of the P300. Reports on lesion effects and responses from implanted electrodes in humans (Knight, Scabini, Woods, & Clayworth, 1989; Valasco, Valasco, & Valasco, 1989) imply a role for the auditory areas in the cerebrum for the P300. On the other hand, ablation studies in animals as well as developmental theories could be interpreted to support the notion that the hippocampus is the P3 generator (Buchwald, 1990).

Nonpathological Factors

One must consider nonpathological factors for the late potentials. A thorough discussion of these factors is beyond the scope of this chapter, and we will mention only a few. Sleep or sedation is well known to affect these late potentials (N1, P2), causing mainly poor repeatability and attenuation of the amplitude of the waveforms (Rapin, Schimmel, & Cohen, 1972). Various states of arousal and alertness also affect the P300, in which attention is vital (Hall, 1992). These late potentials are all influenced by the degree of attention to the stimulus. If the stimulus is ignored, the waveforms are attenuated and possibly delayed (Hall, 1992).

Although the N1, P2, P300, and the MMN (as it relates to the N1) are to some degree endogenous potentials, they remain influenced by stimulus characteristics, such as intensity, frequency, type stimulus (click, tone, or speech), and interstimulus interval (Polich, 1987, 1989; Skinner, 1972). For the P300, random and/or rapid eye movements can contaminate the response; hence, subjects should focus on a target during testing. Difficulty of the task can affect the P300 waveform, with complex tasks yielding a greater latency (Polich, 1987).

Recording the Late Potentials

The N1 and P2 potentials should be recorded from C3, C4, and Cz sites for best use in central auditory assessment. As with the MLR, this can provide comparative electrode measures. The N1 and P2 can also be recorded when measuring P300 using the oddball paradigm. Hence, a variety of potentials can be recorded with little additional time commitment. As mentioned, the P300 is generally recorded from Fz, Cz, and Pz. However, if one wishes also to look at the N1, P2, and P300, a C3, C4, and Cz montage may be useful. If more recording channels are available, Fz, Cz, Pz, as well as C3 and C4 could be used. Reference electrodes can be linked from the ear lobes or positioned at the midline, as discussed in the section on the MLR.

Late Auditory Evoked Responses Indices and Interpretation

The N1 and P2 evoked potentials are most valuable when lateral (C3, C4) and midline (Cz) electrode placements are used (Peronnet & Mickel, 1977). As with the MLR, an electrode effect can be measured, which helps to determine hemispheric involvement.

Ear effects and a total lack of response (with adequate hearing) also can indicate CANS abnormality. Extended latencies of N1 and/or P2 can also be used as an index of central auditory dysfunction (Musiek, Baran, & Pinheiro, 1994).

The P300 does not appear to provide the laterality information seen with the MLR or N1 and P2 (Knight et al., 1989; Musiek et al., 1992). However, the P300 will occasionally show an electrode effect in unilateral disease (Musiek, Baran, & Pinheiro, 1992). Nonetheless, the convention is to use Fz, Cz, and Pz (midline) electrode sites. With these electrode sites, the P300 latencies and/or absence of the P300 can indicate abnormality. The amplitude measure with the P300 is highly variable, which makes the effectiveness of this index uncertain. Latency measures must be adjusted for age, as the P300 begins to increase in latency in the second or third decade of life (Polich, Howard, & Starr, 1985).

If the N1 and P2 are obtained with the P300 using the oddball paradigm, it may be useful to use laterally placed electrodes (C3, C4). This would allow the P300 measurement and a laterality measure from the N1 and P2 (from the nontarget stimuli). In some cases of CNS involvement, if lateral electrodes are used, the P300 also can provide diagnostically significant electrode effects (Musiek, Baran, & Pinheiro, 1992).

Another aspect of interpretation using the P300 is that abnormal responses can be a result of nonauditory abnormalities. For example, Parkinson's disease and some psychopathologies can yield abnormal P300s, and yet these disorders may not affect the auditory system (Knight, 1990).

Late Evoked Responses and Central Auditory Involvement

Few data are available on the sensitivity and specificity of the late potentials for central auditory processing disorders. The data from our 1992 study updated with a few cases would yield sensitivity rates of about 80% and specificity rates of approximately 70% (Musiek, Baran, & Pinheiro, 1992). It is clear from our study that the P300 was more effective diagnostically than were the N1 and P2 potentials. Knight, Hillyard, Woods, and Neville (1980) showed that the N1 is more sensitive than the P2 to focal brain lesions in the temporoparietal region. An electrode effect has been shown for the N1 and P2 potentials in patients with lesions limited to one hemisphere (Peronnet & Mickel, 1977).

In cases with bitemporal lesions, the N1 and P2 have been essentially absent or the latencies were extended and amplitudes decreased (Musiek, 1991; Woods, Clayworth, Knight, Simpson, & Naeser, 1987). In a review by Woods et al. (1987), and with additional cases by Musiek (1991), 19 of 26 (73%) patients with bitemporal lesions demonstrated abnormal N1–P2 potentials. Twelve of the 19 patients had an absence of responses; the remaining patients had latency or amplitude abnormalities. Knight et al. (1988) studied a normal control group as well as nine patients with lesions of the superior temporal gyrus (STG) and six patients with inferior parietal lesions (IPL). In this study the N1 was significantly reduced in amplitude for the STG group, as compared with the control group and the IPL group. The STG group had a definite electrode effect for N1 which was not noted for the other comparison groups of patients. Interestingly, no significant difference was found between these three groups for P2 amplitude and latency characteristics.

Knight et al. (1989) compared six patients with lesions of the temporal-parietal junction with six patients with parietal lesions. For the P300 amplitude index, the temporal group showed markedly reduced waves, as compared with the parietal group which yielded results similar to the normal control subjects. Knight et al. (1989) also used a P300 paradigm involving novel stimuli (stimuli that change in character to keep the subjects' attention) rather than targets, and the results comparing the two groups (temporal and parietal) were similar to those obtained using the standard P300 paradigm as reported by Musiek, Baran, and Pinheiro (1992). Knight et al. found no laterality effect on the patients or normal control subjects. Other studies show increased latencies and/or decreased amplitudes of the P300 in focal brain lesions, most of which involved the auditory areas of the cerebrum. Based on statistical comparisons to various control groups, the P300 was sensitive to either cognitive impairment or focal brain lesions (Ebner et al., 1986; Knight, 1990; Musiek et al, 1992).

Studies also have examined diffuse lesions of the cerebrum or lesions at various sites in the cerebrum. These studies may or may not have had auditory cortex involvement, but are of clinical interest. Obert and Cranford (1990) used the P300 to test 10 patients with neocortical lesions of various sites. They reported that in more than half (53%) of the experimental conditions the patients had absent or delayed waveforms. Significantly delayed P300s also have been noted in patients with traumatic brain injury (Rappaport & Clifford, 1994). Goodin, Aminoff, Chernoff, and Hollander (1990) reported delayed latencies in P300s for patients with HIV who were essentially without symptoms.

Kutus, Hillyard, and Volpe (1990) measured the P300 after commissurotomy in five patients and concluded that the corpus callosum was not needed for the generation of the P300. However, in these commissurotomy patients, there was a larger response over the right hemisphere. Because of this, one cannot rule out the possibility of the contribution of the corpus callosum to the P300. Certainly this asymmetry could also be a result of other kinds of brain dysfunction in this population.

The P300 has also been measured in learning disabled populations. Jirsa and Clontz (1990) used the P300 in a population of normal school-aged children and children who had CAPD. The CAPD group had significantly delayed latencies, but there was no significant difference in the P300 amplitude between the two groups. Squires and Hecox (1983) demonstrated P300 abnormalities and subtle auditory discrimination problems in children with receptive and expressive language disorders. Loiselle, Stamm, Maitinski, and Whipple (1980) used a dichotic P300 paradigm with 11 boys classified as hyperactive. When each group was asked to attend to stimuli in one ear over the other, a latency difference was found between the control and hyperactive groups. However, when this selective listening task was not used, no latency differences were found between groups.

Abnormal P300s have been reported in a number of clinical populations. These abnormal results are probably less closely linked to specific auditory or communication difficulties than those mentioned above. For example, abnormal P300s have been linked to people with Down's syndrome, parkinsonism, and various psychiatric disorders (Knight, 1990; Lincoln, Courchesne, Kilman, & Galambos, 1985). Many studies have shown abnormal P300s (both amplitude and latency) for patients with dementia (McPherson, 1996).

The use of the MMN in defining various clinical populations is in its early stages. Kraus et al. (1993) have shown deficits correlated to an abnormal MMN in patients with CAPD and specific auditory discrimination problems. A recent study on patients with frontal cortex lesions suggested that MMN amplitude was diminished, most notably over the lesioned hemisphere and from the ear ipsilateral to the lesioned hemisphere (Alho, Woods, Algazi, Knight, & Naatanen, 1994).

The late potentials, especially the P300, offer advantages to the professional interested in auditory diagnostics, but there are limitations to using these potentials for understanding various central auditory disorders. To use these potentials to define central auditory lesions, the patient must be carefully defined. The clinician must be sure the patient has no other nonauditory disorders (such as parkinsonism) which could result in abnormal late potentials. If other factors have been excluded, an abnormal late potential can be linked to an auditory problem with greater certainty, especially if the patient has a history consistent with auditory problems. If a patient has a diagnosed nonauditory disorder known to affect the P300, one must consider the disorder as the reason for the abnormal P300. Conversely, patients with known nonauditory disorders and abnormal late potentials could have a concomitant peripheral or central auditory problem. In these complex situations, the use of other auditory tests may prove helpful in defining an auditory disorder.

The N1 and P2 evoked potentials may have a rather long maturational course, which results in changes in latency, amplitude, and general morphology from infancy through the elementary school years (Musiek, Verkest, & Gollegly, 1988). In elderly subjects there may be some latency increase for the P2 wave but not the N1, although more studies are necessary to be certain. The P300 has long been known as a predictor of age. The shortest latency of the P300 is achieved in the late teenage years and early 20s, and its latency increases at a rate of approximately 1.25 msec for every year thereafter (Barajas, 1990).

The MMN response is present early in life and seems to reach adult-like values in the early school-age years (Kraus & McGee, 1994). Few data are available on the MMN response and how it is influenced by age.

THE ACOUSTIC REFLEX AND OTOACOUSTIC EMISSIONS

The acoustic reflex (AR) is not considered a strong measure of central auditory function. However, it is clear that lesions of the low brainstem (pons) alone can result in an abnormal reflex pattern (Hall, 1985). In this regard the AR can be valuable in assessing central auditory integrity in children and adults. However, the AR interacts with only a small portion of the CANS and must be interpreted accordingly.

Reports exist of abnormal ARs in different kinds of CANS or CNS lesions, including multiple sclerosis, head trauma, brainstem vascular disorders, and various types of mass lesions (Hall, 1985). Little sensitivity and specificity data are available on CANS involvement and the AR. The sensitivity of the AR to patients with multiple sclerosis has ranged from 20% to 80% (Jerger et al., 1986; Musiek et al., 1989). The sensitivity of the AR to central auditory lesions depends on the manner in which they are measured. Presence or absence is one way to determine abnormality, but latency and various amplitude analyses also can be used to improve sensitivity (Musiek et al., 1989; Wilson & Margolis, 1991). It is difficult to predict to what extent additional measures will increase sensitivity while concurrently reducing specificity.

The AR appears to be fully developed at birth and is similar in infants and adults (Wilson & Margolis, 1991). Some studies indicate differences in the AR between adults and infants, but these differences can be attributed to the testing instrumentation used, and to the physical differences in the neonatal versus adult ear (Wilson & Margolis, 1991). Findings are mixed about the effects of aging on the AR. These mixed findings may be related to difficulties in matching hearing sensitivity between young and older subjects. Aging appears to have little effect on the AR for frequencies of 2000 Hz and below. At higher frequencies the AR thresholds are slightly elevated for the elderly population.

Otoacoustic emissions (OAEs) are generated by the cochlea but can be valuable in evaluating the CANS. Otoacoustic emissions can help substantiate normal cochlear function, which can be important in the diagnosis of CANS involvement. It is known that cochlear abnormalities can exist with a normal pure tone audiogram. Otoacoustic emissions can be used as another measure to help document that the cochlea is normal.

When OAEs exist in a patient with significant hearing loss, the clinical implication is that the hearing loss may be neural in nature or that the patient is malingering (Musiek, Bornstein, & Rintelmann, 1995; Robinette, 1992). In low-brainstem (cochlear nucleus) involvement or in cases of central deafness, the OAEs should be normal, while pure tone audiometry will indicate hearing loss.

The measurement of OAEs can provide an index of the integrity of the olivocochlear bundle (OCB). The OCB is part of the efferent auditory pathway that originates in the region of the superior olivary complex and terminates at the base of the outer hair cells (medial system) or at the nerve fibers at the base of the inner hair cells (lateral system). The OCB appears to play a role in hearing in noise. Studies have shown that when the OCB is compromised animals cannot hear in noise as well as when this system is intact (Musiek, 1992; Musiek & Hoffman, 1990). Because deficits in auditory performance in noise characterize CAPD, it may be important to know whether the OCB is functioning normally. Otoacoustic emissions are influenced by stimulating the OCB (Collet, Veuillet, Bene, & Morgan, 1992). Clinically, the easiest way to stimulate this system is by introducing noise into the contralateral ear. When this happens in the normal auditory system, the level OAEs are suppressed in amplitude by several decibels. However, in some cases with central or neural involvement this decrease is not evidenced (Berlin, Hood, Cecola, Jackson, & Szabo, 1993).

Because the suppression effect of the OCB on the amplitude of the OAEs is small, its clinical value remains questionable. However, this OCB suppression phenomena is currently under investigation and this procedure may become more valuable as a clinical tool.

BEHAVIORAL AND ELECTROPHYSIOLOGIC TESTS

Using a test battery composed of both behavioral and electrophysiologic tests has advantages and disadvantages. One advantage in using both types of tests is that the sensitivity of the test battery may be better. Different functions of the CANS are tapped when using evoked potentials versus behavioral procedures, which can help the sensitivity of the overall test battery. Also, the clinician's confidence in making a diagnosis of CAPD is increased when abnormalities are shown across both behavioral and electrophysiologic tests.

In some cases, the clinician may want to bias the use of electrophysiologic or behavioral tests (Musiek & Chermak, 1994). An example of biasing is when the clinical question or significant background data pertain to brainstem involvement. In this situation an electrophysiologic test—the ABR—would be used, and its results would be weighted heavily in terms of interpretation. Because the ABR is a more sensitive test of brainstem integrity than are most behavioral tests, and because pretest information indicates the brainstem as a likely site of involvement, the ABR results would be favored in interpreting test battery outcomes. Conversely, if a clinician wants to define an interhemispheric processing problem, behavioral tests, such as dichotic listening, would be preferred to any electrophysiologic test.

Presently, electrophysiological tests, specifically evoked potentials, require more time to administer, more expensive equipment, and cost more than do behavioral tests. Despite these factors, electrophysiologic tests should still be strongly considered in test battery. Many patients with severe CANS problems, such as aphasia or central deafness, cannot be tested behaviorally, and electrophysiologic procedures are the only avenue to use for assessment. Also, we have seen cases where many behavioral tests yield normal results in patients with definite auditory symptoms and CANS involvement but EPs are abnormal (Musiek et al., 1994). If a patient with a strong history of auditory difficulties performs normally on the behavioral test battery, we often will administer an EP test, even if the patient must return at another time.

SUMMARY

Electrophysiologic tests are a welcome addition to the central auditory assessment arena, although they need further development and refinement. The ABR is a valuable tool for the delineation of brainstem lesions, and remains one of the most sensitive and specific audiologic tests for brainstem auditory pathway involvement. The MLR requires multiple electrode sites for optimum effectiveness in central evaluation. Amplitude comparisons across electrode sites in the same patient appear to offer the best diagnostic index. Factors that reduce the effectiveness of the MLR include intersubject variability and sleep and maturation effects. This procedure, however, can provide valuable clinical information relative to the CANS. Of the late potentials, including the N1, P2, P3, and MMN, the latter two hold the most promise for CANS evaluation, primarily because these tests have the capacity and flexibility to assess a variety of processes involved in hearing and cognition.

The P300 and MMN require further study, but they appear to be applicable to the CAPD population. The clinician must be aware that these tests are influenced by a number of other disorders.

The AR can indicate dysfunction of the low pons and should be considered as a measure of central dysfunction. Otoacoustic emissions provide an index of cochlear integrity which can be valuable in CAPD assessment. Also, OAEs can provide a look at the integrity of the OCB which may prove valuable in people who have trouble hearing in noise. More clinical work is necessary to optimize the use of this new procedure.

SUGGESTED READINGS

Chermak, G. (1996). Central testing. In S. Gerber (Ed.), *The handbook of pediatric audiology.* Washington, DC: Gallaudet University Press.

Knight, R. (1990). Neuromechanisms of event-related potentials: Evidence from human lesion studies. In J. Roharbaugh, R. Parasuraman, & R. Johnson. (Eds.), *Event related potentials: Basic issues in applications.* New York: Oxford University Press.

McPherson, D. (1996) *Late potentials of the auditory system.* San Diego: Singular Publishing Group, Inc.

Musiek, F., & Lee, W. (1995). Auditory brainstem response in patients with brainstem or cochlear pathology. *Ear and Hearing, 16,* 631–636.

CHAPTER

7

FUNDAMENTAL CONCEPTS AND CONSIDERATIONS FOR MANAGEMENT

Notwithstanding recent progress in understanding central auditory processes and central auditory processing disorders (ASHA, 1996), efforts must continue to further define and differentiate this heterogeneous group of functional deficits, which shares clinical features with several other perplexing disorders. Although work proceeds to clarify the nature of central auditory processing disorder (CAPD) and its role in the range of language, learning, and behavioral problems with which it is often associated, treatment programs must be implemented to ameliorate the functional difficulties confronting individuals with CAPD.

A number of topics considered basic to intervention are explored in this chapter. Because treatment efficacy generally defines the merit of any clinical approach, the chapter begins with a discussion of efficacy and the related topics of collaboration and generalization. Also discussed are feedback and goal structures, multicultural considerations, and customizing intervention, including life span considerations. The chapter concludes with a delineation of the theoretical foundation of our intervention approach.

EFFICACY

As the health care industry shifts the focus of program evaluation from assessment of structure to assessment of patient outcomes, the challenge to the professions of speech-language pathology and audiology to conduct clinical research demonstrating treatment efficacy is intensified (Olswang, 1990). Third party payers seeking to contain costs increasingly are demanding convincing evidence of the productivity or effectiveness of the treatment process. Apart from the use of data to justify treatment decisions, however, speech-language pathologists and audiologists should recognize the value of data collection as an integral component of the clinical process (Olswang & Bain, 1994).

Indeed, treatment data provide answers to a variety of critical clinical questions and should guide decisions concerning the intervention program. As elaborated by Olswang and Bain (1994), the proactive use of data allows the clinician to reach informed decisions regarding the following clinical questions: "Is the client responding to the treatment program?; Is significant, important change occurring?; Is treatment responsible for the change?; How long should a therapy target be treated?" (Olswang & Bain, 1994, p. 55). The reader is referred to Olswang and Bain (1994) for an excellent review of the principles of data selection and data collection for clinical decision-making.

Motivation and Efficacy

The efficacy of any treatment is contingent on a motivated client. Motivation guides information processing by priming self-regulation of the diverse cognitive and metacognitive operations crucial to listening and learning. As discussed in Chapter 1, individuals with CAPD may present motivational problems resulting from repeated comprehension failure and fatigue in attempting to understand spoken language. Repeated failure leads to a sense of the futility of one's efforts, low self-confidence, maladaptive attributions for both failures and successes, and ultimately poor motivation and low task persistence (Torgesen, 1980; Wong, 1991). Since failure is the likely outcome in the absence of motivation, maintaining motivation toward listening, communication, and learning is essential to successful intervention outcomes. Training tasks must be graded in difficulty to provide challenge, yet ensure sufficient success to maintain motivation.

The keys to maintaining motivation as tasks become more challenging are feedback and collaboration. Reassuring clients that the tasks are difficult and of the importance of persistence, committed effort, and appropriate use of strategies will help maintain motivation. Similarly, collaboration empowers clients, maintains interest, and thereby fosters motivation. (See also subsequent sections on feedback and collaboration.) The reader will find a number of practical suggestions for classroom management of motivational problems, as well as a variety of learning difficulties, in McIntyre (1989).

Documenting Efficacy

Demonstrating treatment efficacy requires documenting that an important change occurred in a client's performance due to the treatment, rather than from maturation or some other uncontrolled factor (Bain & Dollaghan, 1991; Goldstein, 1990). Although it may be convenient to collect valid data addressing changes in central auditory processing, data collected to evaluate clinically significant and important change must be sufficiently broad to encompass the client's progress in the variety of contexts in which that client has opportunity or need to deploy the newly acquired or enhanced processing strategies and/or skills. Multiple measures examining the various dimensions of progress relevant to the client's well-being are needed to evaluate change and thereby document treatment efficacy (Olswang & Bain, 1994). Although factors other than auditory function affect performance in everyday contexts, efficacy of treatment for CAPD should be gauged on the basis of significant change in functionally relevant contexts (e.g., school, home, work) rather than exclusive reliance on improvements in either electrophysiologic or even behavioral performance measures used to assess central auditory processes.

Moreover, the clinician should consider the value of qualitative data used in conjunction with quantitative data to demonstrate functional change. Quantitative data are, by definition, objective and precise and thus are often preferred by clinicians; however, as noted by Olswang & Bain (1994), collection of qualitative data through systematic observation and interviews provides opportunities to examine the client's interaction with the environment, as well as a context within which the question of functional change and efficacy can be assessed. In fact, involving clients in qualitative data collection through the use of diaries and daily logs, for example, not only benefits efficacy studies, but enhances the treatment program by encouraging self-monitoring and executive processes. (These are essential to the metacognitive approaches to intervention detailed in Chapter 8.) And again, although we are not advocating that efficacy be determined on the basis of qualitative data, either primarily or exclusively, it is important to note that, insofar as qualitative data provide a measure of function within the context of the environment, they also are more consistent with the systems-based or ecological perspective underlying our comprehensive intervention program (see Theoretical Foundation). In any case, collection of multiple performance measures involving both quantitative and qualitative data will maximize the prospects for accurately answering the variety of clinical questions necessary to determine best clinical practices.

Theory and Efficacy

Theory helps the clinician understand observed behaviors, explains why a treatment is efficacious, and thereby offers a rational guide for intervention programming (Friel-Patti, 1994b). Documenting treatment efficacy requires empirical examination of the degree to which treatment outcomes reflect the theoretical constructs upon which the intervention is grounded. Hence, articulation of the theoretical constructs underlying treatment programs is fundamental to efficacy research.

Efficacy Research

Unfortunately, efficacy research in communication disorders is limited (Kamhi, 1991). In particular, few studies have been undertaken to examine the efficacy of interventions for CAPD. Several studies have examined the relationship between behavioral performance on auditory processing tasks and event-related auditory potentials (Jirsa, 1992; Jirsa & Clontz, 1990; Kraus & McGee, 1994; Kraus, McGee, Ferre et al., 1993, 1996). A recent report demonstrated the efficacy of temporal processing training for improved auditory discrimination and spoken language comprehension (Tallal et al., 1996). However, most of the evidence demonstrating the efficacy of CAPD intervention has been derived from investigations of FM technology (Blake, Field, Foster, Platt, & Wertz, 1991; Flexer, Millin, & Brown, 1990; Neuss, Blair, & Viehweg, 1991; Ray, Sarff, & Glassford, 1984; Sarff, Ray, & Bagwell, 1981; Shapiro & Mistal, 1986; Stach, Loiselle, & Jerger, 1987a, 1987b, 1991). In addition, several metacognitive approaches have been shown effective in improving language-related and academic problems commonly associated with CAPD (Borkowski, Weyhing, & Carr, 1988; Brown, Campione, & Day, 1981; Chermak, Curtis, & Seikel, 1996; Fabricus & Hagen, 1984; Kendall & Braswell, 1982; McKenzie, Neilson, & Braun, 1981; Moynahan, 1978; Palincsar & Brown, 1984, 1986; Paris, Newman, & McVay, 1982; Paris, Wixson, & Palincsar, 1986; Reid & Borkowski, 1987; Tierney & Cunningham, 1984).

In contrast to the limited number of studies with human subjects, a substantial body of animal research has confirmed both the plasticity of the central nervous system and the impact of training on behavior (Aoki & Siekevitz, 1988; Brainard & Knudsen, 1993, 1995; Brown, Chapman, Kairiss, & Keenan, 1988; Edeline & Weinberger, 1991; Feldman, Brainard, & Knudsen, 1996; Hassmannova, Myslivecek, & Novakova, 1981; Irvine, Rajan, & Robertson, 1992; Jenkins, Merzenich, & Recanzone, 1990; Knudsen, 1987, 1994; Knudsen, Esterly, & du Lac, 1991; Knudsen, Esterly, & Olsen, 1994; Mogdans & Knudsen, 1992, 1993, 1994; Recanzone, Jenkins, Hradek, & Merzenick, 1992; Recanzone, Merzenich, & Jenkins, 1992; Recanzone, Merzenich, & Shreiner, 1992; Recanzone, Shreiner, & Merzenich, 1993; Robertson & Irvine, 1989; Weinberger & Diamond, 1987; Willott, Aitken, & McFadden, 1993). Experience-induced biochemical, anatomical, and physiological central nervous system changes have been observed consistently across species and at various levels in the auditory, visual, and somatosensory pathways (Brainard & Knudsen, 1993; Devor & Wall, 1978; Feldman et al., 1996; Gilbert & Wiesel, 1992; Hassamannova et al., 1981; Jenkins, Merzenich, Ochs, Allard, & Guic-Robles, 1990; Kaas, 1991; Mogdans & Knudsen, 1992; Pons et al., 1991; Recanzone, Jenkins et al., 1992; Recanzone, Merzenich, & Jenkins, 1992; Recanzone, Merzenich, Jenkins, Grajski, & Dinse, 1992; Recanzone, Merzenich, & Schreiner, 1992; Recanzone et al., 1993). These studies demonstrate the power of training to induce cortical reorganization, as reflected in changes in neural representation and response properties and improved performance. The animal research provides a strong foundation on which additional efficacy studies with human subjects can be designed. (See also Cognitive Neuroscience for further discussion of plasticity and cognitive change.)

Human efficacy research employing event-related brain potentials to measure central processing shares with the animal studies the use of electrophysiologic measures to document change. Using both an event-related potential and performance to monitor treatment outcome, Jirsa (1992) reported significant and concomitant changes in P300 latency and amplitude and behavioral measures of auditory processing among a group of children with CAPD who received a structured treatment program, relative to a control group of children with CAPD who did not receive treatment. Jirsa and Clontz (1990) reported significantly delayed P300 latency and reduced P300 amplitude among children with CAPD relative to a control group, although no direct relationship was observed between electrophysiological and behavioral measures. Kraus, McGee, Ferre et al. (1993) demonstrated an association between auditory discrimination deficits under adverse listening conditions and the absence of the mismatch negativity (MMN) event-related potential in a college-age woman with CAPD. Kraus and McGee (1994) presented several case studies documenting the correspondence between an absent MMN response and behavioral auditory discrimination deficits in subjects with central auditory processing problems.

The efficacy of remote microphone technology for enhanced communication ability and academic performance has been documented. Frequency-modulated (FM) sound field amplification has been shown to contribute to improved reading achievement in children with academic deficits (Ray et al., 1984; Sarff et al., 1981). Blake et al. (1991) reported that the use of FM auditory trainers increased attending behavior in children with learning disabilities. Stach et al. (1987) reported similar improvements in academic performance and behavior by children with CAPD who had been fitted with FM technology. Improved word identifcation has been measured when children with developmental disabilities, including minimal hearing impairment, use FM sound field amplification in the classroom (Flexer et al., 1990; Neuss et al., 1991). (See Rosenberg and Blake-Rahter [1995] for a review of the literature.)

Building on research begun in the 1970s, which suggested that some language learning difficulties in children result from temporal processing deficits (Tallal, 1980b; Tallal & Piercy, 1973a, 1973b, 1974, 1975; Tallal & Stark, 1982; Tallal, Stark, & Mellits, 1985), Merzenich et al. (1996) demonstrated marked improvements in the temporal processing skills of children with language impairment following intensive computerized training involving temporal ordering of frequency modulated tone pairs and consonant-vowel pairs. Tallal et al. (1996) demonstrated that intensive computerized training with temporally prolonged speech leads to improved temporal processing thresholds, auditory discrimination, and spoken language comprehension. These results show the linkage between central auditory processes and spoken language comprehension. Moreover, they offer compelling evidence of the efficacy of temporal processing training for ameliorating related central auditory processing deficits (i.e., auditory discrimination), as well as spoken language comprehension deficits. Also corroborating the utility of auditory skills training, Divenyi and Robinson (1989) reported a serendipitous finding of a significant improvement in language comprehension by subjects with aphasia following training on a battery of auditory processing tests (e.g., frequency discrimination, temporal gap discrimination, temporal order discrimination, etc.).

A number of studies of normally developing children and children with learning disabilities have demonstrated improvements in learning, reading, memory, and self-control following metacognitive training (e.g., attribution training, reciprocal teaching, self-regulation training, cognitive strategy training) (Borkowski et al., 1988; Brown et al., 1981; Chermak et al., 1996; Fabricus & Hagen, 1984; Kendall & Braswell, 1982; McKenzie, Neilsen, & Braun, 1981; Moynahan, 1978; Palincsar & Brown, 1984, 1986; Paris et al., 1982; Paris et al., 1986; Reid & Borkowski, 1987; Tierney & Cunningham, 1984). These findings suggest the utility of metacognitive training for mitigating the functional deficits associated with CAPD. Given the moderately strong correlation between listening and reading comprehension (Stanovich, 1993; Sticht & James, 1984), as well as the observed bidirectional transfer between listening and reading comprehension skills, particularly among more experienced subjects (Pearson & Fielding, 1982), it is reasonable to suggest that metacognitive strategies should reduce the functional language and academic deficits frequently seen in individuals with CAPD.

Summary of Efficacy Research

Data from both animal and human studies reveal the potential of behavioral interventions to improve central auditory processing and spoken language understanding. Despite the promise of preliminary reports, the utility of electrophysiologic measures (e.g., P300 and MMN) to assess treatment efficacy remains to be determined. Moreover, efficacy of interventions beyond remote microphone technology must be evaluated. Electrophysiologic measures and narrow behavioral measures may provide preliminary answers to basic efficacy questions pertaining to the appropriateness of treatment targets, treatment techniques, and the client's response to the treatment program; however, broader measures are needed to answer conclusively the central efficacy question as to whether the client is changing (Olswang & Bain, 1994). Improvements in spoken language comprehension following temporal processing training (Tallal et al., 1996) are one example of the type of research which begins to demonstrate such efficacy. However, since the subjects in Tallal et al.'s research were not specifically diagnosed with CAPD, additional research is needed to confirm the efficacy of their approach for treating CAPD.

Efficacy of Our Comprehensive Management Approach

Although the results of controlled clinical trials are not yet available to evaluate the efficacy of all components of the comprehensive management approach presented in Chapters 8 and 9, the limited data reviewed in the preceding section suggest the efficacy of many of our component strategies and techniques. Moreover, our approach is theoretically based and consistent with our knowledge of brain function. (The reader is referred to Chapter 2 for a review of this information.) As delineated below (see Theoretical Foundation), our management approach builds on our understanding of brain function, particularly concepts of brain plasticity, sensory integration/summation, and long-term potentiation, and is framed around the clinical implications of systems theory and information processing theory. Presenting both the theoretical foundation as well as the strategies and techniques comprising our intervention program should allow other researchers and clinicians to join us in assessing the efficacy of our approach. Data revealing treatment outcomes will either substantiate the efficacy of our approach or lead to a revised formulation of our theoretical model and intervention strategies.

COLLABORATION

As emphasized by Rumbaugh and Washburn (1996), optimizing brain plasticity in support of change requires that stimulation be integrated into one's everyday activities and lifestyle. Collaboration among professionals, clients, and families facilitates this integration.

Collaboration involves mutual deliberation in which participants collectively establish or clarify goals and values for the purpose of problem solving (Chermak, 1993). Engaging clients, families, and other professionals as collaborators maximizes problem resolution and successful therapeutic outcomes (Coufal, Hixson, & Stick, 1990; Crais, 1991, Luterman, 1990). The potential adverse impact of CAPD on language, academic performance, and employment underscores the importance of collaboration. As discussed in Chapter 9, the involvement of teachers is crucial to implementing classroom signal enhancement strategies and instructional modifications designed to improve spoken language understanding and academic achievement.

Collaborative consultation should lead to improved diagnostic and treatment strategies, more practical goals for intervention, and increased probability of successfully implementing diagnostic and treatment strategies (Coufal et al., 1991; Crais, 1991). Conversely, failure to involve other relevant professionals and families in planning, decision-making, and program implementation may lead to ineffective intervention (Anderson & Fenichel, 1989; Correa, 1989). Given family involvement in developing goals and designing strategies, and their subsequent motivation to implement treatment activities in the home and other natural environments, collaboration should maximize the transfer of skills (i.e., generalization) from treatment to daily routines (Crais, 1991). (Specific generalization strategies that depend on collaboration are described below.) Because collaboration promotes the client's self-efficacy by emphasizing an active approach to problem solving and encouraging self-regulation, it is a particularly valuable component of the comprehensive management approach delineated in Chapters 8 and 9.

Collaboration Between Audiologists and Speech-Language Pathologists

As discussed in previous chapters, the diagnosis of CAPD is made on the basis of performance deficits demonstrated on valid tests of central auditory processing. Typically, audiologists are responsible for administering and interpreting the audiologic tests and procedures that lead to the CAPD diagnosis; however, other measures, particularly, speech-language measures, provide needed information about language ability and communicative function, which not only assist in the differential diagnosis of CAPD, but also illuminate functional deficits requiring remediation (ASHA, 1996).

The audiologist and the speech-language pathologist each assume a lead effort in implementing one of the two broad and complementary approaches comprising intervention for CAPD (see Chapters 8 and 9). Typically, the audiologist leads the effort to improve signal quality by enhancing the acoustic signal and improving the listening environment. The speech-language pathologist usually leads in enhancing the scope and use of language and other central resources. Confirming the essential role served by speech-language pathologists in both assessment and intervention for CAPD, children and adults suspected of CAPD are often referred first to a speech-language pathologist because of suspected deficits in language-related skills.

Collaboration With Culturally Diverse Families

Collaborative consultation is especially important when working with culturally diverse families. Cultural and language differences may render collaboration more difficult; however, these are the very differences that underscore the importance of collaboration with culturally diverse families (Chermak, 1993). Intensifying the professional's challenge is the additional cultural and linguistic diversity seen among families of similar heritage due to intercultural contact in a multicultural society (N. Anderson, 1991). Nonetheless, sensitive consideration of cultural differences allows clinicians to build partnerships that are both consistent with cultural paradigms and appropriate to the treatment needs of the client. For example, based on their culture's profound respect for teachers and school personnel (Cheng, 1987), Asian families may be less inclined to collaborate, which they might consider as interfering with the educational process. While acknowledging and working to maintain the family's confidence and respect, the clinician might consider gradually providing opportunities to defer to the family, such as, for example, by requesting family input in selecting culturally relevant therapy materials, identifying motivating reinforcers, and designing homework assignments to promote generalization. (See also Considerations for Linguistically and Culturally Diverse Populations for further discussion of cultural values and communication patterns in promoting collaborative partnerships.)

GENERALIZATION

Generalization of newly learned skills and strategies beyond the treatment setting remains a serious concern among speech-language pathologists and audiologists (McReynolds, 1989). Demonstrating generalization of skills and strategies to situations and in contexts not employed during treatment is requisite to documenting change in function and treatment efficacy (Olswang & Bain, 1994).

Frequently, generalization does not occur easily. Failure to generalize may reflect metacognitive deficits and/or limitations of the treatment program (Borkowski, Johnston, & Reid, 1987; McReynolds, 1989). As argued by Borkowski, Estrada, Milstead, and Hale (1989), generalization of even ingrained strategy-specific knowledge to new stimuli and novel situations requires intact executive processing to guide selection and monitoring of strategies. Further, to achieve generalization, specific strategy knowledge and executive processes must be coupled with appropriate attributional beliefs of the likelihood of success (Borkowski et al., 1989). Indeed, the metacognitive emphasis of our comprehensive management approach builds on this understanding by incorporating a number of generalization strategies.

Generalization Strategies

Generalization strategies can be categorized as within-training strategies and environmental support strategies (Guevremont, 1990). As specified by Guevremont (1990), six within-training strategies may be implemented during the course of therapy to promote generalization: "(1) increasing training length; (2) using real-life scenarios and training vignettes; (3) using multiple exemplars and diverse training experiences; (4) incorporating self-monitoring homework exercises; (5) focusing on relevant and pivotal skills; and (6) having booster sessions" (p. 565).

Extending the course of therapy allows for repetition, increased practice, and rehearsal and should promote mastery of skills and automaticity of function. Role-playing and simulation provide opportunities to practice skills in contexts that are meaningful and relevant to the client. Such activities also serve to reduce the differences between the treatment and natural environments, a strategy that has been identified as important to generalization (Stokes & Baer, 1977). Training that allows the client to explore the use of the new skill to be mastered in multiple and diverse contexts expands the client's focus and is among the practices most often suggested to promote generalization of skills (Griffiths & Craighead, 1972; McReynolds, 1989; Murdock, Garcia, & Hardman, 1977; Rumbaugh & Washburn, 1996). Training in diverse contexts, with focus on multiple treatment settings and naturalistic settings including the home, school, and work place, also underscores the importance of collaboration among professionals and families. The clients' active involvement in the therapy process through self-monitoring and ultimately self-regulation forces them to actively consider the use of a particular skill or strategy and is of great value in promoting generalization of behaviors (Guevremont, 1990; Koegel, Koegel, & Ingham, 1986). *Booster* sessions ensure the maintenance of skills over time (Guevremont, 1990). Other suggestions to promote generalization include using functional language to enhance the relevance of therapy activities, gradually increasing task difficulty to force the allocation of resources to the task, and emphasizing induction learning (Connell, 1988, 1989; Washburn, 1993), a particularly effective strategy which we incorporated in our management approach.

Environmental support strategies extend reinforcement for skills learned in the treatment setting to the natural environment and depend on collaboration among professionals and families for successful implementation (Guevremont, 1990). Rules, skills, and strategies learned in the treatment setting must be made salient. Further, contingencies supporting the use of these skills and strategies must be established in the home, school, and/or work place. In addition, the client should be encouraged to seek appropriate reinforcement from peers and authority figures by alerting those individuals when an appropriate strategy is being used, especially when its use results in success (Guevremont, 1990).

FEEDBACK

Although speech-language pathologists and audiologists regularly use reinforcement for mastery and maintenance of skills, less attention has been directed to augmenting the effectiveness of verbal reinforcement via feedback. Since feedback may reinforce as well as instruct, it is important to consider carefully the wording and message conveyed by feedback statements.

Strong feedback is both positive and corrective. Effective feedback statements recognize effort and convey specific suggestions for improvement (Brophy, 1981). Moreover, feedback regarding the value of a strategy yields positive effects on strategy use and generalization (Ellis, Lenz, & Sabornie, 1987; Kennedy & Miller, 1976; Lenz, 1984; Ringel & Springer, 1980). Feedback need not avoid mention of errors. In fact, specific suggestions concerning how one might avoid particular errors further strengthens feedback (Ellis & Friend, 1991).

Feedback should focus on the effectiveness of behaviors, rather than incorporating simple qualitative descriptors such as *good* and *not good*. For example, explaining to an adolescent client that he or she effectively deployed the contextual vocabulary building strategy by examining the words surrounding the unknown target word would be more useful to that client than a simple declaration that his or her behavior was good, or even that his or her behavior was a good use of the contextual vocabulary building strategy.

Communicating with younger clients also requires that words be chosen carefully. Using concrete vocabulary that draws analogies to performance areas in which the client may already experience success (e.g., athletics) may make the feedback more relevant and effective. For instance, asking children to *stretch the muscles of their ears to work harder* to implore exertion of greater listening effort may resonate with the child and elicit the desired response.

Feedback Promotes Metacognitive Control

Feedback serves an important function in promoting executive control; however, it will be most effective when clients understand how their performance is measured. Understanding how performance is assessed enables clients to understand how they must perform and how close they are to the performance criterion. With adolescents and adult clients, the impact of feedback can be augmented by involving them in establishing the goals and the mastery criteria, as well as in tracking their progress toward criterion performance (Ellis & Friend, 1991). Engaging clients in self-monitoring and recording their performance using charts, logs, or other devices is probably more reinforcing than providing extrinsic rewards (e.g., tokens, points, or prizes) (Ellis & Friend, 1991). Self-monitoring renders feedback more effective and develops executive control. Similarly, giving clients an opportunity to elaborate on the clinician's feedback, explaining the shortcomings of their strategies and steps that might be taken to improve their performance, also strengthens feedback, motivates clients, and promotes self-regulation (Adelman & Taylor, 1983; Ellis & Friend, 1991; Pressley, Johnson, & Symons, 1987). Reviewing the clinician's feedback and the client's elaboration prior to the next attempt increases the likelihood that performance of the task will incorporate the appropriate strategies and techniques (Lenz, 1984).

As the client demonstrates greater skill level, the clinician should shift more responsibility for monitoring and adjusting behavior to the client, moving away from directive feedback statements and toward feedback that is more mediative (Ellis & Friend, 1991). Such mediative feedback provides cues to help clients discover and elaborate their own strategies and solutions rather than providing them directly to the client (Ellis & Friend, 1991; Ellis, Lenz, & Sabornie, 1987; Stone & Wertsch, 1984). Again, encouraging clients to monitor and track their progress through maintenance of a diary or log of reflections on strategy successes and failures increases the effectiveness of mediative feedback and promotes executive control. Moreover, encouraging clients to re-establish goals on the basis of feedback strengthens motivation.

Goal Structures

Confidence, task persistence, and motivation can be influenced by the ways in which goals are structured. An impression that failure is an indication of inability, rather than a signal to work harder and more strategically, adversely impacts an individual's motivational level. Attention to goal structuring, or the degree to which individual quality is judged against the performance of others versus judged against one's own past performance (Licht & Kistner, 1986), can alter this impression and is of particular relevance to the classroom.

Of the three distinct goal stuctures—competitive, individualistic, and cooperative (Ames & Ames, 1984)—two are more likely to better serve the student with CAPD. In the competitive structure, the performance of other students serves as the yardstick against which the quality of a particular student's work is judged. Under this structure, the likelihood that a student will succeed and receive praise or other reinforcement is inversely related to the successes of peers. In contrast, in the cooperative structure a group of students works together toward a common goal. The likelihood that a particular student will succeed in a cooperatively structured environment is positively related to the successes of the group members. In the individualistic structure, each student's performance is judged individually such that one student's success is unrelated to the successes of other students.

Given their processing deficits and frequently associated language and academic problems, most students with CAPD will function more successfully under an individualistic structure than a competitive structure, the latter inevitably drawing attention to individual differences in ability and contributions. Individualistic structures allow students with CAPD to focus on their efforts and their resulting achievements. Individualistic structures are most effective when meaningful reinforcement is provided contingent on relative improvement, rather than absolute level of performance (Brophy, 1983).

The cooperative structure may be effective for some students with CAPD, but there are potential difficulties. Since a cooperative goal structure sets a uniform performance criterion for all cooperating group members, it may be as frustrating for the student with CAPD as is the competitive structure. Cooperative goal structures may be employed successfully, however, as long as steps are taken to decrease the salience of individual differences in ability (Ames & Felker, 1979) which cause frustration and low motivation. Most important, feedback and reinforcement should be assigned to each member of the group on the basis of individual contribution and achievement rather than providing feedback to all members of the group on the basis of one group product (Slavin, 1983).

CONSIDERATIONS FOR LINGUISTICALLY AND CULTURALLY DIVERSE POPULATIONS

Over 25% of the U.S. population is non-white (U.S. Department of Commerce, 1991). Presently, an estimated 6 million U.S. citizens of minority heritage have communication disorders (Battle, 1993). The number of persons of minority heritage, as well as the proportion of minorities in the U.S. population, continues to grow rapidly. Projections based on the 1990 U.S. Census suggest that, by the year 2010, one in three Americans will be a person of color, with children from culturally and linguistically diverse groups representing perhaps as many as 65% of school-age children (Battle, 1993; Screen & Anderson, 1994; U.S. Bureau of the Census, 1990). Given these projections for minority population growth, it is clear professionals must be prepared to deliver clinical services to a culturally diverse caseload.

Notwithstanding diversity within a cultural group, reflecting degree of assimilation, mixing of traditional and mainstream values, and individual choices, a general set of values and attitudes seems to characterize groups of people who share a common identity (Helman, 1984; Seligman & Darling, 1990). Professionals have an obligation to gain an appreciation of cultural differences that influence clients' and families' needs, expectations, and opportunities to benefit from professional services; as emphasized by Taylor (1986), the very parameters defining a communication disorder are greatly influenced by one's culture. Indeed, some cultural groups do not believe in intervention for communication disorders (Taylor, 1986). Other groups, while valuing intervention, evidence other cultural values that present implications for the clinical process. For example, in contrast to other groups that may eschew silence, many Native Americans value silence as an integral component of communication (Swinomish Tribal Mental Health Project, 1991; Wilson, 1983). Their interactional style often involves more extended pauses between turn-taking in conversational exchanges, as well as before answering questions (Farkas, 1986; Saville-Troike, 1989). These timing differences might render sound blending programs which require rapid responding to targets (e.g., Phonemic Synthesis program, Katz & Harmon, 1982) more difficult, and, perhaps, inappropriate for Native Americans demonstrating this interactional style. Clearly, to maximize successful outcomes of clinical services, we must become familiar with other cultures' values and traditions, sensitive to linguistic and communication differences across cultures, and employ nonbiased assessment and intervention strategies.

Prevalence

Racial and ethnic differences in the prevalence of auditory dysfunction associated with developmental and acquired diseases and disorders have been reported (Buchanan, Moore, & Counter, 1993; Bush & Rabin, 1980; Forman-Franco, Karayalin, Mandel, & Abramson, 1982; Friedman, Luban, Herer, & Williams, 1980; McShane, 1982; Nuru, 1993; Royster, Royster, & Thomas, 1980; Scott, 1986; Sharp &

Orchik, 1978; Stewart, 1986); however, no systematic investigation of the prevalence of CAPD across racial or ethnic groups has been undertaken (Buchanan et al., 1993). The relationship between CAPD and a history of chronic otitis media (Adesman, Altshuler, Lipkin, & Walco, 1990; Brown, 1994; Gravel & Wallace, 1992; Jerger, Jerger, Alford, & Abrams, 1983; Moore et al., 1991; Silva et al., 1986), combined with the disproportionately high incidence of otitis media among Native American populations (Brody, Overfield, & McAlister, 1965; Cole & Anderson, 1985; Goodwin, Shaw, & Feldman, 1980; McShane, 1982; Nuru, 1993; Stewart, 1986, 1990a, 1990b), suggests that the prevalence of CAPD among Native Americans may be higher than seen in the general population. Similarly, reports of CAPD in conjunction with sickle cell anemia, noise-induced hearing loss, and fetal alcohol syndrome, conditions known to vary in prevalence across racial groups (Buchanan et al., 1993; Bush & Rabin, 1980; Carney & Chermak, 1991; Forman-Franco et al., 1982; Friedman et al., 1980; Gould et al., 1991; McShane, 1982; Morest, 1982; Nuru, 1993; Royster et al., 1980; Salvi, Powers, Saunders, Boettcher, & Clock, 1992; Scott, 1986; Sharp & Orchik, 1978; Willott & Lu, 1982) underscore the importance of determining whether the prevalence of CAPD varies as a function of race or ethnicity.

Cross-Cultural Communication

The clinical process must be guided by mutual respect. Communicating an understanding of, and respect for, cultural differences establishes the foundation for mutual trust among clinicians, clients, and families. Building this relationship begins during the first meeting between clinician and client and is influenced by interpersonal style and communication.

Knowledge of basic cross-cultural communication styles and differences is the key to communicating effectively with culturally diverse families. Differences in both verbal and nonverbal aspects of communication can be confusing and if misunderstood can create tension and jeopardize our best clinical efforts (Payne, 1986). Beyond the obvious obstacles created by native language differences and the difficulties language differences create if not bridged, there are expectations surrounding appropriate topics for discussion between professionals and clients and how communication is conducted. For instance, the same quantity of information presented during a verbal exchange may be seen as excessive in some cultures but thorough in others (Yacobacci-Tam, 1987). Similarly, personal questions considered necessary and relevant by the clinician and raised early in the relationship may be perceived as intrusive and invasive by some cultural groups (Payne, 1986; Yacobacci-Tam, 1987). In nonverbal communication, cultural differences exist as to proper distance between communication partners, appropriate eye contact, dress, posture, and use of gestures (Payne, 1986; Sue & Sue, 1990; Yacobacci-Tam, 1987). For example, visual interaction schedules vary across ethnic groups. In contrast to Anglo-Americans who consider direct eye contact a sign of attentiveness and respect, direct eye contact is considered disrespectful by some Hispanic Americans (Payne, 1986).

Prevention, Assessment, and Intervention

Minority populations present greater incidence and prevalence of many known or presumed risk factors for CAPD (e.g., chronic otitis media, prematurity, low birthweight, alcohol and other drug abuse) (Terrell, 1993). With improved access to health care and education, some of these risk factors can be reduced (Canterbury, 1990).

Assessment must be conducted in a culturally and linguistically nonbiased fashion, ensuring that formal and informal instruments and test procedures and interpersonal interactions are appropriate to the client (Taylor & Payne, 1983). Because few central auditory tests involving speech have been translated from English or developed in other languages, assessing central auditory processing skills apart from language skills in non-English and limited-English proficient speakers requires the administration of a test battery that relies on tonal or other nonverbal stimuli (e.g., frequency and duration patterns, evoked potentials) (Musiek & Chermak, 1994).

As discussed previously, understanding differences in cultural values and behaviors is vital to crafting intervention programs that will best meet the client's needs. Knowledge of communication patterns, child-rearing practices, life styles, attitudes and beliefs about disability, attitudes toward the rehabilitation process, and general health practices should inform the clinical process, culminating in intervention programming that incorporates the best professional practices while meeting with the greatest support and involvement from the client and family (Cole, 1989; Gajar, 1985; Taylor & Payne, 1983).

Also crucial is an understanding of learning style and communication style differences, which vary across individuals and may characterize particular cultural groups (Anderson, 1988; Saville-Troike, 1986). By incorporating preferred learning styles in designing intervention, we maximize opportunities for clients to benefit from the therapeutic process (Anderson, 1991; Clark, 1967; Harris, 1993; Nellum-Davis, 1993; Terrell & Hale, 1992). For example, a preference for a visual learning style exhibited by many Native American children (Harris, 1993) can be used to their advantage in compensating for CAPD. In some instances, however, aspects of a traditional communication style may not coincide with the treatment approach considered optimal by the clinician. The tendency to avoid direct eye contact during communication by some Hispanic Americans would present a special challenge to the clinician, given the importance of visual cues and auditory and visual summation for improving spoken language understanding in individuals with CAPD (see Chapter 9). In such cases, the clinician should acknowledge the traditional communication style, while explaining the importance of incorporating visual cues through direct eye contact. (The reader is referred to Keefe [1987] for an introduction to the theory and applications of learning style.)

Summary

Building collaborative partnerships with families whose culture differs from the clinician's increases prospects for successful intervention. A range of cultural norms and situational variables shape clients and their families (Battle, 1993; Cole, 1989; Taylor, 1986; Taylor & Payne, 1983; Yacobacci-Tam, 1987). Clinicians must be sufficiently flexible in response to cultural differences to ensure effective clinical services. They must deliver services appropriate to the client's needs, yet consistent with the client's cultural paradigms (Chermak, 1993). Although it is imperative that professionals communicate respect for clients of diverse cultures, whose values and behaviors may differ from the clinician's, the clinician's actions must always be consistent with professional ethical standards and judgment regarding best practices.

It is not reasonable to expect that each clinician will become an expert in the values and traditions of every cultural group represented in our society; however, it is necessary for clinicians to expend the effort needed to gain greater understanding of the cultures more frequently represented in their caseloads. Readers are referred to a number of excellent resources to begin the self-education process (Battle, 1993; Pedersen & Ivey, 1993; Screen & Anderson, 1994; Sue & Sue, 1990; Taylor, 1986).

CUSTOMIZING INTERVENTION

Given the heterogeneity of CAPD and its occurrence across the life span in diverse clinical populations (see Chapter 1), it is necessary to ask several questions regarding the distinctiveness of intervention. First, can distinctive intervention strategies be formulated to manage CAPD within a constellation of language or cognitive deficits? Second, should management strategies differ as a function of the client's age? Third, how can we customize intervention to the specific auditory profile? The first question is answered from the perspective of differential diagnosis. The second question is considered from a life span perspective. In addressing the final question, we examine the relevance of clients' test scores to their everyday functioning.

Differential Diagnosis

To formulate distinctive intervention strategies, the relative contribution of the ostensibly concomitant auditory, language, and cognitive processing deficits to the observed spoken language comprehension deficits must be determined. Accurate differential diagnosis must precede efforts to customize therapy; however, notwithstanding careful assessment using an efficient and comprehensive test battery, the relative contributions of auditory, language, and cognitive processes to spoken language comprehension problems may remain uncertain (ASHA, 1996). As clarified by the following examples, formulation of distinctive intervention strategies is limited by our inability to assess the relative contributions of these interdependent processes to a spoken language comprehension deficit.

The fairly typical case of a child who has difficulty understanding spoken language in the presence of competing noise illustrates our dilemma. At least two explanations can be offered to account for this performance deficit. The child may lack control over language resources, which prevents him or her from using language knowledge to compensate for the degraded acoustic signal. Consider the following sentences as examples:

1. Today's stories are about Isaac's many walks through the woods. He walks among trees of different colors.
2. I want to go home.
   I walked home alone.

Notwithstanding redundant references in the first example denoting subject-verb conjugation (i.e., morphological inflection), plurality, and possession, the child with insufficient language knowledge would not be able to take advantage of this linguistic redundancy to fill in the obscured and difficult to hear high frequency "s" masked by the competing background noise. Similarly, unless the child has attained some degree of linguistic sophistication (e.g., metalinguistic and pragmatic knowledge), she or he might confuse the second pair of sentences which should be resolved easily by relying on context, despite acoustic masking. Alternatively, the child may have full command over language resources but a CAPD may cause serious difficulties in analyzing the acoustic signal, resulting in spoken language comprehension problems that cannot be overcome by even full use of language knowledge (ASHA, 1996). Unfortunately, examination of this child's ability to process nonverbal signals does not clarify the situation, as it is not known whether verbal and nonverbal perceptual tasks are equivalent and involve the same auditory processing mechanisms (ASHA, 1996). Indeed, language impairment might still explain this child's difficulty comprehending language in competing noise even if the child were to evidence auditory processing difficulties with nonverbal signals.

Similarly, it is often difficult to determine the relative contribution of cognitive, linguistic, and auditory processing deficits for the language comprehension problems experienced by an adult with cognitive/linguistic disorders (e.g., aphasia) (ASHA, 1996). In fact, it is likely that spoken language comprehension problems in aphasia result from some combination of processing deficits.

Although professionals may disagree whether these cases reflect language disorders, CAPD, or both disorders, it is clear that intervention must be directed toward improving the individual's functional abilities in appropriate contexts. As concluded by the ASHA Consensus Task Force,

> Regardless of the nature of the processing deficit, most persons who have difficulty with the comprehension of spoken language will profit both from procedures that enhance the acoustic signal and from procedures that increase the scope and control of central resources, particularly language resources. . . . Given our current understanding of language disorders and of central auditory processing, techniques that facilitate language competence are likely to improve the auditory processing of language and vice versa (ASHA, 1996, p. 48).

Life Span Considerations

Difficulty understanding spoken language in adverse listening conditions, especially when there is reverberation and the competing signal is speech, is common to younger individuals with CAPD, as well as older adults with presumed central auditory changes (Bornstein & Musiek, 1992; Chermak, Vonhof, & Bendel, 1989; Duquesnoy & Plomp, 1980; Harris & Reitz, 1985; Jerger, 1992; Jerger, Johnson, & Loiselle, 1988; Lasky & Tobin, 1973; Nabelek & Nabelek, 1994; Nabelek & Robinson,

1982; Olsen, Noffsinger, & Kurdzeil, 1975; Prosser, Turrini, & Arslan, 1991). However, like the questions raised regarding the linkage between CAPD and language disorders in children (see Chapter 1), the role of age-related peripheral versus central auditory changes, as well cognitive factors, in causing spoken language understanding difficulties among older adults is somewhat controversial (CHABA Working Group on Speech Understanding and Aging, 1988; Humes, 1996). Although CAPD is prevalent among older adults (Stach et al., 1990) and deficits in central auditory processing have been observed in older adults with normal peripheral hearing and intact cognitive and linguistic abilities (Pichora-Fuller & Schneider, 1991; Rodriquez, DiSarno, & Hardiman, 1990), questions persist regarding whether difficulties understanding spoken language may be explained by age-related peripheral auditory changes and/or age-related decline in cognitive abilities (e.g., working memory, speed of processing). Notwithstanding reports to the contrary (Cohen, 1987; Humes & Christopherson, 1991; Humes & Roberts, 1990; Humes, Watson, Christensen, Cokely, Halling, & Lee, 1994; Lee & Humes, 1992; Marshall, 1981), a significant body of research indicates that age-related decline in spoken language understanding cannot be explained on the basis of peripheral hearing loss or cognitive decline alone (Chmiel & Jerger, 1996; Fitzgibbons & Gordon-Salant, 1996; Grose, 1996; Jerger, 1992; Jerger, Jerger, Oliver, & Pirozzolo, 1989; Jerger, Jerger, & Pirozzolo, 1991; Jerger, Stach, Pruitt, Harper, & Kirby, 1989). Nonetheless individual differences are expected, given the normal variation in brain organization and age-related change across individuals coupled with the variable manifestations of central auditory pathologies (Phillips, 1995). Hence, the sources of CAPD, as well as the effects of central auditory pathologies, are likely to vary across individuals (ASHA, 1996; Phillips, 1995). Therefore, group data implicating or excluding nonperipheral auditory and extra-auditory factors as sources of spoken language understanding difficulties among older adults cannot be used to explain the performance of any one individual. Only comprehensive assessment can determine the ultimate role of these factors in explaining the spoken language difficulties experienced by that individual.

Brain Plasticity, Task Demands, and Central Resources

Beyond individual differences within a cohort, age is one of the most significant sources of individual variability. As discussed in the last section of this chapter (also see Chapter 2), the slow but sustained loss of neurons that begins in adolescence and continues throughout the aging process coupled with some reduction in brain plasticity associated with aging (Kolb, 1995) render neural reorganization and recovery of function following injury or disease less likely in older adults. Indeed, the neural reorganization that occurs (e.g., tonotopic reorganization of frequency maps) may actually *cause* perceptual difficulties for some older adults (Willott, 1996). In contrast, young children may benefit from a great degree of brain plasticity; however, they do not present the wealth of language and world knowledge or the metacognitive knowledge that can mitigate the impact of CAPD.

Moreover, the relative importance of the variety of developmental, situational, environmental, social, and economic factors influencing an individual at various periods throughout life is dynamic, as are the individual's responses to these variables. Children experience increasing and more complex central auditory processing demands as they face more intellectually and linguistically challenging academic and social demands. The central auditory processing demands facing a retired person will differ from the demands facing the ambitious professional just entering the career track. The manifestation of CAPD may vary significantly across the life span as the individual develops and implements compensatory strategies and meets other life challenges, including educational, employment, and family obligations. For some youngsters with CAPD, symptoms attenuate to some degree during late adolescence and adulthood, although for others the full impact of the processing deficit persists.

Implications for Management

In response to whether management strategies should differ as a function of the client's age, we conclude that the reduction in brain plasticity associated with aging necessitates modification of management strategies. It is appropriate to consider management decisions from a life span perspective given the variation in brain malleability, knowledge and skill bases, and continual maturation and growth of the individual within a variety of contexts with divergent demands. Differences in the physiological changes underlying the observed CAPD, degree of inherent neural plasticity, and the prospects for spontaneous or stimulus-induced recovery vary as a function of age. The diminishing plasticity of the older nervous system implies that management strategies in adults and older adults be directed toward compensation rather than recovery of function (ASHA, 1996). However, spontaneous and/or stimulus-induced recovery of function following acute brain injury may suggest a role for remedial approaches as well. Given the inherent neural plasticity of the developing central nervous system, remedial approaches with children should target acquisition or recovery of function; however, compensatory strategies also may prove useful during the period of recovery from neural insult while (re)learning occurs and when recovery is not achieved (ASHA, 1996). Focusing on auditory skills and acoustic signal enhancement, as well as the scope and control of cognitive and language resources, should prove especially beneficial for children whose language comprehension problems may stem from several sources.

Although many of the strategies and techniques described in Chapters 8 and 9 are likely to benefit the great majority of clients with CAPD, specific emphases will vary depending on the nature of the processing deficits identified, the functional consequences of these deficits, the presence of comorbid conditions, and the client's age. At the same time, opportunities to infuse other management strategies developed to address auditory processing deficits for particular client populations (e.g., aphasia, ADHD) should not be overlooked. Common principles guiding intervention across clinical populations include an emphasis on collaboration, self-regulation, and an ecological- and strategy-based orientation. With children, management efforts should be integrated with the academic curriculum.

Customizing Intervention to the Auditory Profile

As our understanding of CAPD increases, it becomes possible to subtype clusters of clients presenting similar symptomatology and formulate treatment programs with emphases directed to those clusters. Consider, for example, the difference in management emphases for individuals diagnosed with CAPD who present similar auditory performance decrements with competing signals, but dissimilar temporal processing abilities. Both individuals would probably benefit from therapy focused on signal enhancement strategies (e.g., FM technology and preferential seating) and linguistic strategies that emphasize use of context to resolve messages. The individual experiencing temporal processing difficulties, however, might also benefit from some attention directed toward the use of prosody to predict degraded messages and recommendations that partners speak more slowly, pause more often, and emphasize key words. Similarly, emphasis directed toward augmenting closure skills would also be particularly appropriate for individuals presenting difficulty resolving degraded acoustic signals (e.g., filtered, reverberant, or compressed speech).

Relationship Between Test Scores and Intervention

Although positive neurologic findings are common in adults diagnosed with CAPD, positive neurologic findings are infrequent in children diagnosed with CAPD (Musiek, Gollegly, & Ross, 1985). The primary goal of central auditory testing with adults is to determine the integrity of the central auditory nervous system. In contrast, given the usually unremarkable neurologic findings in children with CAPD, the ultimate goals of pediatric central auditory testing typically are to ascertain the neuormaturational status of the central auditory nervous system and to quantify functional deficits (i.e., communication, academic, and social) to determine appropriate management strategies (Chermak, 1996; Keith, 1981a, 1981c, 1983; Musiek, Gollegly, & Baran, 1984). These different assessment objectives necessitate some variation in formulating an assessment test battery (Musiek & Chermak, 1994, 1995). In either case, however, assessment data should inform management planning and provide a framework for counseling.

Clearly, assessment data should be used to guide intervention planning. Although remedial programs cannot be designed on the basis of test results alone, understanding the processes underlying successful task performance helps to bridge the gap between data collection and management strategies and techniques (Chermak & Musiek, 1992). Even information gathered from checklists and questionnaires used to identify children at-risk for CAPD can provide insights regarding functional deficits and areas of concern relevant to remedial program planning (ASHA, 1996; Fisher, 1976; Smoski, Brunt, & Tannahill, 1992). As discussed below, however, the practical relevance of data to intervention programming varies considerably across tests.

Task Relevance to Everyday Analogs

Notwithstanding the value of test data to guide intervention, particular tests of comparable efficiency may be preferred for differential diagnosis and monitoring of disease progression or recovery; other tests may be judged more useful in revealing functional deficits and informing intervention (Musiek & Chermak, 1994). We illustrate this point and answer the third question we posed earlier, on customizing intervention to the auditory profile, by comparing the different roles served by masking level differences, speech recognition in competing speech, and the frequency pattern test.

A comparison of masking level differences and tests involving competing message tasks illustrates the relative value of different tests for different purposes. Although each measure provides useful diagnostic insight regarding site or level of dysfunction, the abstract nature of the masking level difference paradigm and the absence of an everyday listening analog renders masking level differences less useful for counseling and management. By contrast, tests involving competing messages reflect everyday functional performance. Reduced performance on these tests would suggest therapy targeting selective or divided attention. Therefore, outcomes of competing message tasks provide more specific direction for auditory and educational management and may also benefit the counseling process by illustrating the impact of CAPD for everyday listening (Chermak, 1996; Musiek & Chermak, 1995).

The frequency pattern test provides another example of a central auditory test that not only informs diagnosis but offers specific direction for intervention. Successful performance on this test is dependent on several auditory and related processes including: pitch discrimination and sequencing (temporal processing), contour (pattern) recognition, linguistic labeling, working memory, and interhemispheric transfer (Musiek & Chermak, 1995; Musiek, Pinheiro, & Wilson, 1980). Since perception of prosody may suffer if temporal processing and acoustic contour recognition are problematic (Blumstein & Cooper, 1974), depressed performance on the frequency pattern test may signal remediation efforts directed toward rhythm recognition and discrimination. (The reader is referred to the Segmentation and Auditory Discrimination, and Prosody sections in Chapter 8 for specific techniques.) Attempts to improve interhemispheric processing may be centered on exercises that require verbal identification of similarly shaped objects which are held in the left hand and recognized through tactile sensation in the absence of visual cues (Musiek & Chermak, 1995). Describing a picture while drawing it also invokes interhemispheric processing and is enjoyable for children who like to draw. Linguistic labeling and sequencing may be targeted through practice in recognizing melodic Morse code and in discriminating temporally similar sound and speech elements (Musiek & Chermak, 1995). (See Auditory Training in Chapter 8 for additional activities promoting interhemispheric processing.)

THEORETICAL FOUNDATION

Systems theory, information processing theory, and concepts from cognitive neuroscience form the cornerstones of our comprehensive management approach. This foundation supports aggressive intervention that is collaborative and ecological or context-based. Viewing listening within an information processing perspective leads to a management approach that emphasizes metacognition. Self-regulation of skills and strategies, both elemental auditory processing skills and higher order linguistic and cognitive skills and strategies, distinguishes the approach. Acoustic signal enhancement aids auditory processing and is considered fundamental to management efforts.

Cognitive Neuroscience

Recent developments in cognitive neuroscience are discussed in great detail in Chapter 2. This brief presentation simply highlights the concepts that directly underlie the clinical practices advocated.

Recent research suggests that the central nervous system is plastic for some time prior to stabilization of neural function (Aoki & Siekevitz, 1988). Although brain plasticity may be greatest and most obvious during development, accumulating data suggest that the brain remains malleable throughout the life span. Plasticity extends to mature nervous systems: significant neural reorganization can occur in response to injury or learning across the life span (Edeline & Weinberger, 1991; Irvine, Rajan, & Robertson, 1992; Kolb, 1995; Moore, 1993; Singer, 1995). In fact, plasticity may account for the maintenance of cognitive control across many decades despite the slow but sustained loss of neurons seen beginning in adolescence and continuing throughout the aging process (Kolb, 1995). (See Efficacy Research in this chapter for related discussion of cortical reorganization.)

Long-term potentiation, the long-lasting increase in synaptic transmission induced by intense synaptic activity (Brown et al., 1988) may be the physiological mechanism underlying a variety of plastic processes in the nervous system (Pascual-Leone, Grafman, & Hallett, 1994; Schuman & Madison, 1994). Studies of long-term potentiation suggest significant opportunity to induce cognitive change through stimulation (Gustafsson & Wigstrom, 1988). Indeed, stimulation enables plasticity and may extend sensitive periods, thereby maximizing potential for successful rehabilitative efforts (Hassmannova, Myslivecek, & Novakova, 1981). Activity-dependent plasticity is thought to underlie learning and memory as the brain changes in response to use and the needs and experiences of the individual (Elbert, Pantev, Wienbruch, Rockstroh, & Taub, 1995; Weinberger & Diamond, 1987). It appears the brain remaps or reorganizes itself to best meet the auditory processing demands (Moore, 1993; Recanzone et al., 1993; Robertson & Irvine, 1989; Willott et al., 1993). Documenting a remarkable example of auditory system plasticity, Allen, Cranford, and Pay (1996) reported normal central auditory processing in an adult with congenital absence of the left temporal lobe.

Hence, plasticity enables the central nervous system to accommodate and offers speech-language pathologists and audiologists the opportunity to improve central auditory processing (Chermak & Musiek, 1992; Musiek, Lenz, & Gollegly, 1991). However, because plasticity is dependent on activity and stimulation, neural plasticity affords opportunity for functional change only insofar as intervention is initiated in a timely manner (Aoki & Siekevitz, 1988; Bolshakov & Siegelbaum, 1995; Hassmannova et al., 1981). Intervention efforts should be aggressive and implemented as early as possible following either confirmed diagnosis or the time the individual, particularly the child, is identified as at-risk for CAPD. Since the absolute time course of the critical or sensitive periods prior to which time neural function begins to stabilize has not yet been established and may extend into adulthood (Merzenich et al., 1984), intervention efforts should never be seen as too late. Conversely, the finite course of critical periods underscores the imperative for early and comprehensive intervention (Chermak & Musiek, 1992).

Bold and aggressive management must be undertaken knowing that neuromaturational development and neural plasticity depend on stimulation. Presenting stimulation in an organized manner that progressively challenges the client with the proper gradation of difficulty level, as well as integrating that stimulation into everyday activities, facilitates change (Rumbaugh & Washburn, 1996). As noted previously, collaboration among professionals, clients, and families fosters this integration. Because the remapping of the brain underlying improvements in auditory function probably requires some as yet unknown period of time that most likely varies widely among individuals and as a function of task demands, the clinician must demonstrate patience and counsel the client similarly, giving the intervention program ample opportunity to activitate the neural processes of plasticity that will lead to change. Indeed, intensive training may accelerate the remapping/relearning process (Merzenich et al., 1996; Tallal et al., 1996). Clearly, our inability to quantify the requisite time period for remapping complicates clinical decisions to maintain or modify a particular therapeutic course based on progress to date.

Systems Theory

Emerging in the 1950s and 1960s in engineering science and computing technology disciplines, the study of systems as entities rather than a conglomeration of parts has received broad application across disciplines, including recent attention in the social sciences, education, and health and rehabilitation sciences (Bartoli & Botel, 1988;

Damico, Augustine, & Hayes, 1996; Duranti & Goodwin, 1990; Weaver, 1993). Systems theory rejects: sequential, linear, cause-and-effect reasoning; dualistic tendencies to separate the knower from the known, the observer from the observed, cognition from motivation, perceptions, and affect; and reductionist views that the whole can be understood from the properties of isolated parts. Rather, systems theory suggests a broad view of *wholeness,* which provides a conceptual framework for understanding the organization, interaction, and dynamicity of elements comprising systems (von Bertalanffy, 1968). A systems perspective considers an individual as a system of interacting cognitive, affective, and physiological subsystems. Environmental events are seen as directly impacting the individual's function. In effect, an individual's behavior is seen as the culmination of numerous transactional interactions between the individual and his or her context (i.e., environment, culture, society).

The face validity of the systems perspective is immediately apparent in considering attention, the most basic level of interaction a person has with the environment. If one understands attention to refer to a conditional relationship between an individual's behavior and the environment, it becomes obvious that the cognitive underpinnings of behavior are contextually dependent (Barkley, 1996). Notwithstanding the neurophysiologic basis of CAPD, we recognize that environmental expectations and demands (e.g., listening to sophisticated language in a noisy classroom) exacerbate the mismatch between internal capacity and external structure and lead to communication dysfunction and academic underachievement.

Consistent with systems theory, individuals are seen as parts of larger social systems, including the family, school, workplace, and community. In contrast to a medical model in which behavioral problems are attributed solely to the neurobiological problems of the individual, a systems approach fosters a broader perspective in which factors external to the individual are seen as interacting with internal neurobiological predispositions and thereby contributing to behavioral deficits. In essence, behaviors are contextualized within a sociocultural context, and the complex array of variables that influence the individual's social, learning, and educational contexts are considered in both reaching diagnoses and planning intervention (Heshusius, 1989). Recent transactional models of development recognize the influence of a child's multiple environments (i.e., home, day care, community) and the interaction of these systems with the child's biological endowment (Sameroff, 1983). Development is affected by the agents in the multiple environments and those agents are influenced by the child. Intervention based on a systems perspective must include attention to interacting internal and external factors.

Systems theory supports an ecological and constructivist perspective of listening and learning. The assumptions of systems theory reinforce the importance of collaboration and empowerment for successful intervention. Systems theory suggests the inadequacy of attempting to understand disability based solely on neurobiological function. Rather, an individual's disability must be understood within a sociological context that recognizes the difficulties an individual faces in responding to the expectations and external demands of the environment (Damico et al., 1996; Weaver, 1993). These assumptions translate into clinical practices that include induction and metacognitive interventions and support treatment of both the individual and the environment (Bartoli & Botel, 1988; Gibson, 1966; Maag & Reid, 1996; Poplin, 1988a, 1988b; Weaver, 1985, 1993). Further, the systems perspective predicts variability in function across settings and within settings across time and confirms the value of employing the collaboration and generalization strategies described earlier. Auditory training and metcognitive and metalinguistic strategies described in Chapter 8 provide interventions directed toward the individual; acoustic signal enhancement and environmental manipulations described in Chapter 9 target the environment.

Information Processing

According to information processing theory, meaning is assigned to audible discourse based on the extraction of information through various processes or stages of cognition, including encoding, organizing, storing, retrieving, comparing, and generating or reconstructing information (Massaro, 1975a, 1975b, 1976). Viewed within the framework of a network processing model (see Chapter 1), these stages involve parallel and distributed operations involving interactions between sensory (e.g., auditory processes) and central processes (e.g., cognitive and linguistic processes) through feedback and feedforward loops (Rumelhart, McClelland, & The PDP Research Group, 1986; Watson & Foyle, 1985). Consistent with this model, listening comprehension involves the analysis, transformation, construction, and reconstruction of input information and requires the interaction of segmentation skills, word knowledge, general knowledge, and metacognitive knowledge. Skilled listeners, actively engaged in discovering what speakers are communicating, use various strategies to monitor their listening and extract information from the spoken message. They must organize and elaborate information and deploy executive strategies and self-regulatory processes to guide the flow of information and coordinate knowledge sources (Borkowski & Burke, 1996; Flavell, 1981; Gibson, 1966).

Conceptualized within this framework in which processes at various sensory and central levels influence information processing, CAPD resulting from specific, sensory processing deficiencies may be exacerbated by higher order (i.e., top-down) deficiencies in regulating or coordinating central auditory and cognitive and linguistic processes (ASHA, 1996; Chermak & Musiek, 1992; McNeil, 1995; Swanson, 1987). In addition to deficits in specific central auditory processes (e.g., auditory discrimination, temporal processing, performance with competing or degraded acoustic signals), individuals with CAPD may lack listening strategies or employ inappropriate strategies and fail to engage in self-monitoring behavior.

Fortunately, practice or learning can modify top-down processes (Watson & Foyle, 1985). Although recent reports suggest that central auditory processes may be remediated through intensive auditory training (Merzenich et al., 1996; Tallal et al., 1996), certain bottom-up, sensory processes may be more resistant to change (e.g., auditory discrimination in competing noise) (Katz & Wilde, 1994). Therefore, comprehensive intervention for CAPD should also include attention to metalinguistic skills (e.g., decoding, segmenting) and techniques to enhance the quality of the acoustic signal (e.g., FM technology, slower presentations, insertion of pauses, augmenting prosodic cues). Even greater success may be realized by coupling these interventions with metacognitive training directed toward coordination and deployment of appropriate strategies as needed (ASHA, 1996; Blumstein, Katz, Goodglass, Shrier, & Dworetsky, 1985; Brown, Bransford, Ferrara, & Campione, 1983; Chermak & Musiek, 1992; Ellis Weismer, & Hesketh, 1993; Harter, 1982; Katz & Harmon, 1982; Keith, 1981a; Kimelman, 1991; Lasky, Weidner, & Johnson, 1976; Meichenbaum, 1976; Reid & Hresko, 1981; Rumelhart, 1977; Ryan, Weed, & Short, 1986; Samuels, 1987; Sloan, 1986; Torgesen, 1988; Wong, 1991). A number of strategies and techniques following from the perspective of information processing theory are discussed in Chapter 8, including auditory training to improve temporal processing, auditory vigilance, and auditory discrimination; attribution retraining to enhance self-systems (i.e., self-efficacy, self-esteem, and self-regulation); cognitive behavior modification to augment use of executive strategies; and context-derived vocabulary building, schema induction, and metamemory to increase word knowledge, semantic relationships, and message comprehension.

SUMMARY

A number of topics considered fundamental to intervention were discussed, beginning with efficacy research and concluding with the theoretical foundation of our management program. Recent data have demonstrated the efficacy of temporal processing training and the potential of metacognitive training in reducing spoken language comprehension deficits; however, additional research is needed to confirm these findings. Since much of the efficacy research has been conducted with subjects with learning disabilities or language impairment, future studies should examine the efficacy of these training programs for subjects diagnosed with CAPD. Moreover, subjects should represent the multicultural populations who comprise a growing segment of our caseloads.

To best serve our culturally diverse caseloads, professionals must become familiar with other cultures' values, traditions, and communication styles and employ nonbiased assessment and intervention strategies. Knowledge of communication patterns, life styles, child-rearing practices, and attitudes and beliefs about disability and the rehabilitation process is important to designing culturally appropriate intervention that meets with the greatest support and involvement from the client and family. By strengthening collaboration, we increase the probability of successful intervention, including the generalization of strategies and skills from treatment to daily activities.

Indeed, the heterogeneous and complex functional deficits associated with CAPD demand the collaborative efforts of speech-language pathologists and audiologists for both diagnosis and intervention. Although it is often difficult to assess the relative contributions of auditory, linguistic, and cognitive processes to deficits in spoken language comprehension, collaborative efforts should be customized as much as possible to the client's auditory profile, age, cultural values and communication style, and any known co-existing conditions. In any case, intervention focused on both auditory skills and acoustic signal enhancement and strategies and techniques that foster language and metacognitive competence should benefit auditory processing of spoken language.

The theoretical foundation of our management approach presented in the final segment of this chapter establishes the basis for the next two chapters in this section. Systems theory, information processing theory, and concepts from cognitive neuroscience support aggressive collaborative intervention conducted in a functional context. The intervention program should be built on challenging activities that emphasize self-regulation of both elemental auditory processing and higher order linguistic and cognitive skills and strategies.

SUGGESTED READINGS

Battle, D.E. (1993). Introduction. In D.E. Battle (Ed.), *Communication disorders in multicultural populations* (pp. xv–xxiv). Boston: Andover Medical Publishers.

Bear, M.F., Kleinschmidt, A., Gu, Q., & Singer, W. (1990). Disruption of experience-dependent synaptic modifications in striate cortex by infusion of an NMDA receptor antagonist. *Journal of Neuroscience, 10*(3), 909–925.

Bindman, L.J., Murphy, K.P.S.J., & Pockett, S. (1988). Postsynaptic control of the induction of long-term changes in efficacy of transmission at neurocortical synapses in slices of rat brain. *Journal of Neurophysiology, 60*, 1053–1065.

Bliss, T., & Lomo, T. (1973). Long-lasting potentiation of synaptic transmission in the dentate area of the anaesthetized rabbit following stimulation of the perforant path. *Journal of Physiology, 232*(2), 331–356.

Cowan, W.M., Fawcett, J.W., O'Leary, D.M., & Stanfield, B. (1984). Regressive events in neurogenesis. *Science, 255*, 1258–1265.

Kalil, R.E. (1989). Synapse formation in the developing brain. *Scientific American, 261*(6), 76–85.

Keefe, J.W. (1987). *Learning style theory and practice*. Reston, VA: National Assocation of Secondary School Principals.

McIntyre, T. (1989). *A resource book for remediating common behaviors and learning problems*. Boston: Allyn and Bacon.

Olswang, L.B., & Bain, B. (1994). Data collection: Monitoring children's treatment progress. *American Journal of Speech-Language Pathology, 3*(3), 55–66.

Pedersen, P.B., & Ivey, A. (1993). *Culture-centered counseling and interview skills*. Westport, CT: Praeger.

Rauschecker, J.P., & Marler, P. (1987). Cortical plasticity and imprinting: Behavioral and physiological contrasts and parallels. In J.P. Rauschecker & P. Marler (Eds.), *Imprinting and cortical plasticity* (pp. 349–366). New York: John Wiley.

Recanzone, G.H., Allard, T.T., Jenkins, W.M., & Merzenich, M.M. (1990). Receptive-field changes induced by peripheral nerve stimulation in SI of adult cats. *Journal of Neurophysiology, 63*(5), 1213–1225.

Recanzone, G.H., Merzenich, M.M., Jenkins, W.M., Grajski, K.A., & Dinse, H.R. (1992). Topographic reorganization of the hand representation in cortical area 3b of owl monkeys trained in a frequency-discrimination task. *Journal of Neurophysiology, 67*(5), 1031–1056.

Scherer, W.J., & Udin, S.B. (1989). N-Methyl-D-Aspartate antagonists prevent interaction of binocular maps in Xenopus tectum. *Journal of Neuroscience, 9*(11), 3837–3843.

Schlaggar, B.L., & O'Leary, D.D.M. (1991). Potential of visual cortex to develop an array of functional units unique to somatosensory cortex. *Science, 252*, 1556–1560.

Schmidt, J.T. (1990). Long-term potentiation and activity-dependent retinotopic sharpening in the regenerating retinotectal projection of goldfish: Common sensitive period and sensitivity to NMDA blockers. *Journal of Neuroscience, 10*(1), 233–246.

Screen, R.M., & Anderson, N.B. (1994). *Multicultural perspectives in communication disorders*. San Diego: Singular Publishing Group.

Sue, D.W., & Sue, D. (1990). *Counseling the culturally different*. New York: John Wiley & Sons.

Taylor, O.L. (1986). Historical perspectives and conceptual framework. In O.L. Taylor (Ed.), *Nature of communication disorders in culturally and linguistically diverse populations* (pp. 1–17). San Diego: College-Hill Press.

CHAPTER

8

MANAGEMENT: AUDITORY TRAINING AND METALINGUISTIC AND METACOGNITIVE STRATEGIES

A comprehensive approach to the management of central auditory processing disorders is necessary given the range of listening and learning deficits associated with this complex and heterogeneous group of disorders (Chermak & Musiek, 1992). Notwithstanding the primacy of auditory processing deficits in central auditory processing disorder (CAPD), cognitive, metacognitive, and linguistic deficits can exacerbate CAPD, compounding the adverse impact of the sensory processing deficit for listening, communication, and learning (ASHA, 1996). Both central auditory processing and spoken language comprehension require the service of cognitive processes (i.e., attention and memory), as well as metacognitive knowledge and executive control.

The involvement of these multiple systems and knowledge bases contributes to the complexity of spoken language comprehension; however, it also offers opportunities for remediation. Metacognitive and metalinguistic systems can be harnessed into remediation strategies to enhance listening and spoken language understanding. Although many of these strategies do not target central auditory processes directly, they can nonetheless promote improved listening and spoken language comprehension through their influence on the metalinguistic and metacognitive systems and knowledge bases. To the extent these strategies improve listening and reading comprehension, they also may reduce learning problems. For example, training in deducing word meaning from context should benefit both listening and reading comprehension, given the robust correlations among vocabulary, reading comprehension, and listening comprehension (Perfetti, 1985; Samuels, 1987; Stanovich, 1993; Sticht & James, 1984; Wigg, Semel, & Crouse, 1973). Similarly, therapy to increase phonological awareness and segmentation skills should aid both reading and listening comprehension (Liberman, Cooper, Shankweiler, & Studdert-Kennedy, 1967; Mann, 1991; Mattingly, 1972; Perfetti & McCutchen, 1982).

CHAPTER OVERVIEW

This chapter provides an indepth presentation of one of two broad intervention approaches. The complementary interventions support both basic skills and executive control strategies. Auditory training and metalinguistic and metacognitive strategies, combined in the first approach, are designed to increase the scope and utilization of auditory and central resources, as described in the following sections. A brief review of theory precedes the clinical application in instances where the reader may be less familiar with the concepts underlying a clinical approach (e.g., schema induction, cognitive style). Specific considerations for younger and older populations are discussed. Signal quality enhancement, the complementary intervention approach, is discussed in Chapter 9.

The reader with some experience in this area may notice the omission of some therapy techniques (e.g., noise desensitization [i.e., auditory-figure ground or selective attention] training, sequential memory training) that have been included in a number of commercially available workbooks for treating CAPD (Bacon, 1992; Barr, 1976; Butler, 1983; Codding & Gardner, 1988; Gillet, 1993; Heasley, 1980; Jeffries & Jeffries, 1991; Kelly, 1995; Lasky & Cox, 1983; Lazzari & Peters, 1994; Rampp, 1976, 1980). As noted in Chapter 1, the traditional, narrow focus directed toward enhancing discrete auditory-language skills has not been particularly effective in reducing the functional deficits associated with CAPD (Chermak, 1981; Chermak & Musiek, 1992; Willeford & Billger, 1978); therefore our management plan is more comprehensive in scope. We target fundamental central auditory processing skills (e.g., auditory discrimination, temporal processing) and particular linguistic (e.g., vocabulary building) and metalinguistic skills (e.g., segmentation, closure) considered amenable to treatment. To complement these remedial efforts, we employ compensatory techniques to address processing deficits considered more resistant to treatment (e.g., acoustic signal enhancement through frequency modulated assistive listening systems to compensate for auditory performance decrements with degraded or competing signals). Concurrently, we also emphasize metacognitive knowledge and strategy development to strengthen self-regulation of spoken language processing.

We acknowledge the work of many others that has influenced our intervention approach. Indeed, we target some of the same areas for intervention recommended by others, albeit in a more comprehensive and metacognitive context. The reader is referred to some of these other sources for both an historical perspective, as well as specific activities to implement strategies discussed in this chapter (Gillet, 1993; Katz & Wilde, 1994; Lasky & Cox, 1983; McIntyre, 1989; Schneider, 1992; Sloan, 1986; Willeford & Burleigh, 1985; Young & Protti-Patterson, 1984).

INTERVENTION GOALS REQUIRE COMPREHENSIVE MANAGEMENT

Improved listening skills and spoken language comprehension are our primary intervention goals. To achieve these goals we must train the listener to actively interact with the acoustic signal, deploying linguistic, cognitive, and metacognitive systems to reconstruct the spoken message. Because listening takes place within the multiple contexts of the acoustic, phonetic, linguistic, and social domains, simultaneous and integrated orchestration of multiple knowledge bases and skills is required for spoken language comprehension.

For successful spoken language comprehension, the listener undoubtedly coordinates various knowledge bases and skills, including auditory vigilance, auditory discrimination, and temporal processing to discern and organize basic acoustic features; segmentation skills to parse the continuous sound stream into constituent phonetic units; language knowledge; general knowledge; and metacognitive knowledge and executive control (Abbs & Sussman, 1971; ASHA, 1996; Chermak & Musiek, 1992; Danks & End, 1987; Fant, 1967; Kintsch,

1977; Massaro, 1975a, 1975b; Ronald & Roskelly, 1985; Samuels, 1987). Effective listeners employ various self-regulation strategies to guide extraction of information and synthesis of the spoken message. Throughout the process, they must continually reflect on the processes and products of their listening. Experience, expectation, and motivation influence both the allocation of resources and the particular meaning derived from the acoustic signal.

Given the number and range of skills and knowledge bases demanding coordination in service of central auditory processing and spoken language comprehension, comprehensive management programs for CAPD must integrate specific skills development and general problem solving strategies. A cognitive functional emphasis is needed to encourage self-regulation of strategy use and motivation. Enhancement of acoustic signal quality coupled with augmented auditory, language, and metacognitive capacities holds promise for improved listening.

A COMPREHENSIVE APPROACH

A comprehensive management approach has been developed based on our current understanding of CAPD (Chermak & Musiek, 1992). Auditory skills training is directed toward improving auditory vigilance, temporal and spectral detection and discrimination, and interhemispheric transfer. Interventions designed to enhance the scope and utilization of central resources focus on improved language and cognitive capacities, auditory-language (metalanguage) skills development, use of compensatory strategies, and deployment of listening and metacognitive strategies (ASHA, 1996; Chermak & Musiek, 1992).

Strategies and techniques employed to mitigate functional deficits commonly observed in CAPD are outlined in Table 8–1. These strategies and techniques support environmental adaptations (e.g., assistive listening devices and acoustic modifications), skills development (e.g., improved memory and vocabulary building), adaptive compensation (e.g., external aids to benefit memory), and metalinguistic (e.g., linguistic closure and contextual derivation of word meaning, segmentation, and mnemonics), and metacognitive knowledge and skills.

AUDITORY TRAINING

Auditory training is directed toward improving the basic auditory skills listed in Table 8–2. These skills encompass both spectral pro-

Table 8–1. Management of Central Auditory Processing Disorders.

Functional Deficit	Strategies	Techniques
Distractibility/ inattention	Increase signal-to-noise ratio	ALD/FM system; acoustic modifications; preferential seating
Poor memory	Metalanguage	Chunking, verbal chaining, mnemonics, rehearsal, paraphrasing, summarizing
	Right hemisphere activation	Imagery, drawing
	External aids	Notebooks, calendars
Restricted vocabulary	Improve closure	Contextual derivation of word meaning
Cognitive inflexibility (predominantly analytic or predominantly conceptual)	Diversify cognitive style	Top-down (deductive) and bottom-up (inductive) processing, inferential reasoning, questioning, critical thinking
Poor listening comprehension	Induce formal schema to aid organization, integration, and prediction	Recognize and explain connectives (additives; causal; adversative; temporal) and patterns of parallelism and correlative pairs (not only/but also; neither/nor)
	Maximize visual and auditory summation	Substitutions for notetaking
Reading, spelling, and listening problems	Enhance multisensory integration	Phonemic analysis and segmentation
Maladaptive behaviors (passive, hyperactive, impulsive)	Assertiveness and cognitive behavior modification	Self-control, self-monitoring, self-evaluation, self-instruction, problem solving
Poor motivation	Attribution retraining, internal locus of control	Failure confrontation, attribution to factors under control

Source: From "Managing central auditory processing disorders in children and youth" by G.D. Chermak and F.E. Musiek, 1992, p. 63. *American Journal of Audiology, 1*(3). Copyright 1992 by American Speech-Language-Hearing Association. Reprinted by permission.

Table 8–2. Auditory Skills Training.

- Vigilance[a]
- Temporal gap detection
- Intensity discrimination
- Frequency discrimination
- Tone glide discrimination
- Phoneme/syllable discrimination
- Temporal gap discrimination
- Temporal order discrimination
- Flutter fusion
- Lateralization
- Interhemispheric transfer[a]

[a]Although vigilance (i.e., sustained attention) and the transfer of information between the two hemispheres via the corpus callosum are not strictly speaking auditory skills, exercises to improve them are included in the auditory training program because successful auditory processing demands vigilance and interhemispheric transfer is pivotal to auditory skills involving binaural interaction, binaural integration, and binaural separation.

cessing (e.g., frequency discrimination) and temporal processing (e.g., gap detection) and underlie phonetic distinctions essential to spoken language processing. A variety of stimuli may be used, although success with nonlinguistic stimuli should precede use of linguistic material as stimuli. Similarly, more demanding psychoacoustic tasks requiring identification, recognition, and production may be constructed once the client achieves criterion performance on the detection and discrimination exercises. Albeit limited, the data available indicate that auditory processing abilities continue to improve in children with normal audition as a function of age, achieving adult-like function between ages 6 to 12 years, depending on the nature of the task (Elliott, 1986; Elliott & Hammer, 1988; Grose, Hall, & Gibbs, 1993; Irwin, Ball, Kay, Stillman, & Bosser, 1985; Jensen & Neff, 1993; Maxon & Hochberg, 1982). This developmental effect must be considered in designing auditory skills training tasks and establishing criterion performance. In our experience clients should perform at a minimum of 70% accuracy before proceeding to these more demanding psychoacoustic tasks. All exercises should be presented at a client's comfortable listening level.

Detection

Trained adult listeners with normal hearing can detect temporal gaps as brief as 1 msec or less (Abel, 1972). Based on this normative data, we train temporal gap detection by asking clients to detect brief gaps inserted within brief bursts of white noise which are progressively shortened approaching the criterion of 1–5 msec gap detection.

Discrimination

Discrimination exercises require the client to decide whether two stimuli are the same or different. Frequency discrimination is trained by requiring clients to discern frequency differences of approximately 5–10 Hz. (A frequency difference of 3 Hz is normally obtained for trained adult listeners [Moore, 1973].)

Trained normal listeners can identify frequency sweep direction for tone bursts with durations of only 1 to 2 msec (Divenyi & Robinson, 1989). Our tone glide discrimination task requires clients to determine the upward or downward direction of a frequency sweep for tone bursts of a few milliseconds. (See Segmentation and Auditory Discrimination for examples of language-related activities that involve auditory discrimination skills.)

Normal trained adult listeners can discriminate temporal gaps of approximately 10 msec (Penner, 1976). In our temporal gap discrimination task, subjects compare the duration of a gap in two consecutive noise bursts. The basic gap is approximately 20 msec, a value typical of a phonetically meaningful distinction, and the comparison gap is approximately 30–40 msec.

In a related task, the client is asked to discriminate between steady-state and interrupted noise. Flutter fusion, or the failure to perceive temporal gaps, is seen in normal listeners when interruption rates exceed 10 per second (Yost & Moore, 1987). Accordingly, our flutter fusion training task involves interruption rates of 5–15 per second.

Temporal order discrimination involves comparing tone sequences in a same-different paradigm. Based on Hirsh's (1959) data showing correct order discrimination for tone durations of about 20 msec, we target order discrimination for tones with durations of approximately 25 msec. Since the tone frequencies are sufficiently separated to ensure their distinctiveness, the client's task is restricted to discriminating tone order. (See Prosody for examples of language-based activities that build on temporal processing.)

Vigilance

As discussed in Chapter 1, vigilance (i.e., sustained attention) is a global neurocognitive process which serves acoustic signal processing. Vigilance is trained using procedures much like those employed in auditory or visual continuous performance tasks (Keith, 1994b; Lindgren & Lyons, 1984; Sergeant & van der Meere, 1990). The client is required to sustain attention to a continuous stream of auditory stimuli, such as environmental sounds, syllables, or words, and to respond (e.g., raising a hand, tapping the table) when a particular stimulus is heard. Failure to detect the target stimulus reflects inattention. False positive errors (i.e., responding to a stimulus other than the target stimulus) may reflect impulsivity.

Interhemispheric Transfer

Interhemispheric transfer via the corpus callosum is employed in tasks requiring interaction between information processed in each hemisphere. As such, it underlies binaural integration (e.g., divided attention) and binaural separation (e.g., selective attention). Tasks useful in promoting interhemispheric transfer include requiring verbal identification through tactile cues of objects held in the left hand; describing a picture while drawing it; singing to music and various music activities; and responding motorically with the left side of the body to a targeted verbal command. (See Task Relevance to Everyday Analogs in Chapter 7.)

METALINGUISTIC STRATEGIES

The metalinguistic strategies discussed in this section include discourse cohesion devices, schema induction, context-derived vocabulary building, segmentation, prosody, and metamemory.

Discourse Cohesion Devices

Discourse cohesion devices are linguistic forms that connnect propositions into more complex messages (Halliday & Hasan, 1976; van

Dijk, 1985), thereby allowing speakers and listeners to more efficiently formulate and resolve messages, respectively. Cohesive ties are used to establish relationships between ideas (e.g., causal relationships signified by *because* or *so*); cohesive chains are built through the use of devices that are either explicit (e.g., pronouns and conjunctions) or must be inferred (e.g., ellipsis). As illustrated in Table 8–3, discourse cohesion devices include referents (e.g., pronouns); substitution (e.g., use of different terminology as coreferent); ellipsis (i.e., deleting rather than reiterating part of a message that can be

Table 8–3. Discourse Cohesion Devices.[a]

Referents		
	Pronouns	Isaac heard a noise. *He* heard *it.*
	Pro-verbs	The rain fell with a vengence. When it *did,* many roads were washed away.
	Comparatives	Alina sings exultantly in the woods; *similarly,* Isaac is exuberant over a symphony.
Substitution		The class designed and painted a mural. The proud parents were not surprised by their *children's* artistry.
Ellipsis		Alina enjoys listening to Mozart. Isaac *does too. [Isaac enjoys listening too.]*
Definiteness		The budget deficit is *an* important issue in this year's election. Unfortunately, the election failed to resolve *the* issue.
Conjunctions[b]		
	Additive	Now is the time for leadership *and* diplomacy.
	Adversative	*Although* she searched for alternatives, no option seemed satisfactory.
	Causal	The college all-star violated the academic honesty code; *therefore,* she was suspended from the team.
	Disjunctive	She chose family medicine *instead* of cardiology despite the substantial difference in earnings potential.
	Temporal	A plan must be formulated *before* resources are committed.

[a] This table provides examples of the major cohesion signaling devices. It is not an exhaustive listing of the various subtypes.

[b] In contrast to the other cohesive devices, conjunctions do not presuppose other elements in the preceding or subsequent text. Rather, they specify relationships within and across propositions.

inferred; definiteness (e.g., activating known versus new information); and conjunctions (e.g., words that connect and specify relationships across a message).

Discourse cohesion devices typically reduce verbiage and therefore increase efficiency of message transfer, but in so doing they place cognitive (e.g., memory) and linguistic processing demands on the listener. To discern subtle differences in meaning, listeners must grasp precisely the relationships signaled by these cohesive devices. Since the primary function of central auditory processing is to aid spoken discourse understanding, improved use of discourse cohesion devices should benefit the spoken language comprehension of individuals with CAPD.

Conjunctions are unique among cohesive devices because they do not presuppose other elements in preceding or subsequent text. Rather, conjunctions specify relationships within and across propositions. While a pronoun can only be unambiguously interpreted in the context of its referent (e.g., The flower wilted. *It* died.), the conjunction *because* links preceding and subsequent clausal ideas. Conjunctions are discussed further in the following sections on schema theory and use.

Schema Theory and Use

Schema is a metacognitive construct used to account for knowledge organization that is invoked when undertaking discrete behavioral or cognitive tasks (Kintsch, 1988; Rumelhart, 1980). A schema is a structured cluster of concepts, a set of expectations, an abstract and generic knowledge structure stored in memory that preserves the relations among constituent concepts and generalized knowledge about a text, event, message, situation, or object, thereby providing a framework to guide interpretation (Mandler, 1984; Miller, 1988; Rumelhart, 1980, 1984). In essence, a schema is a conceptual framework, a multidimensional map connecting interrelated ideas. Schema theory is offered to explain how knowledge and experience are mapped in the mind and how those representations facilitate comprehension and learning (Rumelhart, 1980, 1984).

Schemata have been invoked to explain the ability to theorize, predict, infer, and make default assumptions about unmentioned aspects of a situation. "Schemata are employed in the process of interpreting sensory data (both linguistic and nonlinguistic), in retrieving information from memory, in organizing actions, in determining goals and subgoals, in allocating resources, and generally, in guiding the flow of processing in the system" (Rumelhart, 1980, pp. 33–34). In guiding processing, schemata serve an executive function (see

Chapter 7). Although deploying schemata does not guarantee message understanding, it does maximize the best fit between data and structure (Rumelhart, 1980, 1984).

Schema utilization requires both bottom-up (i.e., data-driven) and top-down (i.e., concept-driven) processing. Although a schema provides top-down guidance to the listener, its activation is dependent on a match between its criterial features and descriptions yielded by lower level analysis (Rumelhart, 1980). (See Cognitive Style and Reasoning for additional discussion of bottom-up and top-down processing in schema activation.)

Developing awareness of spatial, temporal, and causal relationships, children's language shows the use of formal schemata (e.g., *and, then,* and *because*) as young as 2 to 3 years (French & Nelson, 1985; Nippold, 1988). Development continues through adolescence to include more complex conjunctions (Nippold, 1988).

Content Schemata

Schemata operate at two different levels. Formal schemata "give form or structure to experience" (Dillon, 1981, p. 51); they involve knowledge of discourse conventions (Mavrogenes, 1983). Content or contextual schemata provide a generalized interpretation of the content of experience (Dillon, 1981). Content schemata (also referred to as scripts) organize facts, establishing a framework that allows listeners to impose certain structures on events, precepts, situations, and even objects, thereby promoting an interpretation (Rumelhart, 1980).

In the context of spoken language comprehension, listeners use content schemata to interpret messages. For instance, listeners instantiate certain content schemata or scripts that reflect the sequential actions of a common event, prescribing the general direction in which a story should unfold. Having accessed a particular script, the listener would expect that the story setting should precede the major actions of the characters, with a closing following the denouement. Similarly, scripts for eating in restaurants would prescribe a particular action sequence.

Content schemata also evoke inferential elaborations. For example, listeners will construct quite different interpretations of the sentences "The punter kicked the ball" and "The golfer kicked the ball" (Harris & Sipay, 1990, p. 560) depending on the content schema through which the sentence is processed. In addition to eliciting different images of the physical attributes of the balls, listeners will infer that:

> (1) the game being played in the first sentence is football; (2) the punter's team has failed to make a first down or is using the punt as a defensive strategy; (3) the play is probably not a field-goal attempt because place kickers, not punters, are used in such situations; and (4) this is a routine occurrence in a football game. (Harris & Sipay, 1990, p. 561)

In contrast, content schemata would lead a listener to infer that the golfer's behavior was not routine, rather an exhibition of unprofessional behavior, perhaps even cheating, casting aspersions about the golfer's character (Harris & Sipay, 1990).

Formal Schemata

Formal schemata are linguistic markers that serve to organize, integrate, and predict relationships across propositions (Dillon, 1981). They foster the cohesiveness and coherence of messages. Formal schemata include conjunctions (i.e., additive [e.g., *and, furthermore*], adversative [e.g., *although, nevertheless, however*], causal [e.g., *because, therefore, accordingly]*, disjunctive [e.g., *but, instead, on the contrary*], and temporal conjunctions [e.g., *before, after, subsequently]*, as well as patterns of parallelism and correlative pairs [e.g., *not only/but also; neither/nor*]). (See Table 8–3.)

The organizing function of schemata is most salient at the global level, facilitating the integration of ideas across the discourse. This more global organizing function is represented by expressions such as the *first point, and finally,* and *in summary*. These expressions are often coupled with paralinguistic cues, including speaking rate, pauses, repetitions, and inflection and nonverbal cues such as body posture, eye contact, facial expression, and hand gestures which together alert the listener to the organization of the spoken message (Buttrill, Niizawa, Biemer, Takahashi, & Hearn, 1989).

The integrative and predictive functions of schemata operate at local levels (Dillon, 1981). These functions probably demand greater linguistic sophistication as listeners must focus attention on patterns that fuse and foreshadow ideas and facilitate the construction of relationships between the ideas (Chermak & Musiek, 1992). For example, the causal conjunction *because* integrates two propositions and predicts the relationship between them. Similarly, *if-then* constructions activate schemata depicting either causation (prediction) or speculation (via the subjunctive conditional), thereby facilitating comprehension.

The integrative function of schemata also reduces the processing required to comprehend complex sentences in which adverbial or other qualifying language is suspended across clauses (e.g., between the subject and verb). For example, the suspensive constructions in the sentences, "Not only do children listen more effectively when deploying selected strategies, but they also tend to enjoy the process more" and "The youngster, disadvantaged from a life time of neglect and marginalization, invariably faces learning difficulties" are less likely to disrupt comprehension if a listener employs formal schematic knowledge. Given their predictive function, formal schemata assist both literal and figurative interpretation, including inferencing, as discussed below under Cognitive Style and Reasoning.

Perhaps the most important point to remember about formal schemata is that they do not specify meaning. As recurrent patterns, however, they evoke certain expectations, narrow the range of possiblities, and provide the skilled listener with direction in constructing meaning. By activating formal schemata, listeners become aware of the probable message structure, using that knowledge as a framework to form expectations about the organization and relationships among the content; however, the listener must still construct the specific detail to resolve the message.

In summary, schemata provide frameworks that facilitate the organization, integration, and ultimately the understanding of information. Schemata provide extensive networks linking new stimuli with stored knowledge and expectation. In doing so, they render particular perspectives salient, allow for efficient resource allocation, and thereby facilitate comprehension.

Clinical Application

Schema selection, maintenance, and flexibility influence listening comprehension and may account in part for differences between effective and ineffective listeners (Chermak & Musiek, 1992). Processing schemata and other discourse cohesion devices may be more difficult for individuals with CAPD and learning disabilities (Liles, 1985, 1987; Wren, 1983). Clearly, if individuals are unfamiliar with the linguistic structure of a message, they may experience difficulty in determining what is important, what is relevant, as well as the interrelationships among the information presented. They will be forced to allocate resources in a less efficient manner, they will have difficulty guiding the flow of processing in the system, and their comprehension will suffer (Rumelhart, 1980). Because schema utilization depends not only on linguistic facility and cognition (e.g., memory), but also on executive functions (e.g., self-regulation and self-monitoring) and cognitive flexibility as well (Rumelhart, 1984), clinical approaches that enhance metacognitive knowledge and skills will also benefit schema use. The reader should find the metacognitive approaches discussed later in the chapter complementary to the formal schema induction approach we discuss next. The reader is referred to Bergenske (1987), Gerber (1993c), Gordon (1989), Gordon and Rennie (1986), Idol (1987), Pearson (1982), Reutzel (1985), and Wiig and Semel (1984) for approaches to developing use of content schemata.

Translating Theory into a Clinical Approach: Schema Induction

Individuals presenting CAPD may benefit from instruction that emphasizes recognizing and interpreting formal schemata (Chermak & Musiek, 1992). By activating the appropriate formal schemata, the listener invokes a generic framework that illuminates relationships across propositions and thereby assists listening comprehension. Because formal schemata often occur at phrase boundaries, they may help the listener parse larger and more complex messages into smaller units, benefiting both comprehension and retention.

A number of *priming* techniques, which evoke relevant internal representations (Tulving & Schacter, 1990), are useful in activating relevant formal (as well as content) schemata. These priming techniques include: (1) eliciting prelistening mental imagery, (2) preceding a listening task by developing vocabulary and the concepts to be presented in the message, (3) promoting discussion that ties the content of the message to the client's background or experience, (4) using visual aids while presenting a message to help focus attention and reinforce concepts, and (5) asking questions to promote literal or interpretive critical responses. We will discuss a schema induction method that builds on this last technique.

Schema Induction. Induction learning involves an indirect approach to instruction, which emphasizes the central role of discovery for learning. The approach presupposes that induction is natural and that learners come to the learning situation with a predeveloped, perhaps innate, induction capability (Connell, 1988). Consistent with the goal of personal responsibility and metacognitive control, facilitating schema utilization through induction is more likely to lead to generalization of the strategy and its deployment outside the therapeutic setting (Schumaker, Deshler, Alley, & Warner, 1983).

The induction procedure illustrated in Table 8–4 allows clients an opportunity to discover the functions and utility of formal schemata

Table 8–4. Clinical Illustration of Schema Induction.

Objectives: To identify and produce causal conjunctions and constructions.[a]

Step 1 *Clinician:* "A lot of rain fell this morning. The baseball game was canceled. Why do you think the baseball game was canceled?"

Client: "Because the field is wet. It's slippery. If you run too fast, you can break your leg."

Step 2 *Clinician:* "Yes, now let us listen to (look at[b]) what you said." (Clinician plays back client's response.) "Tell me which words tell you why the game was canceled."

Client: "Because I said *because*. I said *if* you run too fast, you can break your leg."

Clinician: "Yes, you are correct. *If* and *because* are the important words which prepare us for the reasons, the answers to the question *why*."

Step 3 *Clinician:* "Listen to this short story and tell me if you recognize any of the same important words you just told me about.

Mother says that I must do my homework. She says that if I study hard, then I will get good grades. If I earn good grades, then I can go to a good college. I will do my homework because I want to be a doctor when I grow up."

Step 4 *Clinician:* "Did you recognize any of the important words?"

Client: "You said that mother said *if* I study hard and *if* I get good grades."

Clinician: "Yes. You are correct. Did you hear any other important key words?" (Clinician may play back the story if the client has difficulty recalling additional words.)

Client: "Yes, the boy said he will study hard *because* he wants to be a doctor."

Step 5 *Clinician:* "Now, I want you to tell me a short story using these important key words and I will try to identify them and explain their function to you."[c]

Objectives: To produce and identify temporal conjunctions.[d]

Step 1 *Clinician:* "Please tell me how your father prepares dinner."

Client: "First he takes the chicken and vegetables out of the refrigerator. Then he cooks the food. Finally, he cuts the food and I eat it."

Step 2 *Clinician:* "Now, let us listen to (look at) what you said." (Clinican plays back client's description.) "Tell me the important key words you said to let me know that your father began by taking food out of the refrigerator?"

Client: "I said, *first* Dad takes out the food."

(continued)

Table 8–4. *(continued)*

Clinician: "Yes, that word *first* certainly gave me a big clue. Now tell me which important word you said so that I would know what happened in the end."

Client: "I said *finally,* I ate."

Clinician: "Yes, that is correct."

[a]The reader will note variations in the sequence of activities supporting the two different objectives. For the first objective (to identify and produce causal conjunctions and constructions), clients listen to a story that is likely to lead them to produce causal conjunctions and constructions. The clinician then asks the client to identify the causal conjunctions/constructions and explain their function. The last step, illustrating reciprocal teaching, requires that the client generate a story which the clinician then analyzes. In the second series of steps supporting the production and identification of temporal conjunctions, the client first produces the organizational words and then identifies them and explains their function. The clinician may then proceed to tell the client a story and ask the client to identify the temporal conjunctions and explain their function. The reader will recognize yet other variations on this induction sequence.

[b]The clinician may wish to exploit the advantage of bisensory processing by using audiovisual presentations. Audiotaping and visual aids (e.g., pictures for younger children and written transcripts for older clients) should improve the effectiveness of this procedure.

[c]This step begins a reciprocal teaching sequence wherein the client assumes the teacher's role and thereby promotes metacognitive control.

[d]This truncated sequence begins with the client generating a story. The clinician may expand this sequence by generating stories for the client to examine.

for listening comprehension. The instructional challenge is to facilitate the client's recognition that a pattern exists in the message and to explain that pattern so that it may be used for message comprehension, as well as message formulation. To achieve these ends, the clinician must structure input so that information necessary to induce the rule governing the pattern is salient and available to the listener (Connell, 1988).

The effectiveness of indirect instruction, as reflected in the induction method, depends on the client's ability and background (Cronbach & Snow, 1981). The discovery element of the inductive method can be very effective, but it also presents the client with a more difficult task. Even the most basic conjunctions (e.g., *and, then, because*) may prove too difficult when presented in the context of the inductive method. Very young clients, those with more serious CAPD, as well as those with associated cognitive, language, or peripheral hearing problems may not succeed with a strict inductive approach.

The approach outlined in Table 8–4 may, therefore, require modification when clients cannot contextually extract the meaning of formal schemata. When prompting, rephrasing, and modeling prove ineffective, it may be necessary to suspend the induction approach and revert to an approach that more directly highlights and draws the client's attention to the formal schemata. Focusing on minimal pairs to underscore schematic contrast serves this purpose (see examples of contrastive pairs in Table 8–5). The semantic absurdities caused

Table 8–5. Contrastive Pairs to Develop Formal Schemata.[a]

1. I eat because I am hungry.
   I eat because I am satisfied.
2. I sleep because I am tired.
   I sleep because I am awake.
3. Before I go to school, I get dressed.
   Before I go to school, I eat dinner.
4. I sleep because I am tired.
   I sleep, but I am tired.
5. I sleep, but I do not want to.
   I sleep because I do not want to.
6. The baseball game was canceled because a lot of rain fell this morning.
   The baseball game was canceled, but a lot of rain fell this morning.
7. After I get off the school bus, I go to school.
   Before I get off the school bus, I go to school.
8. I get dressed before I go to school.
   I get dressed after I go to school.
9. Mom puts the cake in the oven after she puts the batter in the pan.
   Mom puts the cake in the oven before she puts the batter in the pan.
10. I sleep because I am tired.
    I sleep, but I am awake.
11. I eat because I am hungry.
    I eat, but I am satisfied.
12. The first thing I do when I wake up in the morning is brush my teeth.
    The last thing I do when I wake up in the morning is get out of bed.

[a] The contrastive pairs sharing the same conjunction provide a basic and enjoyable starting point (items 1–3). Sentence pairs that contrast conjunctions present greater challenges and may also serve as transition to another conjunction. Altering either the conjunction (items 4–9) or the predicate phrase (items 1–3), presents a more obvious and less difficult contrast than pairs in which both conjunction and predicate are simultaneously varied (items 10–12).

by inappropriate use of a conjunction engages youngsters while providing an opportunity to examine the rule and then return to the induction approach at some later time. Alternatively, the clinician might diverge from the straight induction approach by asking clients to paraphrase conjoined sentences by incorporating conjunctions (see Table 8–6).

The induction approach may be adapted for group work. One means to adapt the approach to group work is through reciprocal teaching in which clients model schema induction for the clinician or for peers with less developed induction skills. As discussed in a later section, reciprocal teaching also provides an effective vehicle to build self-confidence and self-esteem.

Vocabulary Building and Construction of Meaning

Deficits in word knowledge have been reported in individuals with CAPD and learning disabilities. Deficits include limited vocabulary, restrictions in word meaning, difficulties with multiple meaning words, difficulties with comprehension of conjunctions, and deficits

Table 8–6. Paraphrasing and Conjoining Sentences Using Formal Schema.

He studied extensively for the final exam./He earned the highest grade. (He earned the highest grade *because* he studied extensively for the final exam.)
He studied extensively for the final exam./He failed the exam. (*Although* he studied extensively for the final exam, he failed the exam.)
She campaigned aggressively./She won the election. (*Because* she campaigned aggressively, she won the election.)
She campaigned aggressively./She lost the election. (She lost the election, *despite* aggressive campaigning.)
The therapist employed the best clinical practices./The client was cured. (The client was cured *because* the therapist employed the best clinical practices.)
The therapist employed the best clinical practices./ The client continued to experience learning problems. (*Notwithstanding* use of the best clinical practices, the client continued to experience learning problems.)
The exams were graded./Scores were posted. (*After* the exams were graded, the scores were posted. *Before* the scores were posted, the exams were graded.)
I would like to attend graduate school./I have no funding. (I would like to attend graduate school, *but* I have no funding.)

in interpreting figurative language (Ferre & Wilber, 1986; Gajar, 1989; Hoskins, 1983; Houck & Billingsley, 1989; Johnson & Myklebust, 1967; Keith & Novak, 1984; Mann, 1991; Matkin & Hook, 1983; Snider, 1989; Willeford & Burleigh, 1985; Wren, 1983).

Given the central role vocabulary serves in spoken language comprehension (Perfetti, 1985; Samuels, 1987; Stanovich, 1993; Sticht & James, 1984; Wiig, Semel, & Crouse, 1973), it is necessary for clinicians to incorporate vocabulary building from both a quantitative and a qualitative or semantic network perspective. The network perspective broadens vocabulary building to the larger goal of the construction of meaning by focusing on semantic relationships as well as lexicon.

Consistent with the models of central auditory processing and information processing discussed in Chapters 1 and 7, respectively, a number of procedures are presented that promote an active approach to the construction of meaning. Context-derived vocabulary building, word derivation, flexibility with multiple meaning words, and inferencing are among the procedures recommended for extending the breadth and depth of vocabulary knowledge.

Context-Derived Vocabulary Building

Context can be used to derive word meaning and thereby expand vocabulary and enhance message comprehension (Miller & Gildea, 1987). Using the linguistic context of the acoustic signal to resolve vocabulary requires auditory and grammatic closure (Chermak & Musiek, 1992). Like the Cloze procedure employed in reading instruction, context-derived vocabulary building encourages listeners to search their linguistic and world knowledge to determine specific word meaning and ultimately resolve the auditory message (Gerber, 1981). Although relying on context may not always prove effective because some contexts are ambiguous, misleading, or simply uninformative, in many cases context clarifies word meaning and motivates the listener to learn the association between a word and its meaning (Miller & Gildea, 1987). For example, the context surrounding the unknown word *pilfered* in the sentence "The robber pilfered the jewels" is sufficiently informative to enable a listener with basic vocabulary knowledge to derive its meaning. In fact, deducing word meaning from context is more effective than consulting a dictionary, a strategy that requires considerable sophistication if the user is to select the intended meaning from the multiple listings of alternative meanings in dictionaries (Miller & Gildea, 1987). Moreover, context determines the nuances of word meaning, while a dictionary definition provides only minimal clues to word meaning as reflected in the example below borrowed from Samuels (1987, p. 301).

The *baby ate* the steak.
The *executive ate* the steak.
The *dog ate* the steak.

The manner in which the steak is eaten is determined by knowledge of the subject of each sentence (Samuels, 1987). Exercises to develop auditory discrimination skills in context, as discussed in a subsequent section, reinforce context-derived vocabulary building.

Construction of Meaning

Enriching word knowledge and expanding vocabulary can be fostered through a focus on the relationship between root words and derivations (e.g., able/disability, know/knowledge, spirit/inspire, decide/decision). Multiple meaning words (e.g., bank, bark, nature, spring) and homophones (e.g., manner/manor, muscle/mussel, medal/meddle) encourage flexibility in comprehension (Gerber, 1993b) and provide an opportunity to expand semantic networks and increase vocabulary. When placed in context, multiple meaning words also offer the chance to work on context-derived vocabulary building. For example, the sentence "You can *bank* on me to meet you at the river *bank* after I put the money in the *bank*" (Samuels, 1987, p. 300) provides multiple instructional opportunities: to learn word meaning, expand semantic networks, and use context to determine meaning. Similarly, heteronyms (e.g., address/address, content/content, digest/digest), words spelled identically but pronounced differently, provide an excellent vehicle for building vocabulary while also focusing on the role of prosody in spoken language comprehension (Musiek & Chermak, 1995).

In addition to intervention directed toward literal meaning, with the older child, efforts may also be directed in the area of figurative language. Exploration of metaphors, similes, slang, sarcasm, idioms, and proverbs should further build semantic networks (Nippold, 1991; Nippold & Fey, 1983).

Visual imagery offers an alternative sensory modality to strengthen semantic knowledge. Having clients close their eyes and construct mental pictures of words can be incorporated in a variety of activities (e.g., clinician guesses the word on the basis of the client's answers to questions posed regarding what the picture looks like).

Segmentation and Auditory Discrimination

Phonological awareness, the explicit awareness of the sound structure of language, includes the recognition that words are comprised of syllables and phonemes (Catts, 1991). This awareness directs the listener's segmentation of words into their constituent sound segments (Lewkowitz, 1980). Increasing evidence demonstrates the causal linkages between phonological processing ability and reading skill, as well as spoken language comprehension (Adams, 1990; Ball & Blachman, 1991; Stanovich, 1993; Wagner & Torgesen, 1987). Since the development of phonological awareness varies among children, the cognitive and linguistic demands inherent to phonological awareness activities must be considered carefully (Bradley & Bryant, 1985; Catts, 1991). (The reader is referred to Catts [1991] for a review of phonological awareness and segmentation training.)

Auditory Discrimination

Auditory discrimination is perhaps the most fundamental central auditory processing skill underlying spoken language comprehension. The ability to perceive acoustic similarities and differences between sounds is essential to segmentation skills, which require the listener to recognize the acoustic contrasts among contiguous phonemes. Similarly, auditory discrimination is fundamental to phonemic analysis and synthesis. Auditory discrimination and phonemic analysis are so important to spoken language comprehension that treatment programs for CAPD have been constructed around them (Sloan, 1986). (See Auditory Training for additional discussion of auditory discrimination.)

Phonemic Analysis and Phonemic Synthesis

Phonemic analysis and phonemic synthesis (i.e., sound blending or closure) provide two reciprocal approaches to phonological awareness and segmentation training. The primary goal of phonemic analysis is to develop phonemic encoding and decoding skills using either multisyllabic nonsense sequences (Lindamood & Lindamood, 1975) or single syllables and multisyllabic words (Sloan, 1986). The listener identifies which sound is heard and its position in the syllable or word.

Activities to strengthen auditory discrimination and phonemic analysis are detailed in several commercially available treatment programs, including Sloan's (1986) treatment program and the Auditory Discrimination in Depth (ADD) training program (Lindamood &

Lindamood, 1975). Predicated on the linkage among central auditory processing, language learning, and language use, Sloan's (1986) four-part program develops skills in auditory discrimination, sound analysis, and sound-symbol (phoneme-grapheme) association and applies these skills to reading and spelling words. Similarly, the ADD program seeks to increase auditory discrimination for sameness, difference, number, and order of speech sounds, as well as sound-symbol association encoding (spelling) and decoding (reading) skills as prerequisite, and complementary, to reading programs.

Phonemic synthesis involves the blending of discrete phonemes into the correctly sequenced, coarticulated sound patterns. The Phonemic Synthesis program developed by Katz and Harmon (1982) is an example of a program that provides lessons designed to promote mastery of sequential phoneme blending skills.

Unfortunately, most phonemic analysis and phonemic synthesis programs treat the spoken word as a concatenated string of consecutive sounds rather than a system of coarticulated and acoustically and phonetically overlapping and merged sounds (Liberman, Shankweiler, Blachman, Camp, & Werfelman, 1980). It may be more appropriate to work at the level of syllabic segmentation (with the possible exception of nasals and fricatives which, unlike other consonants, can be produced in isolation) and syllabic blending, rather than create artificial sound categories, which create problems in fusing phonemes (Elkonin, 1973). In addition, working at the syllable level allows for syllable prolongation, which may increase its perceptual salience (Leonard, Sabbadini, Volterra, & Leonard, 1988), thereby facilitating phonemic analysis and synthesis (Sloan, 1980a, 1986). Slingerland (1971) and Elkonin (1973) outlined techniques that incorporate syllabic segmentation and blending (e.g., word changing by replacing only one phoneme in a word) using visual aids (e.g., counters, alphabet blocks) to provide concrete representation.

Auditory Discrimination in Context

Auditory discrimination training may be conducted beyond the syllable or word level. Developing auditory discrimination while emphasizing the important comprehension cues provided by context may be accomplished through the use of sentence material like that incorporated in the *Speech Perception in Noise* (SPIN) *Test* (Bilger, Neutzel, Rabinowitz, & Rzeczkowski, 1984; Kalikow, Stevens, & Elliott, 1977). The listener is required to identify the final word of sentences that are preceded by phrases providing high or low test word predictability. High predictability sentences contain high levels of context or *clue words* (e.g., The farmer harvested his crop). Low predictability sentences contain little context from which the final target word can be deduced (e.g., Tom wants to know about the cake). Similarly, auditory discrimination and closure skills may be developed in young children using familiar nursery rhymes and songs (e.g., "Twinkle, twinkle little *star*," "Little Bo Peep has lost her *sheep*").

Prosody

In contrast to segmental analysis, prosody involves the suprasegmental aspects of spoken language. Prosody is the dynamic melody, timing, rhythm, and amplitude fluctuations of fluent speech. Prosodic information is important to spoken language processing: prosody links phonetic segments (Goldinger, Pisoni, & Luce, 1996), guides attention to the more informative parts of a message (Cutler & Fodor, 1979; Cutler & Foss, 1977), and provides information about the lexical, semantic, and syntactic content of the spoken message (Goldinger, Pisoni, & Luce, 1996; Studdert-Kennedy, 1980).

A number of approaches may be used to target perception of prosody in a spoken language context. As mentioned earlier in the section on vocabulary building, heteronyms require focus on prosody (specifically accent or stress) to resolve semantic distinctions. Ambiguous phrases also offer material that draws attention to prosodic detail while training context-derived vocabulary building skills (Chermak & Musiek, 1992). For example, durational contrasts and context allow the listener to disambiguate sentences with identical surface structure, as illustrated in the following sentence pair adapted from Lehiste, Olive, and Streeter's (1976, p. 1200) study of the role of duration in syntactic disambiguation.

> Traveling to new cities can be enjoyable, but *visiting relatives* can be a nuisance./*Visiting relatives* can be a nuisance, especially if they expect to be waited on hand and foot.

In a similar manner, intonation is used as an aid to resolving ambiguous messages where prosody changes meaning. For example, depending on the speaker's intonation and timing, the sentence, "Look out the window," can be parsed and interpreted to mean "Look out!, the window," "Look!, Out the window," or simply the simple imperative statement "Look out the window" (Musiek & Chermak, 1995). Temporally cued sentences (e.g., "They saw the *snow drift* by the window" versus "They saw the *snowdrift* by the window") (Cole &

Jakimik, 1980, p. 159) also may serve to instill an appreciation in the listener for the use of prosody and segmentation knowledge in resolving messages. The reader is referred to Cole and Jakimik (1980) who present a series of temporally cued sentence pairs that contrast one- versus two-word segmentation of the same phoneme sequence.

Reading poetry and noting the location of the emphasis and stress in sentences and words may improve perception of prosody. The listener also may benefit from training with a language master to produce appropriate inflection and prosody in the expressive mode (Musiek & Chermak, 1995).

Metamemory

Given the essential role of memory for spoken language processing and learning, strengthening memory may benefit individuals with CAPD. Metamemory, or knowledge and awareness of one's own memory systems and strategies (Flavell & Wellman, 1977), provides a focus for memory improvement.

Adults demonstrate a substantial understanding of metamemory (Flavell & Wellman, 1977). The developmental literature reveals that children gradually acquire knowledge and appreciation of retrieval cues and effective strategies for coding, organizing, and retrieving items in memory (Howe & Ceci, 1978). By age 6 years, most children begin to demonstrate some awareness of the limitations of memory and of factors affecting memory (e.g., realizing that they cannot remember all information with equal ease) (Kreutzer, Leonard, & Flavell, 1975). By age 8 to 10 years, children demonstrate a planned approach to encoding and retrieval, becoming aware of mnemonics and their benefits (Cavanaugh & Perlmutter, 1982; Harris, 1978; Harris & Terwogt, 1978; Kail, 1990; Kreutzer et al., 1975).

Memory enhancement strategies may be grouped into four categories: pharmacological treatments, internal strategies, repetitive practice, and external devices (Harris, 1992). In addition to the metalinguistic strategies and techniques presented here, the reader is reminded that memory can be enhanced through the influence of executive functions. (See Metacognitive Strategies below, and Executive Function in Chapter 1.)

Pharmacological Treatment

Although some drugs have been shown to improve memory losses associated with neurodegenerative diseases such as Alzheimer's disease (Giacobini & Becker, 1989; Hock, 1995), pharmacological therapies are not available for the treatment of CAPD (Musiek & Hoffman, 1990; Willeford & Burleigh, 1985). This is in direct contrast to the widespread acceptance and predominance of the use of stimulant medication (e.g., methylphenidate or Ritalin) for children whose primary diagnosis is ADHD, many of whom realize positive cognitive effects (e.g., vigilance, memory), decreases in impulsive and inappropriate behavior, and improvement in academic performance and classroom behavior (Rapport et al., 1987; Rapport, Denney, DuPaul, & Gardner, 1994; Swanson, Cantwell, Lerner, McBurnett, & Hanna, 1992). Methylphenidate may also improve central auditory function in children with ADHD (Cook et al., 1993; Keith & Engineer 1991). Given our limited understanding of the neurochemistry of the auditory system (see Musiek & Hoffman, 1990, and Chapter 2) and the absence of a pharmacologic treatment for CAPD, it is appropriate to consider the full range of behavioral interventions.

Internal Strategies

Internal strategies consist of naturally learned strategies and mnemonic devices (Harris, 1992). Naturally learned strategies are used without training and often tacitly without realizing that they are being used. For example, in memorizing a list of dates of important holidays, most adults concentrate on dates they do not already know. Similarly, asking for repetition is another internal strategy used without much notice. The familiar primacy and recency effects in free recall, whereby subjects best recall items that were presented first or encountered last, are other examples of natural internal strategies (Ward, 1937).

Mnemonics refer to *artificial* or contrived memory aids for organizing information (e.g., acronyms, rhymes, verbal mediators, visual imagery, drawing) that operate through the application of basic learning principles (e.g., association, organization, meaningfulness, attention) (Harris, 1992; Loftus & Loftus, 1976). In contrast to naturally learned strategies, mnemonics are consciously learned and used. The majority of mnemonic devices are language-based. Mnemonic techniques and systems have been shown to improve memory in subjects of various ages, including preschool-age children (Levin, 1976) and older adults (Treat, Poon, Fozard, & Popkin, 1977).

Mnemonic Techniques. Elaboration, transformation, chunking, and coding are the four mnemonic techniques encompassing the majority of frequently used internal memory devices.

Elaboration involves assigning meaning to items to be remembered by recasting them in meaningful sentences, analogies, or acronyms. The sentence "Richard Of York Gained Battles In Vain" is an example of elaboration in which the first letter of each word represents the first letter of the colors of the spectrum of light (i.e., red, orange, yellow, green, blue, indigo, and violet). In the same way, "Every Good Boy Does Fine" provides an elaboration used to recall the notes on the treble staff lines. First-letter cueing to form acronyms aids memory for sequences. The acronym *FACE* triggers memory for the notes in the spaces between the lines of the treble staff. Similarly, verbal chaining, or grouping items into sentences, may facilitate memory for otherwise unrelated items. The use of rhymes, such as the one beginning, "Thirty days hath September. . . ." also demonstrates the power of elaboration to benefit memory. Finally, paraphrasing or summarizing are two additional examples of elaborative techniques.

Transformation involves recasting complicated material into a more basic form that can be remembered more easily. For example, transforming Einstein's relativity theory into a simple equation ($E = MC^2$) may give the individual a concise means for storing complicated material. Some types of paraphrasing may also be considered transformations, and thus benefit memory.

Chunking involves organizing items into categories. Organizing a mental shopping list into produce, dairy, meats, and condiments is an example of chunking. Analogously, grouping telephone numbers into parts, a three-digit area code, three-digit exchange, and the final four digits into two-digit pairs also reflects a chunking operation.

Coding involves recasting the form in which the information is presented. Creating mental images or drawing pictures to capture information presented auditorily are examples of coding. Mental images may involve real scenes, absurd mental pictures, or imposed mental charts and diagrams. Drawing may be a particularly useful coding technique for individuals experiencing spoken language processing difficulties, because drawing activates the primary motor cortex of the right hemisphere and thereby applies bihemispheric processing to a verbal memory task (Musiek & Chermak, 1995).

Repetitive Practice

Practice or rehearsal is a necessary and common method employed to improve memory; however, the quantity of practice is secondary to the quality of practice (Bauer & Emhert, 1984; Swanson, 1983; Wong, 1982). Practice is most effective when it is guided by an organized strategy and follows the principles of learning theory (Swanson & Cooney, 1991). Those principles demonstrate the efficiency of distributing practice over time rather than compressing the same amount of practice into a short period of time (Spence & Norris, 1950; Starch, 1912). Tasks should be sequenced to provide opportunities for correct performance and positive reinforcement (Ausubel & Robinson, 1969; Clifford, 1978; Hedge, 1993). Also supported by learning theory, skills and strategies should be overlearned to increase retention (Krueger, 1929). The clinician should follow learning principles in designing opportunities to practice the strategies and techniques reviewed throughout this chapter.

External Aids

External compensatory aids (e.g., prosthetic devices and cognitive orthotic devices) may be preferred over internal strategies by children younger than 11 years old (Kreutzer et al., 1975) because they offer a relatively powerful and immediate means to augment memory. Nonetheless, external devices should not be used to the exclusion of internal aids and repetitive practice. Indeed, internal strategies and repetitive practice are preferable because they require an individual's active control and self-regulation and are therefore more likely to be applied across settings and maintained over time (Borkowski et al., 1989; Guevremont, 1990).

Clearly, attention is basic to any memory enhancement strategy. Alerting a child in a classroom to *follow along* or *listen carefully* is an important first step in implementing an external aid to memory. The reader is referred to Harrell, Parente, Bellingrath, and Lisicia (1992) and Harris (1992) for more explicit discussion of external devices.

Prosthetic Devices. Prosthetic devices are nonelectronic or noncomputerized electronic devices or systems (Fowler, Hart, & Sheehan, 1972). These devices are usually inexpensive and relatively simple to learn to use. Examples of prosthetic devices include alarm clocks, watches, and electronic diaries; pocket tape recorders; signs, icons, or cuing cards; checklists; notebooks; and appointment calendars.

Cognitive Orthotic Devices. Cognitive orthotic devices employ computers and software to perform memory functions for the client. Examples of these devices include telephone answering machines, spelling and grammar checkers, and an ever growing inventory of software and expert systems (Harrell et al., 1992).

METACOGNITIVE KNOWLEDGE AND STRATEGIES

The distinction between process and performance underscores the potential of metacognitive approaches for managing CAPD. Although some central auditory processes may be difficult to change, especially in older adults, improvement in spoken language comprehension may be achieved through the development of listening strategies. Somewhat like the gains in memory seen with increasing age that are attributed to the development of mnemonic strategies rather than capacity (Pressley, 1982), improved spoken language comprehension may be realized through self-regulation of listening strategies. Interventions combining performance strategies (e.g., using context to derive meaning, invoking schemata to guide interpretation) plus self-control training are more successful than either approach in isolation (Brown, Campione, & Day, 1981). Moreover, the prospects for transfer or generalization of strategy use to other appropriate situations are excellent since the metacognitive components trained (i.e., planning, checking, and monitoring) are not task specific, but rather constitute a general strategy for problem solving (Brown, Campione, & Barclay, 1979; Lodico, Ghatala, Levin, Pressley, & Bell, 1983). Implementing executive or metacognitive strategies training in conjunction with auditory process training (e.g., auditory discrimination, temporal processing) provides a powerful intervention approach.

Metacognitive Knowledge

Regulation and deployment of metacognitive strategies require an adequately motivated individual in control of certain executive knowledge and functions. In particular, three types of knowledge (i.e., declarative, procedural, and conditional) are needed to effectively implement metacognitive strategies.

Declarative knowledge refers to knowledge that is known in a propositional manner. For example, an effective listener knows that prior knowledge of the topic and relevant vocabulary facilitate message comprehension. *Procedural knowledge* refers to awareness of the processes underlying effective listening and spoken language comprehension. An effective listener, for instance, knows how to scan the message for main ideas, how to paraphrase the message, and how to incorporate message context to facilitate message comprehension.

Declarative and procedural knowledge are necessary, but not sufficient for effective listening unless employed in conjunction with conditional knowledge. *Conditional knowledge* involves an awareness of conditions that affect listening, knowledge of why particular strategies work, and when to apply those strategies. For example, an effective listener would know that paraphrasing material may not be an optimal strategy when precise detail about the original message is required. Similarly, allocating disproportionate attention to the main idea of a message when the comprehension task requires understanding of a specific chemical reaction described in the message would be less effective and reveal deficient conditional knowledge.

The clinician may find an informal assessment of metacognitive strategies, prior to and during the therapy process, most revealing. By posing questions to the client that tap understanding of metacognitive knowledge bases and processes, the clinician is better prepared to train metacognitive strategy use. The reader may find the items of a metacognitive knowledge and strategies assessment developed for reading (*Index of Reading Awareness*) by Jacob and Paris (1987) easily adapted to explore clients' knowledge of the listening process.

Converting knowledge into practice also requires self-management knowledge. A skilled listener demonstrates planful listening by selectively deploying and coordinating resources and strategies to achieve spoken language comprehension. This process is controlled by the listener's executive processes of planning, evaluation, and regulation. Ongoing self-monitoring ensures the listener opportunities to recognize ineffectiveness and adjust plans and strategies to meet the changing demands and the successes and failures of the listening task. This adjustment process is the executive process of self-regulation.

Metacognitive Strategies

The skills and processes underlying the effective use of metacognitive strategies for listening comprehension include: (1) understanding task demands, (2) appropriately allocating attention, (3) identifying important parts of the message, (4) self-monitoring, (5) self-questioning, and (6) deployment of debugging strategies. Although a number of these processes take place automatically and tacitly in skilled listeners, they may require direct instruction and opportunities for application and reinforcement in clients with CAPD. Through practice, our clients will gain conscious knowledge and take deliberate actions to enhance listening.

A number of metacognitive approaches may be incorporated in CAPD management programs. Notwithstanding differences among these approaches, they promote active, self-regulation and share several distinguishing features. Typically, they provide explicit and detailed instruction regarding the goals of strategies and their application to tasks, as well as training self-regulation and self-monitoring of strategy deployment and outcomes of that deployment (Palinscar & Brown, 1987). Further, they encourage self-identification of strategies employed and the rationale for their use, as well as feedback about the efficacy of strategies for particular tasks (Palinscar & Brown, 1987; Pressley, Borkowski, & O'Sullivan, 1984).

Incorporating several metacognitive approaches in a management program is recommended because elements of one metacognitive approach often reinforce aspects of another. For instance, motivation is fundamental to assertiveness training, and attribution training strengthens motivation.

Eight metacognitive approaches useful in managing CAPD are discussed below. Attribution training, the first approach, targets motivation. The four cognitive behavior modification approaches promote active, self-regulatory listening and learning styles. Reciprocal teaching fosters self-esteem and self-regulation and is highly motivating. Selecting the appropriate cognitive style, yet another metacognitive intervention, is necessary to meet diverse processing demands and listening tasks. Finally, we discuss assertiveness training, which empowers clients and advances therapy goals.

Attribution Training

As explored in Chapter 1, individuals with CAPD are at risk for developing motivational problems as a consequence of chronic listening problems and the often associated academic or workplace failures, as well as the social frustrations attendant to decreased ability to integrate in a peer group or one's family. Indeed, some individuals with CAPD become reconciled to the belief that their listening abilities (and perhaps intellectual abilities as well) are poor and cannot be improved and that their efforts to succeed are futile. These beliefs lead to poor motivation and a deterioration in task persistence (Torgesen, 1980). Paradoxically, these beliefs are likely to infiltrate their perception of their successes as well as their failures. They begin to attribute successes to luck, an easy task, or the benevolence of a teacher, co-worker, or employer (Bryan, 1991; Butkowsky & Willows, 1980; Pearl, 1982; Torgesen, 1980).

Some will not succumb to this vicious cycle. Instead they will invoke a more self-protective explanation of their failings, maintaining confidence by blaming teachers, parents, employers, or other external agents or circumstances for their failures. Others attribute difficulties to insufficient effort (Licht, Kistner, Ozkaragoz, Shapiro, & Clausen, 1985; Speece, McKinney, & Appelbaum, 1985). Indeed, attributions of failure to insufficient effort have been shown to correlate with academic success (Kistner, Osborne, & LeVerrier, 1988).

Attribution (re)training is undertaken to instill causal attributions for failure to factors that are under the individual's control (e.g., insufficient effort) rather than to sensory or intellectual incapacity. Attribution training should lead to higher self-esteem and increased persistence when faced with challenging listening tasks and conditions (Medway & Venino, 1982; Thomas & Pashley, 1982). Although the use of appropriate goal structures and feedback can promote confidence and persistence (see Chapter 7), attribution retraining provides a more direct approach to re-establish self-confidence and persistence in individuals who demonstrate a maladaptive motivational pattern (Licht & Kistner, 1986). Even though children younger than 7 to 10 years of age are less likely to attribute failure to incapacity (Eshel & Klein, 1981; Rholes, Blackwell, Jordan, & Walters, 1980; Stipek, 1981; Stipek & Tannatt, 1984), incorporating attribution training in therapy programs for young children with CAPD offers a preventive approach to motivational problems.

Components of Attribution Training. Attribution retraining is undertaken in two steps. First, the client is confronted with some failure (e.g., an incorrect response to a question posed following an oral-aural story presentation). The second component involves teaching the client to attribute the failure to insufficient effort. In response to the client who incorrectly responds to a question, the clinician might tell the client that his or her answer was not correct, that he or she is working hard but should listen even more carefully. Likewise, successes should be attributed to effort, providing feedback that communicates that the response was correct and acknowledging that the client was listening carefully and trying hard.

The wording of attributional statements is key to the success of this method. Acknowledging hard work while urging even greater effort should motivate the client and result in improved performance and enhanced self-efficacy (Miller, Brickman, & Bolen, 1975; Schunk, 1982). Feedback that fails to recognize efforts already expended, indicating that the clinician perceived no effort or that the client was not indeed already working hard, are less likely to be effective (Miller et al., 1975; Schunk, 1982).

In addition to the specific wording of the attributional statements, the proportion of successes and failures, and scheduling of failures, also influence the effectiveness of attribution retraining. Although confronting failure is integral to attribution retraining, a moderate amount of success is necessary to establish a belief in the method's premise that increased effort will lead to increased success (Clifford, 1978; Dweck, 1975). Tasks must be structured to allow that degree of success. Moreover, persistence is fostered by varying the number of difficult items, which demand increased effort, within an activity (Chapin & Dyck, 1976).

Finally, and perhaps most importantly, attribution retraining must be credible. The validity of the new attributions can be established only if the increased effort does in fact lead to improved performance (Dweck, 1977). In the absence of such a *payoff,* the treatment effects will not persist or generalize (Licht & Kistner, 1986). Metacognitive and metalinguistic strategies must be available to the client and coupled with attribution retraining to maximize the chances that additional effort will lead to improved performance (Reid & Borkowski, 1987).

Advocating the inclusion of attribution retraining in a comprehensive management program should not be interpreted as denying or minimizing the presence of auditory processing deficits in the client with CAPD. Indeed, we recognize that auditory processing deficits are primary to the client's spoken language comprehension problems, compounded by secondary metacognitive deficits resulting from lack of experience with successful listening strategies and limited use of executive function. Further, we recognize that effort alone is not likely to overcome the deficits resulting from CAPD. Our position is that ensuring long-term maintenance and generalization of listening skills requires that the client learn to work harder and more strategically. Knowing how to work harder, through sustained effort coupled with listening strategies, is more likely to lead to permanent improvements in performance and spontaneous deployment of these strategies (Borkowski, Weyhing, & Carr, 1988; Fabricus & Hagen, 1984; Kendall & Braswell, 1982; Moynahan, 1978; Paris et al., 1982). As stated by Reid and Borkowski (1987), "self-attributions about the importance of effort in producing success serve an energizing function in the deployment of available strategies and sustain the cognitive search for alternative strategies in the face of learning obstacles" (p. 306). In the following sections, we present additional strategies to promote more effective listening.

Cognitive Behavior Modification

Cognitive behavior modification moves beyond mere instruction in strategy use. The goal of cognitive behavior modification is to induce self-control through a planful, reflective processing and response style (Lloyd, 1980). Characteristically, executive strategies, as well as task-specific strategies, are involved. Emphasizing the importance of informed and active clients, the client is instructed in the use of a strategy, including how to employ, monitor, check, and evaluate that strategy (Brown et al., 1981).

Cognitive behavior modification is classified into four categories: self-instruction, problem solving, self-regulation, and cognitive strategy training (Whitman, Burgio, & Johnson, 1984). Although there are differences in emphasis and procedures, there is considerable overlap among these categories (Meichenbaum, 1986; Whitman et al., 1984). Common to cognitive behavior modification procedures are: (1) involving clients as active collaborators in the clinical process, (2) modeling of the target strategy during training, (3) focusing on a reflective processing and response style, and (4) focusing on the relationship between the client's actions and task outcomes (Lloyd, 1980; Meichenbaum, 1986).

Demonstrating both the common and divergent foci of the four cognitive behavior modification approaches, self-instruction employs directive self-statements to train task-specific strategies and self-control; cognitive strategy training focuses on the former; and self-regulation training emphasizes the latter. Although incorporating self-instruction, self-monitoring, and self-regulation techniques, cognitive problem solving procedures are focused on yet a different aspect of the cognitive domain—reducing uncertainty and resolving problems. In practical application, procedures from more than one method are often combined to augment training effectiveness (Whitman et al., 1984). For example, Meichenbaum and Goodman's (1971) five-step self-instruction program may be employed across cognitive behavior training regimens. Also shared across the procedures is the use of daily logs or diaries. By encouraging the client to maintain a daily log exploring difficult listening situations and the relative value of strategies deployed to enhance listening, we promote self-monitoring of the effectiveness of listening comprehension strategies. The use of diaries and logs as homework also benefits generalization of executive and task-specific strategies and skills (Guevremont, 1990). (See Generalization in Chapter 7.)

Self-Instruction. Through self-instruction, clients are trained to formulate adaptive and self-directing verbal statements before and during a task or situation. In addition to listening training, self-instruction is particularly useful in addressing academic difficulties and impulsive and hyperactive behaviors (Hart & Morgan, 1993).

Meichenbaum and Goodman (1971) outlined five sequential steps comprising self-instruction: (1) task performance by the clinician while self-verbalizing aloud, (2) performance by the client while the clinician verbalizes, (3) performance by the client while self-instructing aloud, (4) performance by the client while whispering, and (5) performance by the client while self-instructing covertly. Training self-instruction by progressing through Meichenbaum and Goodman's five-step approach should promote inculcation and generalization of the self-instructional routine.

Several problem-solving skills are incorporated in self-instruction, as illustrated in Table 8–7. Steps 1 and 2 elicit planful, reflective responding. Step 2 also focuses the client's attention on relevant aspects of the task. Steps 3, 4, and 5 promote problem solving. The clinician may encourage general or, as in the case illustrated in Table 8–7, more specific problem-solving instructions depending on the nature of the task. Clients should be challenged to ask more sophisticated questions demanding higher level thinking commensurate with the message content and task requirements (Wilson, Lanza, &

Table 8–7. Self-instruction.

Steps	Statements
Attend, Plan, Reflect:	1. How do I listen carefully? I have to pay attention. I must not let myself become distracted. I must listen for important, key words, as well as content.
	2. What is the primary purpose of this message? To tell a story; to describe an event; to explain; to argue a point?
Problem Solving:	3. What key words have been stated? What do these key words tell me?
	4. What about the context? What experience do I bring to this message?
	5. What is the main message? What predictions or inferences are appropriate?
Monitoring, Evaluation, and Feedback:	6. Are my conclusions, predictions, and inferences correct? Do they follow from the spoken words? Are they logical?
	7. Yes, they are correct. I am an effective listener.

Barton, 1988). (The classification system of the cognitive domain developed by Bloom [1956] [i.e., knowledge, comprehension, application, analysis, synthesis, and evaluation] offers a hierarchical taxonomy to guide clients toward more creative, critical, and higher level questioning. Bloom's hierarchical taxonomy is described in Figure 8–1.) The clinician may find it helpful to move problem-solving instructions from the specific to more general as the client's skills increase. Self-monitoring and feedback are provided in step 6. If the client is not successful, it is helpful to include some strategy for coping with failure in step 6. As discussed in the preceding section, coping with failure may be best handled by self-attributions of failure to something under the client's control (e.g., improper strategy selec-

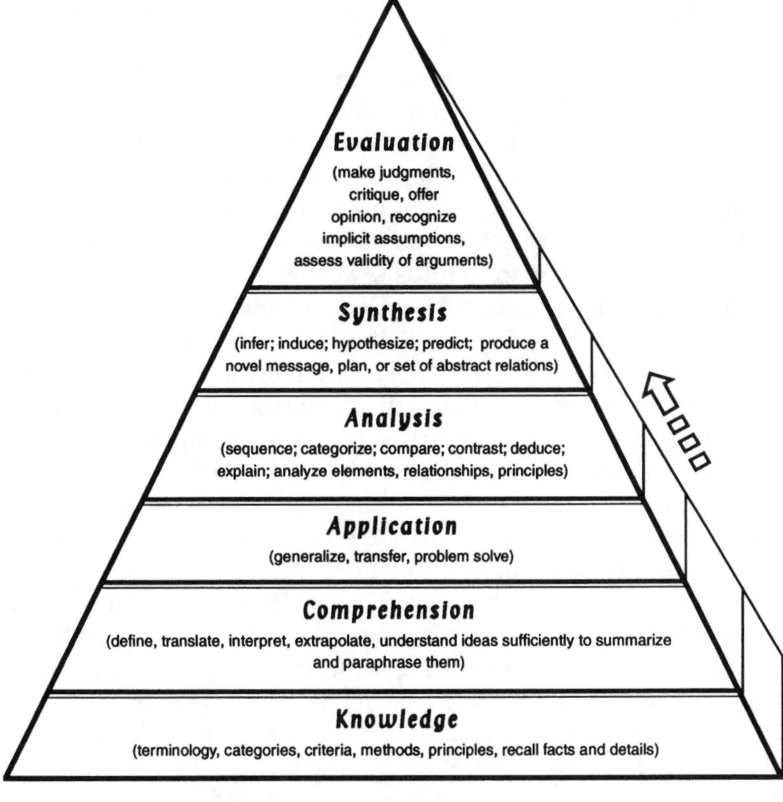

Figure 8–1. Bloom's taxonomy of the cognitive domain.

tion, insufficient effort). Self-reinforcement, the final and quite important step in the self-instruction routine, instills a sense of pride and accomplishment and should increase the client's motivation to transfer the self-instructional technique to novel situations.

Cognitive Problem Solving. Cognitive problem solving is a systematic process that leads clients to resolve problem situations. Basically a five-stage process, the clinician serves as a consultant as the client learns a self-control technique (Haaga & Davison, 1986). Clients with CAPD are taught to reconceive the potentially anxiety-producing listening situation as a problem to be solved. In treating the spoken message as a problem to be solved, listeners deploy executive processes in conjunction with the requisite auditory and language skills. They are taught to analyze situations and generate a variety of potentially viable responses, recognizing and implementing the most effective response. Further, they are helped to confront cognitive distortions (e.g., catastrophizing, jumping to conclusions), which may be sustaining unnecessary anxiety or fear (Hart & Morgan, 1993). Self-regulation procedures (described in the next section) are used to maintain and generalize the productive response (Goldfried & Davison, 1976). Cognitive problem solving is especially therapeutic when working with individuals with anxiety, fear, or phobias (Hart & Morgan, 1993) and has been used successfully in management of patients with tinnitus (Sweetow, 1986).

The clinician may model problem solving using Meichenbaum and Goodman's (1971) five-step self-instruction program, which was outlined in the preceding section. Problem solving begins with preparation or familiarizing oneself with the nature of the problem. Perhaps the most important stage of problem solving, the individual must understand the problem in all its facets (D'Zurilla, 1986). The second stage requires the generation of hypotheses regarding solutions to the problem. In the third stage, one evaluates the solution options, considers their utility and predicts possible costs or consequences, and selects the best one. The fourth stage is bifurcated. If a viable solution is found, it is implemented; if no solution is deemed tenable, the incubation phase begins during which no active effort is expended toward solving the problem (Halpern, 1984). Ironically, it is during this phase that solutions often appear as an epiphany or *out of the blue* (Halpern, 1984, p. 163). A fifth stage in the process involves the monitoring and evaluation of one's performance in relation to solving the problem. Self-monitoring homework assignments are useful in measuring progress. Self-reinforcement for successful problem solving (e.g., spoken language understanding) should lead to enhanced self-efficacy and generalization of the process (Haaga & Davison, 1986). (See Motivation and Efficacy in Chapter 7.) A flow chart illustrating cognitive problem solving in spoken language comprehension is presented in Figure 8–2.

In addition to self-instruction and self-monitoring, cognitive rehearsal is another technique that may be employed throughout the problem-solving process (Haaga & Davison, 1986). For example, by mentally reviewing the listening task prior to completing it, cognitive rehearsal provides a means of identifying potential obstacles, solutions, and preventive steps so that one may listen successfully.

Cognitive problem solving can be adapted for group work. Either the clinician or a group member introduces a problem to the group. The group proceeds systematically through the problem-solving process to reach some resolution. By using a problem that may arise within the group as an exercise for problem solving, the clinician can capitalize on the group dynamic to teach problem solving.

Self-Regulation Procedures. Self-control is the goal of self-regulation training (Brown et al., 1981; Whitman et al., 1984). Self-regulation is a three-stage process involving self-monitoring, self-evaluation, and self-reinforcement (Kanfer & Gaelick, 1991). Training begins by increasing awareness of the behavior targeted for control and proceeds by teaching goal setting and self-monitoring skills for behavioral change (Whitman et al., 1984). The client may be asked to monitor qualitatively and quantitatively, noting aspects of the process and his or her emotional or attitudinal state, as well as quantifying successful performance. If information obtained through self-monitoring matches the individual's standards or listening comprehension goals, a favorable self-evaluation is rendered. This positive outcome is followed by self-reinforcement, which refers primarily to internal satisfaction and heightened motivation rather than self-administered reward (Kanfer & Gaelick, 1991). A working model of self-regulation is depicted in Figure 8–3.

Self-regulation training promotes effective listening by encouraging the listener to monitor comprehension processes to determine whether they are meeting his or her comprehension needs. When comprehension errors, disruptions, or inadequacies are detected, the listener learns to modify strategies to handle ambiguities, inconsistencies, or complexities that might otherwise compromise spoken language understanding (Danks & End, 1987).

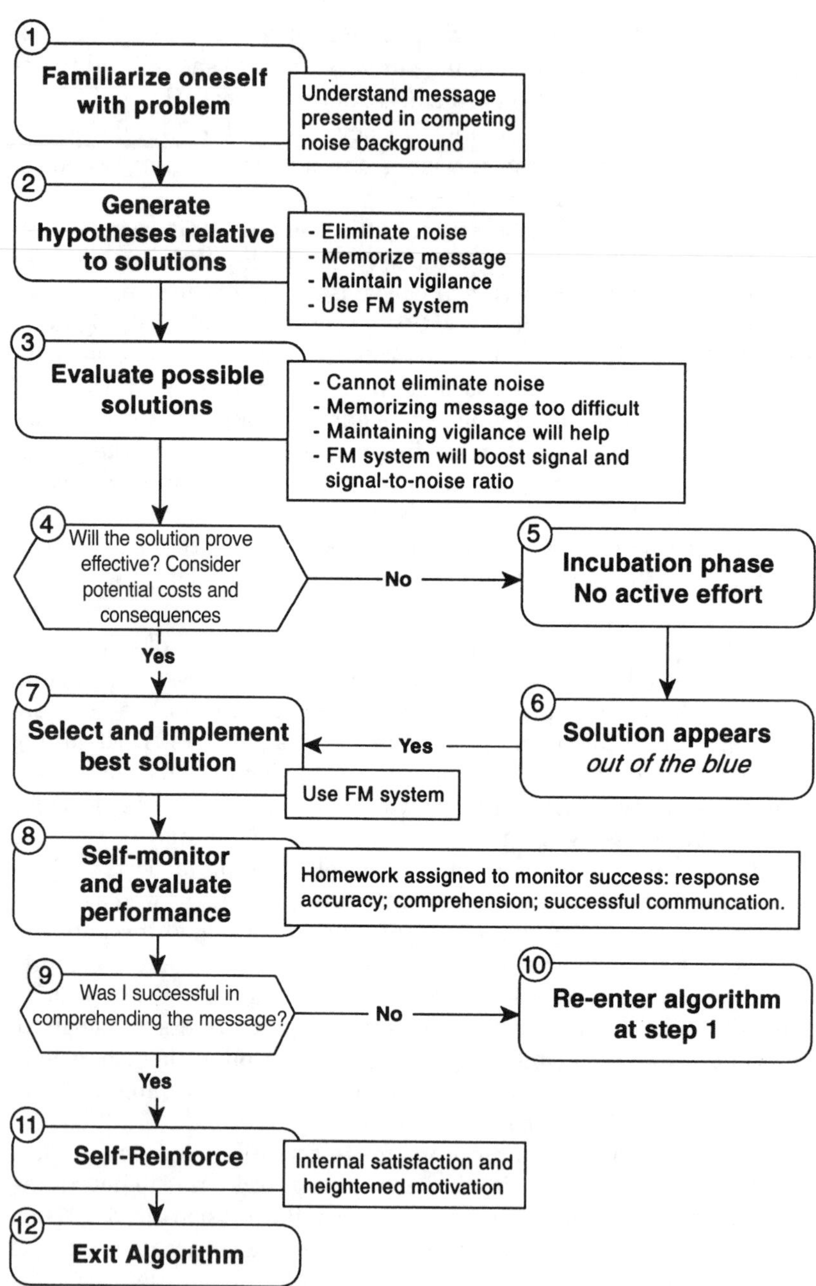

Figure 8–2. Cognitive problem solving in comprehending spoken language.

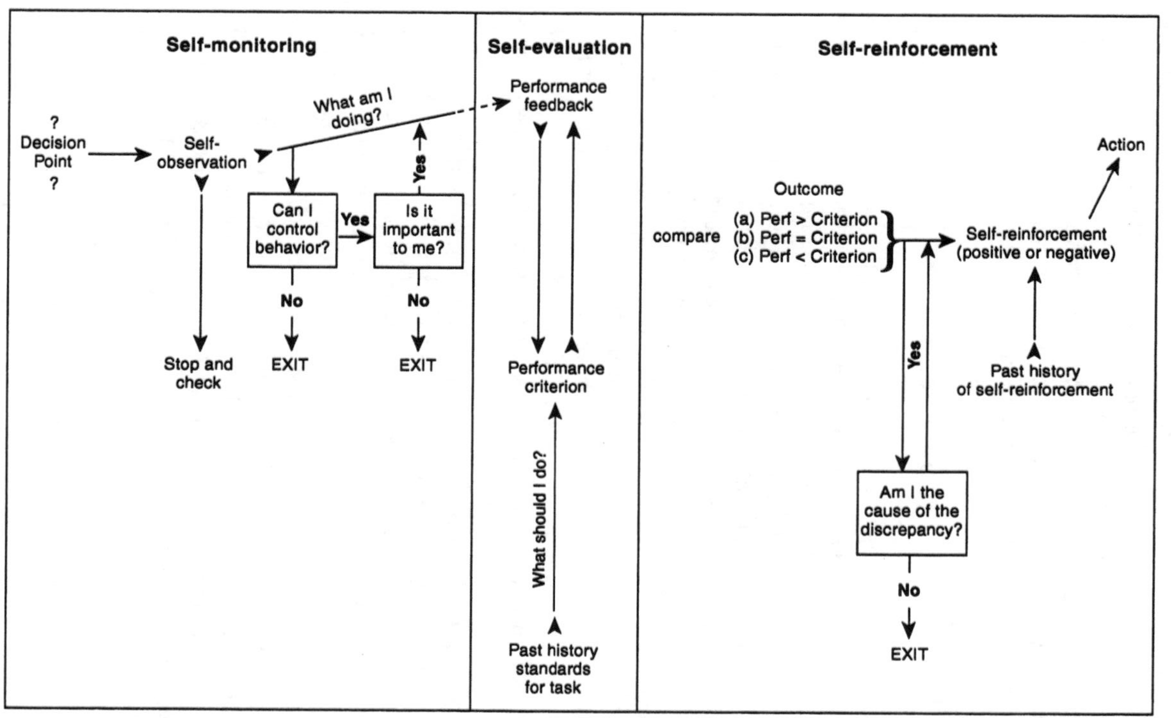

Figure 8–3. Working model of self-regulation. (Perf = performance) (From "Self-management methods" by F.H. Kanfer and L. Gaelick, 1991, p. 311. In F.H. Kanfer and A.P. Goldstein (Eds.), *Helping people change: A textbook of methods* (4th ed.). Copyright 1991, Allyn & Bacon. All rights reserved. Reprinted by permission.

Cognitive Strategy Training. Cognitive strategy training teaches specific strategies underlying effective performance (Brown & French, 1979). The goal is to help clients become skilled in the use of specific task strategies and more aware of their own cognitive processes (Whitman et al., 1984). Cognitive strategies may be trained following Meichenbaum and Goodman's (1971) five-step self-instruction program. Extended training of the strategy and feedback on the strategy's effectiveness are crucial to successful implementation of cognitive strategy training (Whitman et al., 1984).

Reciprocal Teaching

Consistent with the adage that we learn best that which we teach, reciprocal teaching involves alternating roles between the client and clinician, allowing the client to assume the role of teacher as well as student (Casanova, 1989; Chermak et al., 1996; Palincsar & Brown, 1984). In addition to its potential to boost self-esteem and self-efficacy, reciprocal teaching provides an excellent opportunity for clients to anchor their executive process knowledge by making explicit their knowledge and use of strategies. Reciprocal teaching has been demonstrated to be effective in producing gains in reading comprehension, self-monitoring, memory, and health education, including hearing conservation (Chermak et al., 1996; Clarke, MacPherson, Holmes, & Jones, 1986; Palincsar & Brown, 1984, 1986; Paris, Wixson, & Palincsar, 1986).

Reciprocal teaching is based on the following principles and procedures: (1) the clinician-teacher actively models the desired behavior, making the processing strategies overt, explicit, and concrete; (2) strategies are modeled in context; (3) discussions focus on the content of the message as well as the client's understanding of the strategies being used for message comprehension; (4) the clinician provides feedback appropriate to the client's level of mastery; and (5) responsibility for comprehenion is transferred from the clinician to the client as soon as the client demonstrates an adequate success level (Harris & Sipay, 1990). Reciprocal teaching can be expanded to include peer tutoring.

Cognitive Style and Reasoning

Reasoning involves the evaluation of arguments, drawing of inferences and conclusions, and generation and testing of hypotheses (Nickerson, 1986). Effective listening requires reasoning to critically evaluate and ultimately reconstruct the messages we hear, as well as the flexibility to invoke the cognitive style that best meets changing task demands. Inflexible reasoning and sole reliance on any one cognitive style is ineffective in meeting the variety of processing demands and listening tasks, especially given the imprecision and ambiguity inherent in acoustic and linguistic signals. Evidence of that ambiguity and imprecision is seen in auditory illusions such as phonemic restoration and verbal transformation effects; polysemy, including homonyms and heteronyms; and figurative language such as metaphors, idioms, and proverbs (Bard, Shillcock, & Altmann, 1988; Marslen-Wilson & Tyler, 1980; Warren & Warren, 1970). The inadequacy of a single cognitive style can be seen in the failure to infer due to overreliance on literal interpretation. This overreliance leads to misunderstanding a message's content.

Similarly, overreliance on the cognitive style of top-down processing may cause schema inflexibility, biasing interpretation and impeding comprehension. As noted earlier (see Schema Theory and Use), schema activation demonstrates the complementary function of bottom-up and top-down processes (Rumelhart, 1980). Through top-down processes the listener recognizes patterns and evidence supporting a schema and upholds the interpretation supported by the schema. Schema inflexibility would prevent the listener from incorporating accumulating data that are incompatible with the activated schema; the listener would choose instead to discard inconsistent data rather than use the emerging pattern to support the activation of an alternate and more appropriate schema (Rumelhart, 1980).

The model of central auditory processing presented in Chapter 1 illustrates the necessity for the operation of complementary cognitive styles for spoken language comprehension. The importance of accessing multiple cognitive styles is amplified for persons with CAPD whose deficient auditory processes render them less able to cope with degraded acoustic signals and for whom sole reliance on bottom-up processing would leave them extremely vulnerable to comprehension problems. Although we train our clients with CAPD to take advantage of information revealed through bottom-up processing (e.g., auditory discrimination, including changes in prosody), we also emphasize the benefits of top-down processing for *reading between the lines*, recognizing conceptual nuances, reaching auditory and grammatic closure, and inferring or abstracting meaning.

Although skilled listeners often unconsciously and automatically adjust their cognitive style to meet the processing demands of the task, less skilled listeners must be instructed to make these smooth transitions and reach a level of automaticity. For example, our clients with CAPD may benefit from opportunities to recognize the benefits of analysis and reflection prior to synthesizing information and converging on an interpretation of a complex message, which may contain new vocabulary and require complicated reasoning.

Cognitive style is subject to change through training. For example, children become more reflective following training in the use of a verbal self-control strategy (Craighead, Wilcoxon-Craighead, & Meyers, 1978). Given the importance of cognitive style flexibility for spoken language comprehension and the opportunity for change, instruction promoting cognitive flexibility should benefit individuals with CAPD.

Deductive and Inductive Inferencing. Effective reasoning, and therefore effective listening, requires the range of cognitive approaches to information processing, including both deduction and induction and analysis and synthesis. Inductive inferencing involves generalization, reasoning from the particulars to the general; deductive inferencing involves reasoning from the general to the particular (Nickerson, 1986). Relative to spoken language comprehension, it is clear that individuals infer information not specifically presented in the message, but which may be implied and induced or deduced from the available patterns of information.

Inferencing skills can be developed through the context-derived vocabulary-building technique described earlier. Short stories requiring inferencing on the basis of perceptual information, logic, and/or evidence (see Gerber, 1993c) also are useful. Activities that require the drawing of inferences can be entertaining and appropriate for younger clients. For example children's poetry requiring inferencing for interpretation can be read to younger children and discussed. In addition to promoting cognitive style flexibility, inferencing also challenges memory, as stored knowledge is essential to the inferencing process.

Attention to the appropriate use of other cognitive styles (e.g., divergent/convergent, impulsive/reflective, adaptive/innovative, synthetic/analytic, field dependent/field independent) should also be introduced in therapy.

Assertiveness Training. Assertion can be defined as "self-expression through which one stands up for one's own basic human rights without violating the basic human rights of others" (Kelley, 1979, p. 14). The goal of assertion is to attain personal effectiveness by communicating what one feels, thinks, and wants. Assertive behavior is self-enhancing and empowering, promoting good feelings about one's self, as well as furthering attainment of desired goals (Alberti & Emmons, 1978). Assertiveness can be learned (Bornstein, Bellack, & Hersen, 1977; Rehm, Fuchs, Roth, Kornblith, & Romano, 1979); however, self-confidence and self-esteem are prerequisite (Kelley, 1979). Motivation drives assertiveness; without a desire to succeed, one is not likely to assume the personal responsibility inherent to assertiveness. Similarly, command of basic interpersonal and communication skills is necessary to effective assertiveness.

It has been our clinical experience that a client's assertiveness is directly related to more successful treatment outcomes. Because assertive clients tend to be more actively involved in planning and directing their own therapy, they tend to derive greater gain. Moreover, they tend to generalize new strategies and skills to everyday life contexts.

Integral to assertion are verbal and nonverbal skills and a positive cognitive *mindset* (Kelley, 1979). Assertion typically involves a verbal exchange; the individual must formulate and deliver an assertive message (Kelley, 1979). In addition to the actual words used to express the assertion, the effectiveness of the assertion will be influenced by the nonverbal aspects of the message's delivery, including paralinguistic elements (e.g., vocal intensity, intonation, rhythm), kinesics (e.g., facial expression, posture, gestures), and proxemics (e.g., distance between parties, seating arrangements). Nonverbal cues that fail to corroborate the verbal message will weaken the effectiveness of that message.

A positive cognitive set reinforces one's confidence in the value and right to assert and motivates one to persist (Kelley, 1979). Since anxiety can interfere with assertion, training in anxiety-reduction skills may be a necessary precursor to work on the verbal and nonverbal dimensions of assertion.

Assertiveness training techniques may involve modeling; guided practice; coaching; homework and self-management; readings; and small group discussion (Kelley, 1979). Anxiety reduction techniques include relaxation, imagery, self-talk, coping, and desensitization (Kendall, 1992). The reader may consult Kelley (1979) for detailed discussion of assertiveness training techniques and Kendall (1992) for discussion of procedures used for coping with and managing anxiety.

CONSIDERATIONS FOR PRESCHOOL AGE CHILDREN

Early identification and diagnosis of CAPD in children is especially important given the significant adverse impact CAPD can have on communication, academic achievement, and social function (Musiek & Chermak, 1995; Keith, 1981b; Willeford, 1985). Unfortunately, with the exception of the *Pediatric Speech Intelligibility* (PSI) *Test* (Jerger & Jerger, 1984), criterion measures of CAPD with sufficiently documented reliability and validity are not yet available for this age group (Musiek & Chermak, 1994). Efficiency data, even for screening measures of CAPD, are sparse for this population (Stach, 1992). Since a firm diagnosis of CAPD may be impossible to obtain with this age group, it is probably prudent to involve preschool children suspected of, or at-risk for, CAPD (e.g., children with histories of recurrent and persistent otitis media with effusion) in programs designed to promote development of auditory perceptual skills.

Programs for these children should build on the philosophy of whole language, which emphasizes the principles of natural language learning (Norris & Damico, 1990). The development of auditory perceptual and auditory-language skills may be facilitated through a highly responsive language environment involving planned activities that are interesting to the child and provide natural opportunities for listening and communication. Repetition of daily routines creates a sense of familiarity, allowing the child to focus attention on new auditory information. Collaboration between speech and hearing professionals, preschool teachers, and families maximizes the transfer of skills to daily routines and other settings (Chermak, 1993).

Because listening is fundamental to learning at all levels, children should benefit from experiences early in life that encourage careful listening. Creating an optimal listening environment is crucial to the success of early intervention/prevention. Strategies used to enhance the acoustic signal and the listening environment for individuals with hearing impairment are also appropriate for children suspected of, or at risk for, CAPD. Presenting visual information (e.g., pictures, facial expression, gestures and other nonverbal cues) to support and reinforce auditory information also will enhance the saliency of the acoustic signal.

Strategies to enhance the acoustic signal include reducing the distance between child and speaker (e.g., preferential seating, one-on-one or small group activities); gaining the child's attention before speaking to her or him; speaking slowly, clearly, at a comfortably loud level, and with natural intonation; using appropriate vocabulary; repeating key words and rephrasing important information; allowing adequate time for processing and responding; and using frequent comprehension checks to ascertain that information was understood

(Roberts & Medley, 1995). In addition, personal or sound field FM amplification may prove useful in group situations in providing a clearer, louder signal over unwanted background noise (Flexer, 1994).

Strategies to enhance the listening environment include reduction of noise background through decreasing or eliminating noise (e.g., turning off televisions, radios, dishwashers), architectural modifications (e.g., using partitions to separate spaces, retrofitting appliances), and furnishings (e.g., carpet, drapes, upholstered furniture, and acoustic ceiling tiles). (Strategies to enhance the acoustic signal and the listening environment are elaborated more fully in Chapter 9.)

The following activities provide opportunities to reinforce good listening skills through bottom-up (e.g., discriminating sounds) and top-down processes (e.g, being read to) and may be used with older children, as well as with 3- to 5-year-olds. An activity to nurture emerging executive functions is also described. Activities also may be designed to promote the development of metalinguistic skills (e.g., rhyme play, knock-knock jokes) (van Kleeck, 1994). Gillet (1993) provides numerous exercises designed to develop auditory perceptual and listening skills and lists relevant commercially available products.

Listening to Stories

Reading aloud to children serves several purposes, including concept learning, vocabulary building, and practice in selective listening (Musiek & Chermak, 1995). To encourage selective listening, target words, for which the child should listen, should be designated before beginning the story. For example, children might be instructed to raise their hands each time a word is read that represents an animal. Focusing on target words may also encourage the child to listen for subtle prosodic cues (e.g., intonation, stress). To ensure that the child listens to the story and not only to individual words, comprehension questions should be posed at the end of the story to promote listening for meaning. A story grammar might be used to formulate questions (e.g., where and when did events in the story take place [setting]; what did the main character do [action]; what happened as a result of the main character's action [consequences]). Posing questions that require tracking of both the story context and the designated target words promotes auditory closure and comprehension. Multisensory integration can be fostered by allowing the child to examine the accompanying pictures and words as the story is read aloud. Joint book reading, wherein the caregiver and child elaborate on the pictures in a book or sections of the text that are of particular interest to the child seems to foster vocabulary development and reading skills (Ninio, 1980; Teale, 1984; Wells, 1985).

Following Directions

In addition to providing authentic contexts in which the child must follow sequenced directives to successfully complete the task, games can be organized that require the child to follow directions presented auditorily (e.g., *Simon Says*) (Musiek & Chermak, 1995). The child can be asked to repeat the directive before acting to enhance reauditorization and transference to a motor activity (the directive should require some motor task). *Telephone* and other games requiring children to repeat what they have heard to other people and barrier games in which the child must follow directions presented auditorily to create something (e.g., building or drawing) also are effective activities to promote listening.

Directives may range from simple to complex, involving one or multiple sequenced actions. Oral directives may be made more complex by inserting adjective sequences (e.g., "Touch the big blue circle and the small red circle"), prepositions (e.g., "Pick up the blue crayon and place it beside the book"), a number of facts (e.g., "Find the two pictures of animals in a stack of photographs. Find the picture of the teacher. Find five pictures of toys"), or using more sophisticated linguistic concepts (e.g., "After I point to my nose, you point to yours"). The barrier game offers a particularly challenging opportunity to focus on listening as the child attempts to replicate a configuration of objects on the other side of the barrier without the benefit of visual cues by asking questions and listening to the responses.

Group actions requiring cooperation among the children may be used, and children can be given the chance to act as clinicians (i.e., reciprocal teaching) by generating directives for others to follow, thereby building confidence and self-esteem.

Discriminating Sounds

For most preschool children, discriminating differences among sounds is a challenging, yet engaging, task. Environmental sounds differing in intensity, frequency, duration, and quality can be used to develop auditory discrimination. For example, a child might be asked to state which of three bells of different pitches has the highest, middle, and lowest pitch. Identifying different but familiar voices is also an excellent exercise. To increase task difficulty, the speakers can alter their voices, speak quickly, say short words or consonant-vowel combinations, or use a combination of these three modifications (Musiek & Chermak, 1995).

Planning

By age 5 years, children have begun to develop metacognitive knowledge and executive strategies (Kreitler & Kreitler, 1987). Given the importance of these strategies to listening comprehension (as discussed briefly in the introductory sections of this chapter and elaborated upon in Chapter 1), activities to reinforce and nurture these strategies are advisable. Short scenarios and follow-up questions that require planning knowledge can provide material for such activities (Kreitler & Kreitler, 1987), as illustrated in the following scenario.

> Isaac and Alina were both planning birthday parties for the same day. Due to uncomfortably high temperatures in the mid-afternoon, both children wanted lunch-time parties. Dinner parties would be too late in the day. They both wanted their parties at *McDonald's*. The management said they could both have parties at *McDonald's,* but they would have to share the space. If you were Alina or Isaac, how would you plan your party so that it did not interfere with the other child's celebration?

CONSIDERATIONS FOR ADULTS AND OLDER ADULTS

The adult and older adult with CAPD present a different clinical profile than that of a younger person with CAPD. A neuromorphological disorder is suspected in the majority of youngsters with CAPD, particularly when associated with learning disabilities; in contrast, the central auditory processing deficits of adults are likely the result of fairly circumscribed and identifiable lesions of the central auditory nervous system (Musiek & Gollegly, 1988; Musiek, Gollegly, Lamb, & Lamb, 1990). The central auditory processing deficits of older adults, although perhaps less circumscribed, have a neurologic basis, resulting from accumulated damage or deterioration to the central auditory nervous system due to aging, neural insult, and/or neurodegenerative disease (Baran & Musiek, 1991). Moreover, adults and older adults are experiencing loss or disruption of processing functions that were previously intact, while children with CAPD may never have developed efficient processing skills.

Whereas efforts to acquire or recover normal (or equivalent) function in children should prove fruitful due to the inherent plasticity of their developing brains, interventions for adults and older adults will usually focus on compensation rather than recovery of function due to the reduced plasticity inherent to their mature central nervous system (ASHA, 1996). Remedial approaches may still be appropriate with adults and older adults who have suffered acute brain insults where opportunity for spontaneous recovery and/or stimulation-induced recovery of function presents itself (ASHA, 1996). Likewise, compensatory strategies may be appropriate for children during periods of (re)learning and for skills not amenable to functional adequacy. In any case, the prognosis for effective utilization of compensatory or remedial strategies will be determined in large part by the source of the CAPD (i.e., circumscribed lesion or pervasive neuropathology). An older adult suffering from aphasia is less likely to benefit as much from CAPD treatment as would an otherwise normal older adult with presbycusis who is experiencing CAPD as a result of the aging central auditory nervous system (ASHA, 1996). Clearly, the group and individual differences resulting from variation in intellectual, cognitive, linguistic, and psychosocial state will influence treatment outcome and must necessarily influence treatment delivery.

Older adults experience difficulty understanding speech in competing noise backgrounds (CHABA Working Group on Speech Understanding and Aging, 1988). Although peripheral reductions in sensitivity, particularly at the high frequencies, account for some of these difficulties, other factors including central auditory nervous system changes and/or senescent changes in cognition may also contribute to reduced speech understanding in noise among older adults (CHABA Working Group on Speech Understanding and Aging, 1988). Notwithstanding results to the contrary, a significant body of research demonstrates that age-related decline in spoken language comprehension cannot be explained on the basis of peripheral hearing loss or cognitive decline alone (Jerger, 1992; Jerger, Jerger, Oliver, & Pirozzolo, 1989; Jerger, Jerger, & Pirozzolo, 1991; Jerger, Stach, Pruitt, Harper, & Kirby, 1989). Positive correlations between perceived degree of hearing handicap and central auditory nervous system status (Fire, Lesner, & Newman, 1991) underscore both the role of CAPD in compromising spoken language understanding and the importance of intervention to improve central processing function. (See Life Span Considerations in Chapter 7.)

There is little doubt, however, that peripheral deficits and cognitive decline or differences could exacerbate the effects of a CAPD. For example, older adults with peripheral and central auditory deficits receive less benefit from hearing aid use (Stach, Loiselle, & Jerger, 1991). Moreover, even age-related cognitive style differences affect processing outcomes. For example, Craig, Kim, Rhyner, and Chirillo (1993) found that older adults required longer duration segments to correctly identify monosyllabic word targets. They interpreted these results to suggest that older adults may impose greater lexical restraint than younger adults, displaying less flexible lexical searching behavior. Older adults may present differences in decision-making strategies and reduction in the overall speed of processing, which exacerbate difficulties resolving spoken language (Craig et al., 1993).

Given the older adult with CAPD's primary complaint of difficulty understanding spoken language in the presence of background noise, as well as the frequent co-occurrence of peripheral and central auditory deficits among older adults (Stach et al., 1991), management of CAPD in older adults must begin by considering amplification, preferably a personal frequency-modulated (FM) system. The remote microphone technology employed in FM systems is more effective than hearing aids in reducing the background competition, which interferes with the older adult's ability to understand spoken language (Stach et al., 1991; Stach, Loiselle, Jerger, Mintz, & Taylor, 1987). The management program should also include development of strategies to enhance utilization of central resources (e.g., auditory discrimination in context, flexible cognitive style, etc.). (See Frequency-Modulated [FM] Assistive Listening Systems in Chapter 9.)

SUMMARY

Improved listening ability and spoken language comprehension are the goals of intervention for CAPD. To achieve these goals, we must encourage listeners to regulate their listening strategies. Coupling auditory process training with metalinguistic and metacognitive strategy training helps listeners structure auditory input and orchestrate information processing. Moreover, structuring therapy to support induction or discovery learning, as well as direct instruction, empowers clients to invoke complementary strategies to meet the variety of processing demands and listening tasks. Based on the data available, we believe our approach provides a powerful intervention program likely to lead to generalization of skills across settings. Additional study of our methods is needed, however, to ascertain their efficacy.

SUGGESTED READINGS

Bergenske, M. D. (1987). The missing link in narrative story mapping. *The Reading Teacher, 41,* 333–335.

Catts, H.W. (1991). Facilitating phonological awareness: Role of speech-language pathologists. *Language, Speech, and Hearing Services in Schools, 22*, 196–203.

Cole, R., & Jakimik, J. (1980). A model of speech perception. In R. Cole (Ed.), *Perception and prediction of fluent speech* (pp. 133–160). Englewood Cliffs, NJ: Lawrence Erlbaum.

Gerber, A. (Ed.). (1993). *Language-related learning disabilities: Their nature and treatment*. Baltimore: Paul H. Brookes.

Gillet, P. (1993). *Auditory processes*. Novato, CA: Academic Therapy Publications.

Gordon, C.J. (1989). Teaching narrative text structure: A process approach to reading and writing. In K.D. Muth (Ed.), *Children's comprehension of text* (pp. 79–102). Newark, DE: International Reading Association.

Gordon, C.J., & Rennie, B.J. (1986). Restructuring content schemata: An intervention study. *Reading Reseach and Instruction, 26*, 162–188.

Harrell, M., Parente, F., Bellingrath, E.G., & Lisicia, K.A. (1992). *Cognitive rehabilitation of memory: A practical guide.* Gaithersburg, MD: Aspen.

Harris, J.E. (1992). Ways to help memory. In B. Wilson & N. Moffat (Eds.), *Clinical management of memory problems* (pp. 56–82). San Diego: Singular Publishing Group.

Idol, L. (1987). Group story mapping: A comprehension strategy for both skilled and unskilled readers. *Journal of Learning Disabilities, 20*, 196–205.

Jacob, J.E., & Paris, S.G. (1987). Children's metacognition about reading: Issues in definition, measurement and instruction. *Educational Psychology, 22*(3/4), 255–278.

Katz, J., & Wilde, L. (1994). Auditory processing disorders. In J. Katz (Ed.), *Handbook of clinical audiology* (4th ed., pp. 490–502). Baltimore: Williams & Wilkins.

Kelley, C. (1979). *Assertion training: A facilitator's guide.* San Diego: University Associates.

Kendall, P.C. (1992). *Anxiety disorders in youth.* Boston: Allyn and Bacon.

Lasky, E.Z., & Cox, L. C. (1983). Auditory processing and language interaction: Evaluation and intervention strategies. In E.Z. Lasky & J. Katz (Eds.), *Central auditory processing* (pp. 243–268). Baltimore: University Park Press.

McIntyre, T. (1989). *A resource book for remediating common behaviors and learning problems.* Boston: Allyn and Bacon.

Pearson, P.D. (1982). Asking questions about stories. *Ginn Occasional Papers*, No. 15. Columbus, OH: Ginn.

Reutzel, D.R. (1985). Story maps improve comprehension. *The Reading Teacher, 38*, 400–404.

Schneider, D. (1992). Audiologic management of central auditory processing disorders. In J. Katz, N. Stecker, & D. Henderson (Eds.), *Central auditory processing: A transdisciplinary view* (pp. 161–168). St. Louis: Mosby.

Sloan, C. (1986). *Treating auditory processing difficulties in children.* San Diego: College-Hill Press.

Wiig, E.H., & Semel, E. (1984). *Language assessment and intervention for the learning disabled.* Columbus, OH: Charles E. Merrill.

Willeford, J.A., & Burleigh, J.M. (1985). *Handbook of central auditory processing disorders in children.* Orlando, FL: Grune & Stratton.

Young, M.L., & Protti-Patterson, E. (1984). Management perspectives of central auditory problems in children: Top-down and bottom-up considerations. *Seminars in Hearing, 5*(3), 251–261.

CHAPTER

9

ENHANCING THE ACOUSTIC SIGNAL AND THE LISTENING ENVIRONMENT

The second of two complementary approaches to managing central auditory processing disorders is discussed in this chapter. Following the presentation of auditory training and metalinguistic and metacognitive strategies in Chapter 8, this chapter describes a variety of means to improve the quality of the acoustic signal and the listening environment. These interventions serve to reduce stimulus uncertainty and thereby enhance spoken language understanding. The application of these techniques to group listening environments, and in particular to the classroom, is emphasized. Use of personal and sound field FM technology and physical space alterations to benefit listening in noisy or reverberent environments, as well as modification of instructional strategies for the classroom, are discussed. Also emphasized is the role of the speech-language pathologist in evaluating individuals with central auditory processing disorder (CAPD), qualifying youngsters with CAPD for special education services, and implementing classroom management strategies.

DIAGNOSING CENTRAL AUDITORY PROCESSING DISORDERS AND ASSOCIATED COMMUNICATION PROBLEMS

As discussed in previous chapters, CAPD can adversely impact language learning and language use and often presents in association with diverse clinical conditions (e.g., attention deficits, developmental language disorder, aphasia, traumatic brain injury). Differential diagnosis requires a team approach, involving complete audiologic and speech-language evaluations to assess auditory and communicative performance and determine a diagnosis reflecting the primary factors, as well as secondary deficits, contributing to the observed functional deficits (ASHA, 1996). Further, neuropsychological and psychoeducational evaluations are needed to ascertain the status of cognitive and metacognitive systems and determine academic achievement levels.

A thorough understanding of primary and secondary deficits influences treatment decisions; however, the importance of comprehensive evaluation and differential diagnosis with school-age children is magnified because eligibility for special education services and, thus, effective intervention programming, depends on documentation of the nature and extent to which CAPD impacts a child's attention and learning. Diagnosis of CAPD in the absence of concurrent diagnosis of learning disability or attention deficit disorder may not be sufficient to qualify a student for special educational services. (See Qualifying Youngsters With CAPD for Special Education Services.)

Speech-Language Assessment

The speech-language pathologist is an essential member of the interdisciplinary team responsible for the differential diagnosis of CAPD. The speech-language pathologist administers a battery of tests to evaluate speech and language ability and communicative function of children and adults suspected of having CAPD. The evaluation should assess both expressive and receptive language, as well as metalinguistic abilities (Friel-Patti, 1994a; Sloan, 1980b; van Kleeck, 1994).

Although comprehensive evaluation is required, certain components of the evaluation should be emphasized, given their potential to inform management of CAPD. For example, assessment of vocabulary is particularly relevant because of the strong correlation between vocabulary and listening comprehension (Perfetti, 1985; Samuels, 1987;

Sticht & James, 1984). Similarly, examination of grammatical morphology is especially important since grammatical inflections (e.g., plural *-s*, past tense *-ed*), which are typically unstressed and of shorter duration, are less perceptually salient and more perceptually challenging for the youngster with CAPD who has temporal processing deficits and limited language experience (Leonard, Sabbadini, Volterra, & Leonard, 1988; Sloan, 1992).

Although the language profiles of youngsters with CAPD are highly variable (Sloan, 1980a, 1980b), metalinguistic deficits, including segmentation and sequencing deficits which can impact reading and spelling (Sloan, 1986; van Kleeck, 1994), often are evident (Friel-Patti, 1994a). It is essential, therefore, that the speech and language evaluation include assessment of metalanguage. So, for example, the *Test of Language Competence* (Wiig & Secord, 1985) might be useful in illuminating difficulties in understanding ambiguous sentences and drawing inferences. The Formulated Sentences Subtest of the *Clinical Evaluation of Language Fundamentals-Third Edition* (CELF-3) (Semel, Wiig, & Secord, 1996) may provide some information concerning understanding of conjunctions (e.g., *and, because, but, before, after*), which comprise the formal schemata discussed in Chapter 8. Selected tests of metalanguage are listed in Table 9–1.

Neuropsychological and psychoeducational evaluations are also useful for differential diagnosis and intervention planning. Neuropsychological assessment ascertains the status of cognitive and metacognitive systems. For example, instruments such as the *Swanson-Cognitive Processing Test* (Swanson, 1996), *Auditory Continuous Performance Test* (Keith, 1994b), *Visual Continuous Performance Test* (Rosvold, Mirsky, Sarason, Bransome, & Beck, 1956), and *Wisconsin Card Sort* (Heaton, 1981) provide systematic measures of executive function, the self-control system that regulates behavior. Psychoeducational assessment determines academic achievement level. Although many speech-language pathologists refer to psychologists for these assessments, pertinent information also may be obtained through administration of standard speech-language instruments. For example, some understanding of working memory may be inferred through the ability to follow directions contained in the embedded language of the *Revised Token Test* (McNeil & Prescott, 1978). The reader is referred to Obrzut and Hynd (1991) for in-depth discussion of neuropsychological assessment methods.

Observations of an individual's behavior during test administration also are revealing. Dynamic assessment, an interactive assessment approach, provides a model and framework to guide observation. By focusing on the means and strategies by which individuals

Table 9–1. Selected tests of metalanguage.

Analysis of the Language of Learning
Auditory Conceptualization Test
Clinical Evaluation of Language Fundamentals-3rd Ed.
Denver Auditory Phoneme Sequencing Test
Detroit Tests of Learning Aptitude
Flowers-Costello Test of Auditory Abilities
Goldman-Fristoe-Woodcock Auditory Skills Test Battery
Language Processing Test
Lindamood Auditory Conceptualization Test
Phonemic Synthesis Test
Practical Test of Metalinguistics
Revised Token Test
Swanson Cognitive Processing Test
Test of Auditory-Perceptual Skills
Test of Awareness of Language Segments
Test of Language Competence
Test of Phonological Awareness
Test of Word Knowledge
Word Test

achieve scores rather than the scores achieved, dynamic assessment provides a good estimate of an individual's potential for change when given assistance (Campione & Brown, 1987; Palincsar, Brown, & Campione, 1994). The clinician systematically assists the client experiencing difficulty by modifying the format, providing feedback on successful strategies, and/or offering more direct cues or prompts. Information obtained through dynamic assessment may illuminate pragmatic aspects of language use, as well as the metacognitive (i.e., executive) planning, monitoring, and evaluating functions so important to effective listening and spoken language understanding (Heyer, 1995). Because of the window it provides on strategy knowledge and use, the information derived from dynamic assessment can be particularly useful to strategy training discussed in Chapter 8.

Because dynamic assessment provides a vehicle to assess an individual's potential for acquiring skills, rather than simply determining which communicative skills have already been mastered, it is also useful in assessment of non-English and limited-English proficient individuals and others from culturally diverse backgrounds. It provides a means of gaining insight into processing rather than a language-specific product (Erickson & Iglesias, 1986).

The reader is referred to Damico and Simon (1993), Friel-Patti (1994a), Gerber (1993a, 1993b), van Kleeck (1994), and Wiig and Semel (1984) for discussion of speech-language evaluation in the differential diagnosis of learning disabilities and CAPD.

QUALIFYING YOUNGSTERS WITH CAPD FOR SPECIAL EDUCATION SERVICES

Although prevalence estimates of CAPD among school-age youngsters are not available, a large number of youngsters with symptoms or diagnoses of CAPD present their special needs to teachers, school speech-language pathologists, and educational audiologists. The challenges these youngsters present to their families and professionals are exacerbated by the difficult and too often unsuccessful efforts to qualify these youngsters for school-based special services. As many youngsters do not quite meet the requirements of some federal legislation and state codes that mandate services to students with disabilities, parents, teachers, speech-language pathologists, and audiologists often are frustrated in their efforts to provide youngsters with CAPD with equal educational opportunities. Fortunately, several approaches may be pursued to qualify youngsters with CAPD for educational services.

Two federal laws specifically mandate special educational services for youngsters with disabilities who *qualify* for such services. The 1975 Education for All Handicapped Children Act (PL 94-142) and its reauthorized and renamed 1990 version, the Individuals with Disabilities Education Act (IDEA, PL 101-476), provide the vehicles that ensure that children with *qualifying* disabilities will receive the special education and related services, at no cost to parents, necessary to provide a free and appropriate public education. Because eligibility for services is determined at the state level and states vary greatly in the way they choose to operationalize their identification procedures, students deemed eligible in one state may not be eligible in a neighboring state (Doris, 1993).

In most states, youngsters are not qualified for school-based special services on the basis of a diagnosis of CAPD. Rather, they must be qualified under some other category to receive special services. Given the overlapping symptomatology, if youngsters with CAPD are qualified for services at all, it is most commonly on the basis of a *specific learning disability* or under the category of other *health impairment* due to the concurrent diagnosis of attention deficit disorder (ADD). Although a substantial number of youngsters with CAPD experience significant learning problems, they may not be of the severity or in the areas specified by law for diagnosis as learning disabled. Similarly, a diagnosis of ADD is not sufficient to qualify for special education and related services. Rather, youngsters diagnosed with ADD may be qualified under the other health impairment category only when a comprehensive evaluation by a multidisciplinary team documents that the condition imposes limited alertness that adversely affects their educational performance. The speech-language pathologist frequently leads the professional teams evaluating youngsters for learning disabilities and attention deficits.

In a few states, some youngsters with CAPD may qualify for services under the *hearing impairment* category due to a fluctuating hearing loss (often related to chronic otitis media) associated with the CAPD or because the category is written broadly enough to include those with *listening* problems, which may or may not be related to a peripheral hearing loss. For children with CAPD who do not qualify under the specific learning disability, other health impairment, or hearing impairment categories, two other federal laws offer protection.

Americans With Disabilities Act and the Rehabilitation Act of 1973

Even if a child with CAPD does not qualify for services under IDEA, the requirements of the Americans With Disabilities Act (PL 101-336) and Section 504 of the Rehabilitation Act of 1973 (PL 93-112) may provide viable bases for qualifying youngsters with CAPD for special education services. In contrast to IDEA, which is a funding law, the Rehabilitation Act of 1973 is a civil rights law, which prohibits agencies receiving federal funds from discriminating against otherwise qualified individuals simply on the basis of the disability.

The Americans with Disabilities Act (ADA), which was signed into law in 1990, is a comprehensive civil rights law that ensures people with disabilities access to all facets of American society. Broader in scope than the Rehabilitation Act, the ADA provides protections in both the public and private sectors, regulating employment; state and local government services (including the public school system and public transportation); public accommodations, including private transportation; and telecommunications (Williams & Carey, 1995). Indeed, the ADA covers all public school system programs and activities including those not covered by the IDEA (e.g., activities or programs open to parents or the public, graduation ceremonies, parent-teacher organization meetings, plays, and adult education classses) (Kilb, 1993). Because disability is defined more broadly in both Section 504 and the ADA—to include any person who has (or in the case of the ADA has a history or is regarded as having) a physical or mental impairment that substantially limits one or more major life activities (including learning)—the protections of Section 504 and the ADA extend to some youngsters who do not fall within the disability categories specified in IDEA. Under Section 504 and the ADA, youngsters with disabilities must be provided a free and appropriate public education, which may consist of *regular or special education and related services* designed to meet an individual student's unique needs. Hence, if it is determined following a comprehensive speech-language and psychoeducational evaluation that a youngster with CAPD experiences difficulty in learning (a major life activity), Section 504 and the ADA would require that the youngster receive either special education services *or regular education services with appropriate adaptations and interventions* to ensure access to an appropriate education. These interventions might include supplementary aids such as a frequency-modulated (FM) assistive listening system, as well as pedagogical adaptations, including audiovisual aides, use of tape recorders, note-takers, and tutorials (see Instructional Modifications).

Although neither Section 504 nor the ADA provide federal funding to agencies to implement necessary accommodations for persons with disabilities, state or local education agencies must still comply with these laws whether or not they accept educational funds provided through the education acts. Section 504 and the ADA entitle youngsters with disabilities, regardless of the nature, diagnosis, or severity of their disabilities, to full and equal educational opportunities and access (Chermak, 1981; Flexer, 1994). Regular education funds may be used to cover costs of services provided under Section 504 or the ADA.

In essence, youngsters with disabilities need not meet eligibility criteria for educational services under Section 504 or the ADA. Youngsters with CAPD who are not deemed eligible for services under IDEA may still be eligible for services on the basis of protections afforded by Section 504 and ADA. The audiologist must demonstrate, however, that the younster with CAPD does not have acoustic access to instruction and must therefore, at minimum, be furnished with assistive technology (e.g., an FM system) to achieve access to auditory information (Flexer, 1994).

Documenting Inadequate Acoustic Access

To argue convincingly that a youngster with CAPD is being denied an appropriate public education because the disability impedes acoustic access to instruction requires careful documentation of hearing and listening problems. Although a number of standardized tests and procedures are available to support the diagnosis of CAPD (see Chapters 3, 4, and 5), these instruments may not provide the performance data needed to establish a basis for educational accommodation. Rather, the educational audiologist must supplement the diagnostic test battery with measures of functional listening in contexts commonly found in classrooms. In addition to behavioral measures such as speech recognition in noise, several rating scales are useful in this regard.

The Children's Auditory Processing Performance Scale (CHAPPS) (Smoski, Brunt, & Tannahill, 1992), for example, is a clinical tool that can be used to document the observed listening performance of children with CAPD in a variety of listening conditions, including conditions of quiet, background noise, and competing visual inputs. In addition, the observer is asked to rate the youngster's ability to attend to and recall spoken information. The Screening Instrument for Targeting Educational Risk (SIFTER) (Anderson, 1989) is a rating scale completed by teachers that provides information concerning a youngster's attention, communication, academic achievement, and classroom behavior. The SIFTER may be used to identify youngsters at risk for educational problems due to peripheral or central auditory disorders. On the basis of data obtained from these instruments, the audiologist may be able to demonstrate diminished acoustic access to instruction and succeed in demanding at least an opportunity to use FM technology on a trial basis in the classroom.

CLASSROOM ACOUSTICS

Spoken language comprehension is essential to successful communication and learning. The acoustic and linguistic redundancy of spoken language (Denes & Pinson, 1993; Fletcher, 1953; Liberman, 1970; Liberman, Cooper, Shankweiler, & Studdert-Kennedy, 1967) is of tremendous benefit to listeners with deficient central auditory function; however, benefiting maximally from this highly redundant signal requires a high-fidelity listening environment.

The intelligibility of speech is affected by a number of acoustic characteristics, including the intensity of background sound competition relative to the signal and reverberation (i.e., the persistence of sound within an enclosed space due to multiple reflections off hard walls and surfaces), as well as the distance between speaker and listener. Not unlike other physical spaces, the acoustic characteristics of the classroom can substantially affect a student's ability to understand spoken language and learn (ASHA, 1995; Berg, 1987, 1993; Crandell & Smaldino, 1994, 1995b; Crum & Matkin, 1976; Finitzo-Hieber & Tillman, 1978; Flexer, 1994).

Noisy, often crowded classrooms present a less than optimal acoustic environment for listening and learning (ASHA, 1995; Berg, 1993; Crandell, 1993a; Crandell & Smaldino, 1994; Finitzo-Hieber & Tillman, 1978; Flexer, 1994; Ross, Brackett, & Maxon, 1991). The multiplicative distortions involving background noise and reverberation create a degraded and demanding listening situation: reflected noise increases overall noise level and creates a more uniform noise, both spectrally and temporally (ASHA, 1995; Bornstein & Musiek, 1992; Harris, 1960). In addition, the student's distance from the speaker and poor acoustic design of many classrooms also reduce the quality of the acoustic signal. Moreover, loss of high speech frequencies because the teacher is speaking while facing the blackboard (Bornstein & Musiek, 1992), as well as at a fast speaking rate (McCrosky & Thompson, 1973), further contribute to listening difficulties.

Poor classroom acoustics can impede listening for students with normal auditory and language function; however, their intact internal processes may enable them to cope with unfavorable listening conditions by exerting extra effort. Nonetheless, they probably suffer fatigue (Downs & Crum, 1978). For the student with either peripheral or central auditory deficits, however, the degradations to the message caused by poor room acoustics results in an arduous challenge (Finitzo-Hieber & Tillman, 1978; Bornstein & Musiek, 1992). Given the reduction or *smearing* of temporal cues caused by the multiple sources of distortion (Bornstein & Musiek, 1992), as well as the sheer level of background competition, it is not surprising that youngsters with CAPD, in whom we have noted temporal processing deficits, deficits performing with competing or degraded signals, and often depressed language abilities as well, find the classroom inhospitable for listening.

Noise

Background noise impedes spoken language recognition by masking acoustic features of the signal and thereby reducing the redundant cues available to the listener (Cooper & Cutts, 1971; Miller, 1974; Miller & Nicely, 1955). Ambient room noise of approximately 60 dBA has been reported in traditional classrooms (when occupied) of average size, location, and acoustics, and levels as high as 73 dBA have been reported in open plan classrooms (Bess, Sinclair, & Riggs, 1984; Finitzo-Hieber, 1988; Nober & Nober, 1975; Ross & Giolas, 1971; Watson, 1964; Webster & Snell, 1983). More important than the absolute noise level is the signal-to-noise ratio (SNR). Classroom SNRs range from +5 dB to -7 dB; the speech signal is, at best, only 5 dB greater than the background noise (Berg, 1993; Finitzo-Hieber, 1988; Markides, 1986; Sanders, 1965).

Numerous investigations have demonstrated greater decrements in speech recognition in noise performance among listeners with peripheral hearing impairment, non-English and limited-English proficient listeners, children, older adults, and individuals with CAPD and learning disabilities relative to normal hearing adults (Bergman, 1980; Chermak, Vonhof, & Bendel, 1989; Crandell, 1991, 1993b; Elliott, 1979, 1982; Elliott et al., 1979; Finitzo-Hieber & Tillman, 1978; Katz & Illmer, 1972; Lasky & Tobin, 1973; Nabelek & Robinson, 1982a; Olsen, Noffsinger, & Kurdziel, 1975; Takata & Nabelek, 1990). Skinner (1978) argued that even children with normal hearing require about a +30 dB SNR to maximally use spoken language information. Even more conservative estimates requiring an SNR of +6 to +12 dB for normal hearing children (Crandell, 1991; Finitzio-Hieber & Tillman, 1978) nonetheless demonstrate the potential for noise levels commonly reported in classrooms to adversely impact spoken language understanding in children with CAPD.

Reverberation

Reverberation degrades signals and impedes spoken language recognition by masking direct sound energy with temporally delayed, reflected sound energy (Bolt & MacDonald, 1949; Houtgast, 1981). Generally, spoken language recognition ability decreases as reverberation time (i.e., the time required for an acoustic signal to decay 60 dB from its initial level) increases (Finitzo-Hieber & Tillman, 1978; Nabelek & Nabelek, 1994; Neuman & Hochberg, 1983). Reverberation times in typical classrooms, reported to range between 0.4 second to 1.2 seconds (Bradley, 1986; Crandell & Smaldino, 1994, 1995b; Finitzo-Hieber, 1988; Kodaras, 1960; McCrosky & Devens, 1975), often exceed the times known to impact speech recognition (Finitzo-Hieber & Tillman, 1978). Although a 0.4 second reverberation time may not substantially degrade the speech recognition performance of children with normal hearing in relatively quiet environments, longer reverberation times cause significant degradation for many listeners (Finitzo-Hieber & Tillman, 1978). These reverberation times pose greater challenges for individuals with peripheral or central auditory impairment, learning disabilities, non-English and limited-English proficient listeners, and older adults who experience greater difficulties understanding spoken language in reverberant environments than individuals with normal auditory function (Bergman, 1980; Bess, 1985; Crandell, 1991, 1992; Finitzo-Hieber & Tillman, 1978; Bornstein & Musiek, 1992; Nabelek & Donahue, 1986; Nabelek & Nabelek, 1994; Nabelek & Pickett, 1974a, 1974b; Nabelek & Robinson, 1982a; Neuman & Hochberg, 1983; Takata & Nabelek, 1990).

Distance

In addition to noise and reverberation, distance between the listener and sound source influences spoken language recognition. Because the intensity of the signal at the listener's ear decreases as a function of distance from the source (i.e., inverse square law which, strictly speaking, is applicable only in free-fields), spoken language recognition generally decreases as distance between listener and source increases (Crandell & Smaldino, 1995b). Crandell (1993a), for example, reported a 24% reduction in children's mean speech recognition scores in a typical classroom as the speaker-listener distance doubled from 6 to 12 feet. Crandell and Bess (1986) suggested that even children with normal hearing sensitivity experience greater difficulty understanding spoken language when seated in the middle to the rear of a typical classroom. In contrast to the spoken language signal level, which decreases with increased distance, noise is often distributed homogeneously throughout a room (Nabelek & Nabelek, 1994); therefore, the SNR, as well as the absolute level of the signal, decreases as distance from the source increases. Hence, preferential seating for students with CAPD, which allows them more direct access to a louder and less reverberant signal, as well as to visual cues (as discussed below), is appropriate and necessary.

Multiple Distortions

Noise and reverberation rarely occur in isolation; therefore, the synergistic effects of these two distortions must be considered. The interaction of noise and reverberation causes greater decrements in speech recognition than the sum of both distortions operating independently (Finitzo-Hieber & Tillman, 1978; Nabelek & Pickett, 1974a, 1974b). As with noise and reverberation in isolation, individuals with CAPD, hearing impairment, or other *special listeners* (including children with normal audition but fewer listening strategies and still developing language skills) experience greater difficulty understanding spoken language in noisy and reverberant conditions than adult subjects with normal hearing (Bornstein & Musiek, 1992; Finitzo-Hieber & Tillman, 1978; Nabelek & Nabelek, 1994; Yacullo & Hawkins, 1987). Even a favorable SNR of +12 dB paired with a short reverberation time of 0.4 seconds leads to reduced speech recognition performance for normal hearing children (Crandell & Smaldino, 1995b).

METHODS TO IMPROVE CLASSROOM ACOUSTICS

Clearly, noise and reverberation degrade the acoustic signal and adversely affect spoken language comprehension. The effects are exacerbated for listeners with CAPD in whom auditory system deficits compound the difficulties presented by a degraded signal with decreased redundancy. Although complete elimination of noise and reverberation is probably impractical and, in the case of reverberation, perhaps undesirable since some degree of reverberation gives speech and music a natural quality, modification of the physical characteristics of the classroom can improve the listening environment for all students, especially those with CAPD.

Classroom Design

Designing a classroom conducive to listening requires attention to background noise levels, reverberation, distance between listener and source, and access to visual cues. Classroom SNRs should exceed +15 dB; reverberation levels should not exceed 0.4 seconds (ASHA, 1995; Crandell & Smaldino, 1994, 1995b; Finitzo-Hieber & Tillman, 1978; Nabelek & Robinson, 1982a; Neuman & Hochberg, 1983). Students with CAPD (as well as those with peripheral hearing loss) may require even more favorable SNRs and shorter reverberation times to maximize their access to acoustic information (Crandell & Smaldino, 1995b). Control of both airborne (e.g., produced by sources directly radiating to the air, such as traffic, music, classroom activity) and structure-borne noise (e.g., noise transmitted through floors and walls of buildings) is necessary to meet these design criteria. Noise originating in the classroom, external to the classroom but within the school building, and external to the school must be controlled.

Of course, the most effective means of reducing noise levels and limiting reverberation is through proper planning and architectural design. Schools should be built in quieter sections of communities; and classrooms within these schools should be located away from noise sources, such as the cafeteria, gymnasium, auditorium, and playground. Double-walled construction, double doors, double-paned windows, and properly sealed doors and windows attenuate noise transmitted into the school building and into the classroom. Installation of quiet heating and cooling systems, ventilation systems, and other equipment can lessen unwanted structural and airborne noise.

Unfortunately, consideration of noise levels prior to building construction is not typical (Crandell, 1991, 1992). More typically, rooms and buildings are acoustically modified by installing carpeting, curtains, and acoustical paneling on the walls and ceilings to reduce noise levels. Inexpensive modifications that reduce noise levels include placing rubber tips on chair legs and desks, placing sound-absorbing rubber or felt insulation around windows and doors, using bookshelves as room dividers to produce quieter spaces for one-on-one communication and instruction, and using corkboard as bulletin boards. Acoustic modifications that cover hard, reflective surfaces with absorptive material (e.g., ceiling tiles, carpeted floors, cushioned chairs, curtains, cork bulletin boards or bookshelves on walls, positioning mobile bulletin boards at an angle [i.e., not parallel] relative to the wall) also reduce reverberation. Some of these modifications (e.g., curtains, carpets) also reduce glare which can impede access to visual cues, which provide supplementary information to maximize spoken language comprehension and learning for the youngster with CAPD. Creative landscaping, including strategic placement of shrubs, trees, and earthen berms or banks may reduce noise transmission into the classroom by absorbing and diffracting sound (Crandell & Smaldino, 1994).

The reader is directed to Nabelek and Nabelek (1994) for an overview of the relationship between room acoustics and speech perception. Beranek (1986), Crandell and Smaldino (1995b), Knudsen and Harris (1978), and Lawrence (1970) describe acoustical methods to reduce noise and reverberation.

Visual Cues

Maximizing access to visual information necessitates attention to lighting, as well as distance and angle between speaker and listener.

The classroom environment should be well lighted and free of glare from reflective surfaces such as glass tabletops and waxed floors (Harley & Lawrence, 1977). Materials written using large print, double-spaced, and on contrasting backgrounds are more visible. As noted above, a number of methods employed to reduce noise and reverberation also benefit lighting. For example, carpeting and curtains reduce glare, as well as noise levels and reflection.

Seating in the classroom offers another means to reduce noise levels, improve SNR and the ratio of direct to reverberant sound energy, and maximize the listening environment for a student with CAPD. Offering preferential seating to students with special listening needs within the direct sound field of the teacher and away from noise sources such as ventilation fans, heating ducts, and air conditioners improves the SNR and minimizes interference from reflected energy, thereby positioning these students to access important visual information. The student with CAPD should be seated near the teacher or other sound source with full, face-to-face view. Reducing the distance between speaker and listener provides a louder, less reverberant signal, as well as the opportunity to take advantage of visual instructional aids and visible cues accompanying spoken language (e.g., speechreading). As many students do not maintain regular eye contact, teachers may need to modify this behavior to enable them to fully utilize visual cues.

Instructional Modifications

Collaboration between speech-language pathologists, audiologists, and teachers is a key dimension of management programming for youngsters with CAPD. Collaboration typically involves adjustments in instructional format and presentation, as well as cooperation in auditory and language skills training. Pivotal to this collaboration is understanding the superiority of bisensory (auditory-visual) speech recognition (Dodd, 1977, 1980; Erber, 1969; Massaro, 1987; Sanders & Goodrich, 1971). Hence, it is imperative for teachers to incorporate visual cues as supplements to auditory information. The benefits of auditory and visual summation can then be achieved to derive maximal information integration (Chermak & Musiek, 1992). Likewise, audiologists and speech-language pathologists should support the educational curriculum by using academic concepts and materials as content for therapy (e.g., new vocabulary from the student's academic coursework in the vocabulary-building techniques described in Chapter 8).

As with the design modifications discussed in the preceding section and sound field technology discussed in the following section, pedagogical adaptations can improve the listening environment for all students, including those with CAPD who might not qualify for special education services (including the use of personal FM systems). Insofar as these adaptations enhance access to the acoustic signal, which serves as a primary instructional vehicle, they reduce the burdens attendant to listening in the typically noisy classroom and thereby provide particular benefit to students with CAPD or minimal hearing loss.

Encouraging students to use visual and auditory input for better comprehension is central to the modified instructional approach. For example, relieving youngsters with CAPD of note-taking allows them to concentrate on available auditory and visual information: to listen and watch, but not write. Note-taking precludes watching the teacher, forcing students with CAPD to rely solely on their compromised auditory system for all information. Because these youngsters are often poor writers, their pedestrian note-taking skills exacerbate an already difficult situation as their transcription lags behind the spoken message (Chermak & Musiek, 1992). The resulting antagonism between writing and listening leads to division of attention; instead of summating information across auditory and visual modes, confusion ensues as attention is diverted from the already less than adequate auditory system. Providing lecture notes to youngsters with CAPD prior to the class presentation, having another student take notes for them, or using a tape recorder for later transcription enables students with CAPD to attend to and process both auditory and visual information (Chermak & Musiek, 1992). Similarly, supplementing verbal instructions with visual instructions and using computer-aided instruction and other audiovisual equipment benefits students with CAPD. Concurrently, audiologists, speech-language pathologists, and teachers can collaborate to improve note-taking skills by encouraging students' use of prosodic cues, formal schemata, and metamemory strategies to gauge the relative importance of information, guide organization and outlining, and enhance retention.

The advantages of auditory-visual summation were reflected in two programs discussed in Chapter 8, including the phonemic analysis programs of Sloan (1986) and Lindamood and Lindamood (1975). Two particularly creative, visually based approaches merit specific mention.

Paris, Wixson, and Palincsar (1986) suggested the use of concrete metaphors as a component of their strategy-based reading program. Easily adapted to promote strategic listening, concrete metaphors, colorfully illustrated in large posters and placed on classroom bulletin boards, can provide a visual reminder of listening goals. For example, the metaphor *Turning on the Meaning* illustrated using light bulbs reinforces the notion that effective listening is active and constructive (Paris et al., 1986). Similarly, the metaphor *Searching for Reading [Listening]* Treasure reminds youngsters that listening is difficult and demands persistence, but is aided by paying careful attention to all clues.

Mind mapping, the second innovative, visually based approach, involves the drawing of pictures, usually supplemented by words, as an alternative to note-taking or outlining (Margulies, 1991). These maps provide a nonlinear means of recording information and reflecting relationships among concepts and ideas.

As elaborated in Table 9–2, a number of additional techniques can be used to enhance signal quality and ease the listening burden for individuals with CAPD in the home, classroom, and other contexts. These techniques include having communication partners modify temporal aspects of their speech by speaking more slowly; inserting more pauses, particularly at appropriate clausal or phrasal boundaries; augmenting prosodic cues by emphasizing key words; and increasing response time (Blumstein, Katz, Goodglass, Shrier, & Dworetsky, 1985; Ellis Weismer & Hesketh, 1993; Keith, 1981b; Kimelman, 1991; Lasky, Weidner, & Johnson, 1976; Saville-Troike, 1989). The latter recommendation may be of particular significance when working with certain multicultural clientele, as discussed in Chapter 7. Berg (1993), Edwards (1995), Flexer (1994), and Rosenberg and Blake-Rahter (1995a) discuss room design and instructional strategies to facilitate listening in the classroom.

FREQUENCY-MODULATED (FM) ASSISTIVE LISTENING SYSTEMS

Even when coupled with instructional modifications, rarely will acoustic modifications ensure an optimal classroom listening environment for the student with CAPD. Fortunately, the audibility of the teacher's voice can be increased with assistive listening systems. These technological advances, coupled with legislation mandating access to technology for reducing communicative and learning barriers in the classroom, have led to an increase in the availability and use of assistive listening systems in the classroom (ASHA, 1994).

The most commonly used amplification device for individuals with normal hearing is the frequency-modulated (FM) assistive lis-

Table 9–2. Suggestions for alleviating difficulties associated with central auditory processing disorders and minimal hearing loss.

1. Gain the individual's attention prior to presenting auditory information. Remind the individual to "listen," call her or him by name, use a common carrier phrase, or use a visual or motor prompt such as lightly touching the shoulder. Be sure that she or he is looking directly at you when you give instructions. Whenever possible, speak at the child's eye level, get close to the child, and face the child to provide clear visual and auditory information.
2. Speak slowly, clearly, at a comfortably loud level, with a natural intonation pattern. Use words within the individual's vocabulary. Emphasize important information using intonation and stress and repeat important words when necessary.
3. Arrange the environment to minimize extraneous noise (both auditory and visual distraction). Noise interferes with reception of auditory information and distracts the individual from the complex task of processing (i.e., organizing and interpreting) information.
4. Position the individual away from noise sources (e.g., street traffic, hall noise, air conditioning or ventilation noise, other competing voices, etc.) and near the place from which the teacher or speaker will present auditory material.
5. Allow flexible seating so that the individual can change his or her position or seat to obtain the greatest advantage as the speaker or primary source changes.
6. Avoid *open classroom settings.* Reduce distractions by using sound barriers (e.g., bookshelves, flannel boards) and other modifications to improve the listening environment (e.g., carpeted floors, curtains over windows).
7. Keep doors and windows closed to reduce the amount of external noise entering the classroom.
8. Consider allowing the individual to wear sound attenuating earmuffs/earplugs when working individually to help minimize background noise and thereby reduce distraction and foster concentration. Earplugs/earmuffs also may be appropriate in the car or in other noisy situations where conversation may not be not expected.
9. Present information in ways that provide redundancy and facilitate auditory processing. Monitor rate of speech. Repeat, rephrase, and paraphrase auditory information and offer examples, illustrations, and demonstrations. Present only a few tasks or directions at one time.
10. Use step-by-step instructions. All new information should be presented in small, well-defined packets. Limit the amount of information in any one statement or instruction and distribute the information across several short

Continued

Table 9–2. *continued*

sessions rather than one long session in which a massive amount of information is presented for processing.

11. Allow for completion of one task prior to beginning another. Incorporate breaks between tasks.
12. Prevent fatigue by alternating activities requiring greater auditory processing with those that are less demanding.
13. Maintain interest by presenting material in a meaningful context. Preview new material and relate new material to an individual's previous experience and environment. Where possible, provide an active, experiential approach to learning (i.e., field trips, discovery activities).
14. Preassign readings and home assignments. Review material before gradually presenting new information.
15. Structure and organize the environment. Arrange for expected and predictable routines and use consistent vocabulary and formats.
16. Complement new concepts and information with visual aids, including overheads, computers, and blackboards. Explain and show. Give directions (or chores) both in writing and orally. With young children, point to objects, pictures, or people as they are talked about.
17. Encourage comprehensive listening. Suggest that all available cues be utilized: auditory, visual, language context, experience, knowledge. Listen for meaning, look at a speaker's face, and relate information to one's own experience and knowledge.
18. Assign another student to take notes for the student with a central auditory processing disorder so that the visual system can be devoted to supplementing or complementing auditory processing, rather than being divided between the requirements of simultaneous writing and listening.
19. Check the individual's auditory comprehension by requiring feedback. Remind her or him to wait until all of the information is presented before beginning to inference, draw conclusions, make judgments, and so on. Ask for verbal accounts of what was said rather than whether she or he understood the materials, which requires only a yes-no response. Reinforce listening for meaning rather than exact repetition.
20. Ask specific and short, structured questions.
21. Provide ample opportunity for thinking and assimilation of information prior to requesting a response.
22. Use a *buddy system* in the classroom so that another student can help with class notes, assignments, and instructions.
23. Consider use of radio frequency FM personal auditory trainers or FM sound field system to enhance the relative level of the wanted signal over the background noise.

24. Communicate a positive attitude, praise generously, and reinforce for even small successes and minimal improvement. Maintain sensitivity to the individual's strengths and weaknesses and help to make her or him aware of the nature of the auditory processing problems and their academic and social ramifications.
25. Encouragement and support are key factors for success. Assist the individual in developing and employing coping and compensatory strategies. Encourage the individual to ask questions, to request repetition or paraphrasing of messages, and to request assistance.
26. Provide some challenge, but do not burden the individual with tasks for which she or he is not yet able to cope.

---

tening system. These systems, once used exclusively by individuals with significant hearing impairment, are now recommended as a component of a remediation program for individuals with CAPD, fluctuating or minimal hearing loss, learning disabilities, phonological and language disorders, and head injury (ASHA, 1996; Blake, Field, Foster, Platt, & Wertz, 1991; Casterline, Flexer, & DePompei, 1989; Flexer, 1989; Flexer, Millin, & Brown, 1990; Hodson & Paden, 1983; Loose, 1984; Neuss, Blair, & Viehweg, 1991; Ray, Sarff, & Glassford, 1984; Sarff, Ray, & Bagwell, 1981; Shapiro & Mistal, 1985, 1986; Shriberg, 1983; Smith, McConnell, Walter, & Miller, 1985; Stach, Loiselle, & Jerger, 1987a, 1987b, 1991; Stach, Loiselle, Jerger, Mintz, & Taylor, 1987). We consider the personal or sound field FM system a cornerstone intervention for most clients with CAPD.

By placing a remote microphone near the speaker's mouth and transmitting the signal via FM radio waves to a receiver on or near the listener, the effects of noise, reverberation, and distance are largely overcome (Lewis, 1995). Personal FM systems enhance the speech signal by approximately 15 to 20 dB at the listener's ear relative to the background noise (Hawkins, 1984). In essence, FM systems preserve the fidelity of the signal and reduce the effects of background noise and reverberation by enhancing the SNR. By improving the SNR in noisy and reverberant environments, it is anticipated that attention to the speech signal will be increased and distractability decreased (ASHA, 1991; Blake et al., 1991; Flexer, 1989; Ross, 1992; Stach, Loiselle, & Jerger, 1987a, 1987b, 1991). Indeed, improved spoken language understanding, academic achievement, and on-task behavior have been reported consistently for a wide variety of clinical populations, including CAPD, when using FM systems (Blair, Myrup, & Viehweg, 1989; Blake et al., 1991; Flexer, 1989; Flexer et al., 1990;

Neuss et al., 1991; Ray et al., 1984; Ross, Giolas, & Carver, 1973; Sarff et al., 1981; Stach , Loiselle, & Jerger, 1987a, 1987b, 1991). (See also Efficacy in Chapter 7.)

Fitting Personal FM Systems

Candidates for FM technology must be evaluated by an audiologist to ensure optimal fitting (ASHA, 1994, 1995). Recently published FM fitting and monitoring guidelines should be considered carefully (ASHA, 1994). Individuals with CAPD are fitted with mild gain, low output units in either a traditional body-worn or, more recently, a behind-the-ear configuration. The body-worn FM system is coupled to the listener's ears using headsets, earbuds, or button receivers/earphone assemblies coupled to custom snap-ring, vented earmolds; the ear-level FM system usually is coupled to the listener's ear using an open earmold. The open mold coupling is comfortable and allows the listener to monitor environmental sound.

In an effort to reduce interference caused by environmental noise, low gain, behind-the-ear FM systems do not employ an external microphone, which is commonly found in the traditional body-worn systems. Although some body-worn FM systems allow independent adjustment of the gain of the external microphone relative to the FM transmitter microphone (Yuzon, 1994), concurrent activation of internal and external microphones (i.e., FM plus environmental microphone) may still cause a distorted signal due to the temporal delay of the acoustical signal received at the external microphone relative to the electrical signal transmitted instantaneously through the internal microphone. Unfortunately, the absence of an external microphone may limit the user's ability to monitor the environment or interact with anyone (e.g., other students) not speaking into the FM transmitter. Use of a conference microphone, which enables the listener to hear several different speakers, may minimize this limitation and be a particularly effective option for small group work (Lewis, 1995).

The behind-the-ear FM system's more restricted range of function relative to the traditional body-worn system (i.e., approximately 100 feet outdoors versus 300 feet) may limit its use in contexts where distance is a factor (e.g., playgrounds, outdoor recreation, large auditoria); however, this restricted range also reduces the risk of interference among systems when more than one unit is transmitting on the same channel (Lewis, 1995). Because the behind-the-ear FM system may be more cosmetically appealing and less stigmatizing than the traditional body-worn system, it may be the preferred fitting for children and teenagers struggling with peer pressure.

In fitting either system, the audiologist must carefully consider the type of microphone worn by the speaker (e.g., lavalier, lapel, head-worn boom). Although a boom microphone positioned in front of the lips may be optimal in noisy environments, this placement may obscure visual cues and impede speechreading. A lavalier microphone, worn around the neck or attached to clothing, may be more comfortable and less obstructive.

Other Considerations

Although the efficacy of FM technology for individuals with CAPD has been demonstrated, several factors can compromise its effectiveness. First, personal FM technology is expensive. Since insurance carriers are less likely to cover purchase of FM systems, individuals and families must be prepared to shoulder the purchase cost. As discussed previously, qualifying youngsters with CAPD for school services and securing appropriate intervention, including the use of a personal FM system, often is difficult.

FM systems require careful handling, daily monitoring, and regular maintenance. Audiologists must educate users, parents, and teachers about the function and operation of the system. They must understand how to use the equipment properly, check its functioning daily, and troubleshoot minor problems. Since this cooperation can be compromised if the system is seen as too *high-tech* and difficult to operate, audiologists must make certain they offer clear and compelling presentations to users, parents, and educators on the use of FM systems to increase compliance. In addition, cosmetic concerns can jeopardize the success of a fitting, particularly for teenagers. The audiologist must work with the teenager to demonstrate the benefits of the technology in meaningful contexts (e.g., ease of listening in the classroom, following friends' conversations in competing noise backgrounds) to encourage its acceptance and use.

Sound Field FM Systems

Although not optimal, sound field FM systems may provide an alternative in cases where a personal FM unit cannot be obtained. The sound field FM system provides a cost-effective means to improve the listening environment for all participants and has been well received in school settings (K. Anderson, 1991; Berg, 1993; Crandell & Smaldino, 1995b; Flexer, 1994). Basically a public address system, the sound field FM system requires placement of an FM wireless microphone by the speaker's (e.g., teacher's) mouth. The signal is transmitted to an amplifier and then delivered to all listeners via several loudspeakers strategically placed throughout the room.

A number of studies have shown the benefits of this system, particularly improved speech recognition and academic achievement, for students with normal hearing as well as students with hearing impairment (e.g., unidentified or fluctuating hearing loss, unilateral hearing loss, minimal hearing loss, high frequency hearing loss) or other developmental disabilities (Berg, 1987; Flexer et al., 1990; Neuss et al., 1991; Ray et al., 1984; Sarff, 1981; Sarff et al., 1981). No active cooperation is required of students, who nonetheless benefit from the enhanced sound provided by the sound field FM system. Because students need not wear a special receiver, the sound field system is seen as less stigmatizing than the traditional FM system (Lewis, 1994). Teachers also may feel more comfortable with the sound field system because there are no student receivers to monitor and troubleshoot (Lewis, 1994). Because of these benefits and the fact that the system is inexpensive on a per capita basis relative to other electronic methods of improving classroom acoustics, the sound field FM system is the most rapidly expanding component of the FM market, with systems being installed in classrooms across the country (Crandell & Smaldino, 1995b).

Notwithstanding its relative ease of operation, audiologists still must educate teachers about the FM sound field system's benefits, basic function, and features. Audiologists must also educate teachers and administrators about the limitations of this technology, ensuring that they understand that it is not a panacea or a substitute for other necessary interventions. The reader is referred to Rosenberg and Blake-Rahter (1995a) for discussion of FM training for the classroom teacher and to Allen and Anderson (1995) for marketing considerations.

Limitations

As noted by Lewis (1995), sound field FM systems present some limitations, particularly in comparison to personal FM systems. Unlike the 15 to 20 dB signal enhancement relative to the background noise experienced by the listener wearing a personal FM system (Hawkins, 1984), the sound field alternative provides only a 10 to 15 dB boost (Crandell & Smaldino, 1995b; Flexer, 1994). Moreover, if a sufficient number of loudspeakers is not placed in appropriate locations in the room, signal enhancement may not be obtained uniformly throughout the classroom (Flexer, 1992; Leavitt, 1991). In fact, improper installation can result in increased reverberation and a poorer signal than that obtained in the absence of amplification (Flexer, 1992; Leavitt, 1991; Lewis, 1994). Careful attention to installation is crucial, given the physical differences in room size and shape, as well as variations in seating arrangements and teaching style (Lewis, 1994). Even if properly installed, the 10 to 15 dB amplification may not be sufficient in particularly noisy or reverberant classrooms (Crandell & Smaldino, 1995b) or for students with more than mild degrees of hearing loss (Blair et al., 1989). In addition, sound field systems are not portable and, therefore, do not support field trips or outdoor activities. Further, unless a sufficient number of systems are installed, older students who typically change classrooms during the day may find themselves in an unamplified classroom. A personal FM system may be a more appropriate fitting for these students.

For in-depth reviews of FM technology and its applications, the reader is referred to Berg (1987, 1993), Crandall, Smaldino, and Flexer (1995), Flexer, (1994), Lewis (1995), Ross (1992, 1994), and Yuzon (1994). Manufacturers of FM systems are listed in Table 9–3.

Table 9–3. Manufacturers of frequency-modulated (FM) systems.

ANCHOR AUDIO. 913 West 223rd Street, Torrence, CA 90502; (310) 533-5984

AUDIO ENHANCEMENT. 12613 South Redwood Road, Riverton, UT 84065; (801) 254-9263.

AUDIOLOGICAL ENGINEERING. 35 Medford Street, Sommerville, MA 02143; (617) 623-5562.

AVR SONOVATION. 1450 Park Court, Chanhassen, MN 55317; (800) 462-8336.

COMTEK. 357 W. 2700 S., Salt Lake City, UT 84115; (800) 496-3463.

CUSTOM AUDIO DESIGN. Box 597, Wenatchee, WA 98807-0598; (800) 355-7525.

LIFELINE AMPLIFICATION SYSTEMS. 55 South 4th Street, Platteville, WI 53818; (800) 236-4327.

PHONIC EAR. 3880 Cypress Drive, Petaluma, CA 94954; (800) 227-0735 USA, (800) 263-8700 Canada.

SENNHEISER ELECTRONICS. 6 Vista Drive, Old Lyme, CT 06371; (203) 434-9190.

TELEX COMMUNICATIONS. 9600 Aldrich Ave. S., Minneapolis, MN 55420; (612) 884-4051.

WILLIAMS SOUND. 10399 W. 70th Street, Eden Prairie, MN 55344-3459; (800) 328-6190.

Infrared Systems

Although FM assistive listening devices are the most commonly used amplification devices, especially in the educational setting, other assistive technology is available and is finding application in a variety of settings. Infrared systems are an alternative to the sound field FM system for personal and area listening for individuals with CAPD.

Infrared systems transmit acoustic signals via infrared light. A modulator processes the acoustic signal for transmission. This processing includes amplitude limiting and expansion, pre-emphasis of high frequencies, and modulating the acoustic signal onto a radio frequency subcarrier (Lieske, 1994). An infrared emitter transmits the radio frequency signal via infrared light. An infrared receiver demodulates the radio frequency signal back to an acoustic signal. The receiver is coupled to the listener's ear using headphones or earbuds. (The receiver output can be coupled to a hearing aid through electromagnetic induction using neckloops or silhouettes, or through direct audio input.)

Comparison of Infrared and FM Systems

Both infrared and FM systems provide excellent sound quality. The major advantages of infrared systems are that they are impervious to radio interference or other electromagnetic disturbances, the same receiver can be used with any infrared transmitter, and any number of infrared systems can be used in contiguous rooms without interference from one another (Ross, 1994). Large-area infrared systems, however, generally are more expensive per square foot of coverage, and they are more difficult to install than FM systems. They are not as portable as FM systems and cannot be used outdoors (Lieske, 1994). Because line of sight between transmitter and receiver is crucial, persons or other obstructions can impede infrared transmission; however, line of sight transmission can be used to secure privacy of communication. Clearly, the choice of assistive listening system will depend on listening requirements and available resources.

SUMMARY

Interventions to improve signal quality and enhance the listening environment were presented in this chapter. These interventions involve boosting signal intensity and improving the signal-to-noise ratio through the use of assistive listening devices such as personal FM and sound field FM amplification systems, proper design and physical space modifications to reduce environmental noise and reverberation, and instructional strategies to benefit listening and learning in the classroom. The package of acoustic and pedagogic accommodations is crucial to the youngster with CAPD whose compromised internal auditory processing system can be easily overwhelmed by the multiplicative distortions of noise and reverberation.

Unfortunately, in a number of states, restrictive eligibility criteria exclude many youngsters with CAPD from special education services. Audiologists and speech-language pathologists must continue their efforts to work with parents and school districts to qualify youngsters with CAPD for special education services or *regular education services with appropriate adaptations and interventions* to ensure access to an appropriate education. By delivering a signal with greater fidelity, use of sound field FM systems in regular classrooms accommodates students with CAPD, while benefiting all students. Nonetheless, innovative instructional methods are needed to ensure that listeners with CAPD obtain maximum advantage from the enhanced acoustic signal and listening environment.

SUGGESTED READINGS

Allen, L., & Anderson, K. (1995). Marketing sound-field amplification systems. In C. Crandell, J. Smaldino, & C. Flexer, *Sound-field FM amplification* (pp. 201–211). San Diego: Singular Publishing Group.

Beranek, L. (1986). *Acoustics.* Woodbury, NY: Acoustical Society of America.

Berg, F.S. (1987). FM equipment. *Facilitating classroom listening: A handbook for teachers of normal and hard of hearing children.* Boston: College-Hill Press.

Berg, F.S. (1993). *Acoustics and sound systems in schools.* San Diego: Singular Publishing Group.

Crandell, C., & Smaldino, J. (1995). Acoustical modifications in classrooms. In C. Crandell, J. Smaldino, & C. Flexer, *Sound-field FM amplification* (pp. 83–92). San Diego: Singular Publishing Group.

Crandell, C., Smaldino, J., & Flexer, C. (1995). *Sound-field FM amplification.* San Diego: Singular Publishing Group.

Damico, J.S., & Simon, C.A. (1993). Assessing language abilities in school-age children. In A. Gerber (Ed.), *Language-related learning disabilities* (pp. 279–299). Baltimore: Paul H. Brookes.

Edwards, C. (1995). Listening strategies for the classroom teacher. In C. Crandell, J. Smaldino, & C. Flexer, *Sound-field FM amplification* (pp. 83–92). San Diego: Singular Publishing Group.

Flexer, C. (1994). *Facilitating hearing and listening in young children.* San Diego: Singular Publishing Group.

Friel-Patti, S. (1994). Auditory linguistic processing and language learning. In G.P. Wallach & K.G. Butler (Eds.), *Language learning disabilities in school-age children and adolescents* (pp. 373–392). New York: Charles E. Merrill.

Gerber, A. (1993a). Interdisciplinary language intervention in education. In A. Gerber (Ed.), *Language-related learning disabilities: Their nature and treatment* (pp. 301–322). Baltimore: Paul H. Brookes.

Gerber, A. (1993b). Intervention: Preventing or reversing the failure cycle. In A. Gerber (Ed.), *Language-related learning disabilities: Their nature and treatment* (pp. 323–393). Baltimore: Paul H. Brookes.

Knudsen, V., & Harris, C. (1978). *Acoustical designing in architecture.* Washington, DC: The American Institute of Physics for the Acoustical Society of America.

Lawrence, A. (1970). *Architectural acoustics.* Amsterdam: Elsevier Publishing Company.

Lewis, D.E. (1995). Orientation to the use of frequency modulated systems. In R.S. Tyler & D.J. Schum (Eds.), *Assistive devices for persons with hearing impairment* (pp. 165–184). Boston: Allyn and Bacon.

Nabelek, A.K., & Nabelek, I.V. (1994). Room acoustics and speech perception. In J. Katz (Ed.), *Handbook of clinical audiology* (4th ed., pp. 624–637). Baltimore: Williams & Wilkins.

Obrzut, J.E., & Hynd, G.W. (Eds.). (1991). *Neuropsychological foundations of learning disabilities.* San Diego: Academic Press.

Rosenberg, G., & Blake-Rahter, P. (1995). Inservice training for the classroom teacher. In C. Crandell, J. Smaldino, & C. Flexer, *Sound-field FM amplification* (pp. 149–190). San Diego: Singular Publishing Group.

Ross, M. (1992). *FM auditory training systems: Characteristics, selection and use.* Timonium, MD: York Press.

Ross, M., (1994). FM large-area listening systems. In M. Ross (Ed.), *Communication access for persons with hearing loss* (pp. 51–69). Baltimore: York Press.

Van Kleeck, A. (1994). Metalinguistic development. In G.P. Wallach & K.G. Butler (Eds.), *Language learning disabilities in school-age children and adolescents* (pp. 53–98). New York: Charles E. Merrill.

Wiig, E.H., & Semel, E. (1984). *Language assessment and intervention for the learning disabled.* Columbus: Charles E. Merrill.

Yuzon, E. (1994). FM personal listening systems. In M. Ross (Ed.), *Communication access for persons with hearing loss* (pp. 73–101). Baltimore: York Press.

CHAPTER 10

RESEARCH NEEDS AND FUTURE DIRECTIONS

Diagnosis and management of central auditory processing disorders (CAPD) have improved dramatically in recent years. Nonetheless, important questions remain regarding the neurobiology of central auditory processing, the linkage among central auditory processing, language, and cognition and their attendant disorders; and the efficacy of clinical practices. A clearer understanding of CAPD will advance all dimensions of our professional interests, including clinical services, advocacy, and scientific study.

More precise conceptual and scientific understanding will provide a context for interpretation of research outcomes and clinical observations. A robust foundation of knowledge and skills reflected in positive clinical outcomes should enhance professional credibility and provide a respected platform from which we may advocate on behalf of our clientele. No less important, this expanded knowledge base will further professional autonomy and recognition from contracting agencies and third party payers, which is vital in the tumultuous health care arena in which we must compete to continue to deliver our professional services.

Some of the controversies that have beset the area of CAPD may be attributed to the youth of this label and field of inquiry. As reviewed in Chapter 1, although reports of central auditory nervous system dysfunction in adults have been reported since the 1950s (Bocca, Calearo, & Cassinari, 1954; Bocca, Calearo, Cassinari, & Migliavacca, 1955), it was not until a 1977 conference on CAPD in children (Keith, 1977) that this term became prominent and interest in research on pediatric CAPD was stimulated (Katz & Illmer, 1972; Manning, Johnson, & Beasley, 1977; Martin & Clark, 1977; Sweetow & Reddell, 1978; Willeford, 1977). It is imperative that we exploit the momentum that has taken us to our current level of understanding and clinical practice, as described in the preceding chapters.

The ASHA consensus report delineating the status of research and clinical practices in CAPD (ASHA, 1996) may be the watershed event, heralding a renewed commitment to research, professional training, and professional service provision in this area. In this final chapter, we identify a number of the unresolved issues and research priorities, as well as technological applications and future directions that should benefit our clients.

RESEARCH PRIORITIES

The following research priorities, identified in the 1996 ASHA consensus report, are elaborated on following this extract from the report.

Basic Science

Elucidate the anatomical, physiological, and behavioral correlates of audition.

Determine the influence of peripheral hearing on central auditory processing and the influence of central auditory processing for peripheral processes.

Determine the neuropharmacological influences for diagnosis and treatment of central auditory processing disorders.

Explore the role of genetics and heredity as causal agents of central auditory processing disorders. Investigate the prevalence of central auditory processing disorders in multicultural populations.

Determine whether central auditory processing disorders in children result from neurologic abnormality, neuromaturational disorder, developmental delay, or some combination of factors.

Determine the interrelationships among central auditory processing, attention, cognition, and language.

Explore the influence of temporal characteristics of real-time speech signals and the real-world demands placed upon on-line temporal processing mechanisms.

Assessment

Establish efficiency (i.e., sensitivity and specificity) of behavioral and physiologic measures of central auditory processing. Psychometric rigor of tests purporting to assess central auditory processing must be established for both adults with known lesions and children with suspected diffuse neural dysfunction and documented listening problems.

Develop improved audiologic measures to ascertain the listener's use of both acoustic-phonetic and linguistic-contextual information for spoken language understanding.

Develop minimal test batteries of physiological and behavioral measures necessary and sufficient for identification and assessment of central auditory processing disorders.

Develop tests using verbal stimuli in other languages for assessment of central auditory processing on non-native listeners, as well as tests that evaluate the particular spoken language understanding problems facing non-native listeners.

Delineate the effects of neuromaturation on measures of central auditory processing.

Delineate the effects of aging on measures of central auditory processing.

Establish guidelines for the identification of children at risk for central auditory processing disorders.

Develop guidelines for knowledge and skill competencies in the administration and interpretation of tests of central auditory processing.

Management

Establish guidelines for knowledge and skill competencies in the development and implementation of management strategies.

Develop guidelines for management strategies and techniques, including use of FM systems, in treating central auditory processing disorders.

Examine the efficacy of treatment methodology related to effectiveness and acceptability of treatments.

Ascertain the effects on central auditory processing of medication frequently prescribed for management of attention deficit hyperactivity disorder.

Determine the interrelationships among central auditory processing disorders, attention deficit hyperactivity disorder, and cognitive and language disorders.

Explore the applicability of new real-time speech rate conversion technology for the treatment of central auditory processing disorders.

Professional Practice

Develop guidelines for a team approach to the identification, assessment, and management of children and adults with central auditory processing disorders focused on collaborative exchange with other disciplines and professionals.

Establish Common Procedural Terminology (CPT) codes to facilitate reimbursement for assessment and treatment services related to central auditory processing disorders. (ASHA, 1996, pp. 50–51)

FUTURE DIRECTIONS

The concerted efforts of researchers and clinicians are needed to accomplish the preceding research priorities and firmly establish CAPD as a viable diagnostic category labeling a biologically based group of disorders. Answers to the questions underlying or stated in the foregoing research priorities will provide evidence confirming the neurobiologic etiology of CAPD and differentiating CAPD from other related disorders, and thereby lead to improved diagnostic and treatment protocols. These priorities presage a number of directions for the future, as described in the following sections.

Professional Education

The quality of clinical services provided by practitioners determines society's valuation of their clinical specialty. Recent data indicating underpreparation of speech-language pathology and audiology graduates in the area of central auditory processing confirms the urgency to develop guidelines for knowledge and skill competencies in assessment and management of CAPD (Henri, 1994). The guidelines should be developed by university educators and clinicians to reflect the demands of the workplace while recognizing the resource constraints of today's graduate education programs. Appropriate coursework and clinical experiences in assessing and managing CAPD must be included in training programs. Perhaps most important, university faculty and clinical supervisors must conceptualize audiological evaluation and rehabilitation more broadly, teaching students that comprehensive evaluation and effective management programming require careful attention to both the peripheral and central auditory systems.

Assessment and Management

A number of research priorities identified by the ASHA Task Force on Central Auditory Processing (ASHA, 1996) converge on the development of improved assessment measures and treatment strategies. Persistent questions concerning linkages among CAPD, attention deficit disorders, and cognitive and language disorders reveal the importance of a comprehensive and thorough evaluation using sensitive measures to discern more subtle variations in performance. Clinicians must accept the challenge to evaluate the integrity of underlying perceptual, linguistic, and cognitive systems to determine the predominant and primary deficits, as well as secondary problems (McFarland & Cacace, 1995). Meeting this challenge requires the interdisciplinary efforts of audiologists, speech-language pathologists, teachers, psychologists, and physicians. The extensive clinical profile developed through such collaboration should improve differential diagnosis and maximize the potential for effective intervention. For example, determining the degree to which secondary metacognitive deficits preclude active deployment of listening strategies and thereby exacerbate spoken language processing deficits in individuals with CAPD will allow us to refine the balance between auditory processing skills and metacognitive strategies in intervention programming.

Collaboration, Systems Approach, and Dynamic Assessment

Professional collaboration is pivotal to the systems (i.e., ecological) approach to assessment and management that we have advocated throughout this book. Individuals cannot be evaluated without an analysis of the contexts in which they interact because environmental factors influence development, learning, and performance (Barkley, 1996; Bartoli & Botel, 1988; Heshusius, 1989; Palincsar, Brown, & Campione, 1994; Poplin, 1988a, 1988b; Sameroff, 1983; Weaver, 1985, 1993). Although performance deficits noted on a battery of central auditory processing tests may justify a diagnosis of CAPD, comprehensive assessment of CAPD demands evaluation of functional deficits in the variety of contexts in which the individual operates. Information regarding home, school, and employment settings, as well as interactions with family, teachers, peer group, and co-workers should be obtained through case history and/or systematic observation to appropriately evaluate the client and plan effective treatments. The presence of central auditory processing deficits in association with language and/or cognitive deficits (e.g., aphasia, traumatic head injury, learning disabilities) underscores the need for collaboration among audiologists, speech-language pathologists, and other professionals responsible for assessment and management.

A dynamic assessment approach focused on the processes, rather than exclusive reliance on the products (i.e., scores) of performance, will enhance our understanding of an individual's central auditory abilities. A dynamic approach to assessment, including information obtained from an extensive case history and systematic observation, should provide insight regarding factors that exacerbate or mitigate the performance difficulties noted on the central auditory test battery, as well as influence prognosis and treatment outcomes. Hence, new assessment measures and treatment strategies should be developed within a systems framework.

In considering the potential benefits of collaboration, we urge collaboration between clinicians and scientists to gain the clearest understanding of central auditory processing and CAPD, an expansion of the multidisciplinary professional exchange recommended in the ASHA consensus report. Collaboration combining the clinician's firsthand knowledge of client needs with the researcher's expertise in the scientific method provide a potent approach to asking the right questions and obtaining enduring answers.

Test Battery

Notwithstanding significant advances in tests of central auditory processing, continued efforts must be directed toward developing efficient behavioral and electrophysiological measures of central auditory functions. Test batteries that are powerful yet not overly time consuming to administer should be developed. The multiple purposes served by central auditory tests (e.g., differential diagnosis, site-of-lesion testing, identifying deficient processes and functional deficits, determining neuromaturational status, monitoring recovery from insult/injury, planning intervention, monitoring intervention) and the diverse populations to whom these tests are administered (e.g., multicultural, pediatric, older adult populations; populations with either documented or uncertain central nervous system pathology) underscore the need for an adequate array of tests and procedures to allow flexibility in designing a test battery to meet the particular purpose(s) of testing and the client's level of function.

Incorporating electrophysiologic procedures (e.g., middle-latency and event-related auditory evoked potentials) within the central auditory test battery will elucidate the neurobiologic substrata of CAPD, providing more definitive diagnostic information and leading to more focused intervention programming. In particular, event-related auditory evoked potentials that assess physiological and behavioral activity simultaneously (e.g., P300, mismatch negativity potential [MMN]) should be investigated further. Preliminary reports have documented that event-related potentials reveal electrophysiologic correlates for auditory discrimination (i.e., MMN) and selective auditory attention deficits (P300) (Jirsa, 1992; Jirsa & Clontz, 1990; Kraus, McGee, Ferre et al., 1993; Musiek, Baran, & Pinheiro, 1992). Electrophysiologic procedures, as well as the neuroimaging techniques discussed below, may provide a better understanding of the interdependent functions of the peripheral and central auditory systems in integrating and processing information and help differentiate among disorders presenting overlapping clinical profiles. For example, youngsters with CAPD present significantly delayed P300 latencies and reduced P300 amplitudes compared to youngsters with ADHD whose P300 latencies and amplitudes do not differ from those of normal control subjects (Jirsa & Clontz, 1990; Sangal, Sangal, & Persky, 1995).

Further research also is needed to examine the performance of individuals representing the spectrum of diagnostic labels associated with CAPD on a common test battery (Cook et al., 1993; Gascon, Johnson, & Burd, 1986). Inclusion of comparable auditory and visual behavioral processing tasks and electrophysiologic procedures in the test battery should clarify the modality-specific versus supramodal nature of attention deficits presumed in CAPD and attention deficit disorders, respectively (McFarland & Cacace, 1995). Because the event-related potentials are not modality specific, they may be particularly useful in illuminating the relationship between CAPD and the more global attention deficit disorders. New procedures recently adapted for audiology also present promise. Insofar as they reveal processing interactions between the physical and linguistic dimensions of a stimulus, the traditional visual Stroop and Garner tasks administered in conjunction with their auditory analogs have potential for elucidating the relationship between spoken language processing and auditory processing (Jerger, Elizondo, Dinh, Sanchez, & Chavira, 1994; Jerger, Stout et al., 1993).

Also offering immense potential are neuroimaging techniques that illuminate the structure and function of the central nervous system. The further development of these procedures will profoundly expand our understanding of the neurobiological linkages and distinctions among the spectrum of comorbid disorders presenting overlapping symptomatology (Chermak, 1996; Duffy, Denckla, Bartell, & Sandini, 1980; Finitzo & Pool, 1987; Frumkin, Potchen, Aniskiewicz, Moore, & Cooke, 1989; Galaburda, 1989; Galaburda & Eidelberg, 1982; Galaburda & Kemper, 1978; Galaburda, Sherman, Rosen, Aboitz, & Geshwind, 1985; Hynd & Semrud-Clikeman, 1989; Hynd, Semrud-Clikeman, Lorys, Novey, & Eliopulos, 1990; Hynd, Semrud-Clikeman, & Lyytinen, 1991; Lou, Henriksen, & Bruhn, 1984; Lou, Henriksen, Bruhn, Borner, & Nielsen, 1989; Mann, Lubar, Zimmerman, Miller, & Muenchen, 1992; Voeller, 1991; Zametkin et al., 1990). Functional magnetic resonance imaging, for example, may clarify the relationships between neural structure and function, including the sites where different stimuli are processed.

Efficacy

Among the research priorities delineated in the ASHA report, none is more fundamental and crucial to our ability to continue to serve clients with CAPD than establishing the efficacy of our treatments. As discussed in Chapter 7, preliminary reports are encouraging; however, additional studies are needed. Carefully designed clinical studies, controlling threats to internal validity and incorporating appropriate outcome measures, are needed to establish treatment efficacy. Outcome measures must be sufficiently broad (e.g., improved spoken language comprehension) to demonstrate significant change in functionally relevant contexts (e.g., school, home, work). Controlling subject selection and precisely defining subject characteristics are necessary given the comorbidity and possible linkage among a number of related disorders (e.g., CAPD, attention deficit disorder, learning disability). Such controls will enable us to determine how treatment programs affect well-defined CAPD and which treatment strategies and programs are most efficacious in meeting the needs of clients with particular CAPD profiles at particular life stages. Indeed, greater precision in identifying and classifying subjects selected for research should lead to clarification regarding the relationships among the spectrum of conditions manifesting central auditory processing deficits.

Regarding the call to establish guidelines for use of FM systems in treatment programs, the safety and efficacy of amplification devices with individuals with normal peripheral hearing must be ascertained. Although preliminary reports are encouraging (Blake, Field, Foster, Platt, & Wertz, 1991; Flexer, 1989; Ray, Sarff, & Glassford, 1984; Sarff, Ray, & Bagwell, 1981; Stach, Loiselle, & Jerger, 1987a, 1987b, 1991), research design limitations (e.g., lack of control group, subject selection and subject characteristics, specifics regarding characteristics of amplification systems and environments in which they are used), cast some questions on the validity of reported outcomes (ASHA, 1991, 1996). Questions surrounding potential for iatrogenic noise-induced hearing loss and monitoring of assistive listening systems also must be addressed (ASHA, 1991).

Classification and Prevalence

The heterogeneous nature of CAPD, as manifested in diverse clinical populations and the overlapping symptomatology across CAPD, attention deficit hyperactivity disorder, and language disorder, require continued examination of our approach to classification. In particular, we may wish to assume a polythetic approach to classification, an approach that has become dominant in a number of psychiatric and educational classification schemes (Blashfield, 1993).

According to the polythetic classification model, a positive classification of a disorder does not require the presence of all characteristics or any one characteristic used to define that disorder; rather, classification may be based on the presence of a subset of characteristics (Blashfield, 1993). Given the heterogeneous nature of CAPD, the polythetic classification model would seem appropriate as diagnosis of CAPD typically is confirmed on the basis of some subset of processing deficits.

As we continue to refine the definition of CAPD and identification and diagnostic batteries, it is important to consider that subsets or clusters of behavioral characteristics may then be used to further understand and possibly subtype CAPD into groups sharing similar symptoms. Such subtyping will necessarily influence treatment plans. For example, it is well known that some individuals with CAPD present with language impairment, but others do not; some experience academic and social difficulties, while a smaller group shows no language or academic deficits despite difficulties performing the tasks of central auditory processing tests (Efron, 1963; Jerger, Johnson, Jerger, Coker, Pirozzolo, & Gray, 1991; Kraus, McGee, Ferre et al., 1993; Ludlow, 1980; Medwetsky, 1994; Tallal, Stark, Kallman, & Mellits, 1980; Willeford & Burleigh, 1985). The recently proposed four category subtyping system based in part on performance patterns on the *Staggered Spondaic Word* (SSW) *Test* provides an example of a polythetic approach to classification (Katz, 1992; Katz & Smith, 1991). The validity of this system, however, has not been established.

Prevalence

The classification model accepted as the professional standard will influence prevalence estimates. As stated in Chapter 1, prevalence data for CAPD are lacking. Establishing the prevalence of CAPD in pediatric, adult, and older adult populations awaits the refinement of classification efforts.

Neuropharmacologic Management Of CAPD

Efforts to understand the neurochemistry of the auditory system have intensified based on preliminary reports suggesting the potential for clinical intervention. A number of studies have demonstrated that pharmacologic intervention can alter physiologic and behavioral aspects of audition (Feldman, Brainard, & Knudsen, 1996; Musiek & Hoffman, 1990; Sahley, Kalish, Musiek, & Hoffman, 1991; Sahley, Musiek, & Nodar, 1996; Sahley & Nodar, 1994). For example, reported decrements in neurotransmitter levels in the auditory areas of the brains of aged animals suggest that central auditory processing deficits among older adults may respond to pharmacologic intervention (Banay-Schwartz, Laztha, & Palkovits, 1989; Caspary, Milbrandt, & Helfert, 1995; Caspary, Raza, Lawhorn-Armour, Pippin, & Arneric, 1990). Pickles and Comis' (1973) finding that injected atropine sulfate raised noise thresholds more so than quiet thresholds suggests that this drug affects the olivocochlear system, the system posited to improve neural signal-to-noise ratios and enhance the detection of signals in noise (Dewson, 1968; Dolan & Nuttall, 1988; Nieder & Nieder, 1970; Wiederhold, 1986). Research suggesting an even broader role for the olivocochlear system, influencing selective auditory attention, improving the clarity of sound, and modulation of auditory nerve activity, as well as signal in noise detection (Art & Fettiplace, 1984; Wiederhold, 1986), underscores the potential of pharmacologic intervention for treatment of CAPD. Preliminary reports suggesting some therapeutic efficacy for a number of pharmacologic agents (e.g., pentoxifylline, physostigmine, piracetam, propentofylline, vinpocetine) in reducing cognitive, learning, and communication deficits of older adults with organic brain disease may presage the development of similar drugs for treatment of the same deficits frequently associated with CAPD (Hock, 1995; Huber, Kittner, Hojer, Fink, Neveling, & Heiss, 1993; Ikeda et al., 1992; Moller, Maurer, & Saletu, 1994; Nicholson, 1990; Parkinson, Rudolphi, & Fredholm, 1994; Saletu, Moller, Grunberger, Deutsch, & Rossner, 1990; Sano et al., 1993; Torigoe et al., 1994). Promising alternatives to stimulant medications now under investigation for attention deficit disorder (e.g., clonidine, guanfacine [Tenex]) may also prompt research of pharmacologic treatment options for youngsters with CAPD (Chappell et al., 1995; Hunt, Arnsten, & Asbell, 1995; Hunt, Minderaa, & Cohen, 1985). We may soon witness discoveries that will revolutionize the treatment of CAPD and related disorders in children and adults (Campbell & Cueva, 1995; Caspary et al., 1990; Hock, 1995).

Recovery of Function

Several long held presumptions in neurobiology recently have been challenged. Under question are the presumptions that neurogenesis (i.e., the generation of neurons) in the mammalian central nervous system ends soon after birth and that the production, migration, and differentiation of cochlear hair cells occur embryonically and/or immediately postnatally (Ruben, 1967). The previously accepted resignation to the irreversible nature of hair cell and neural losses that followed from these questionable presumptions also has come under scrutiny (Ruben, 1996). It now appears theoretically possible to restore auditory function following damage or injury if the proper neurotrophic mechanisms (i.e., mechanisms that promote the regeneration and survival of neurons) are activated (Ruben, 1996; Van De Water, Staecker, Apfel, & Lefebvre, 1996). Greater understanding of the genetics of audition and auditory disorders should provide crucial information needed to stimulate neural and hair cell regeneration and mitigate the effects of gene mutations on audition (Steel & Kimberling, 1996).

Recent demonstrations of regeneration of cochlear hair cells in birds (Corwin & Cotanche, 1988; Cotanche, 1987; Cruz, Lambert, & Rubel, 1987; Jacobsen, 1991; Rubel, Oesterle, & Weisleder, 1991; Ryals & Rubel, 1988), hair cell and neuronal regeneration in the mammalian ears of chinchillas, guinea pigs, rats, and humans (Bohne & Harding, 1992; Forge, Li, Corwin, & Nevill, 1993; Lambert, 1994; Lefebvre, Malgrange, Staecker, Moonen, & Van De Water,

1993; Sun, Bohne, & Harding, 1995; Warchol, Lambert, Goldstein, Forge, Corwin, 1993), and the proliferation of nerves of the central nervous system of mice (Reynolds & Weiss, 1992) and fish (Eitan et al., 1994) offer an exciting prospect for restoration of hearing sensitivity and perhaps recovery of processing function in CAPD. The consistent finding that cochlear pathology can alter temporal processing (Florentine, Fastl, & Buss, 1988; Gengel, 1972; Green, Birdsall, & Tanner, 1957; Watson & Gengel, 1969; Wright, 1968; Zwicker & Wright, 1963), coupled with the recent finding of recovery of auditory discrimination of bird vocalizations following hair cell regeneration in birds (Dooling, Manabe, & Ryals, 1996), suggests that recovery of certain central auditory processing functions might follow restoration of cochlear function, perhaps even in the absence of completely restored neural function. Certainly, significant neural reorganization in response to injury or learning across the life span demonstrates the plasticity of mature nervous systems and the potential for restoration of neural function (Edeline & Weinberger, 1991; Irvine, Rajan, & Robertson, 1992; Kolb, 1995; Moore, 1993; Schwaber, Garraghty, & Kaas, 1993; Singer, 1995).

Prevention of Central Auditory Processing Disorders

Understanding the genetics of audition and auditory disorders and the molecular mechanisms of neural regeneration may lead to therapies to prevent deterioration and loss of function (Steel & Kimberling, 1996; Van De Water et al., 1996). Significant progress has been achieved in identifying genes causing auditory disorders (Duyk, Gastier, & Mueller, 1992; Guilford, Ayadi et al., 1994; Guilford, Ben et al., 1994; Steel & Brown, 1994; Steel & Kimberling, 1996). Moreover, the growing body of literature documenting the acquired resistance or *toughening* of the auditory system to intense noise exposure offers hope that one day we may be able to prevent this most common type of acquired hearing loss. Auditory resistance to temporary threshold shift and noise-induced hearing loss has been observed rather consistently following *conditioning* or *priming* exposures to noise (Campo, Subramaniam, & Henderson, 1991; Canlon, Borg, & Flock, 1988; Canlon, Borg, & Lofstrand, 1991; Clark, Bohne, & Boettcher, 1987; Hamernik, Ahroon, Davis, & Lei, 1994; Henderson, Campo, Subramaniam, & Fiorino, 1992; Henselman, Henderson, Subramaniam, & Sallustio, 1994; Miyakita, Hellstrom, Frimanson, & Axelsson, 1992; Ryan, Bennett, Woolf, & Axelsson, 1994; Subramaniam, Campo, & Henderson, 1991; Subramaniam, Henderson,

Campo, & Spongr, 1992; Subramaniam, Henderson, & Spongr, 1993). Albeit, not completely understood, the mechanisms responsible for increased resistance to noise appear to involve fundamental changes in cochlear physiology (Henderson, Subramaniam, Spongr, & Attanasio, 1996; Lim, Jenkins, Myers, Miller, & Altschuler, 1993; Neely, Thompson, & Gower, 1991; Ryan, 1988), although a possible role for the olivocochlear system in diminishing the impact of intense noise exposure has not been excluded (Cody & Johnstone, 1982; Handrock & Zeisberg, 1982; Rajan, 1988; Rajan & Johnsone, 1983, 1988, 1989). Involvement of the olivocochlear system might offer opportunity to preserve central auditory processes (e.g., auditory performance in competing signals), given the purported role of the olivocochlear system in enhancing neural signal-to-noise ratios and modulating auditory nerve activity (Art & Fettiplace, 1984; Dewson, 1968; Dolan & Nuttall, 1988; Nieder & Nieder, 1970; Wiederhold, 1986). Although additional or different mechanisms might underlie prevention of central auditory processing disorders, the knowledge gained regarding both neural regeneration and conditioning in modulating auditory sensitivity may someday lead to means to preserve and repair the central auditory nervous system.

APPLIED TECHNOLOGY

The real-time speech rate conversion technology listed among the ASHA research priorities is an excellent example of the application of our increasing understanding of the role of temporal cues for spoken language recognition. Although the recognition of speech had been thought to depend on spectral (frequency-specific) cues, recent work suggesting a larger and more primary role for temporal cues (Shannon, Zeng, Kamath, Wygonski, & Ekelid, 1995; Van Tassell, Soli, Kirby, & Widin, 1987) has led to improvements in expanded speech technology. For example, a real-time speech rate conversion system that decreases the presentation rate of real-time speech without disturbing voice quality or other important aspects of the speech signal and simultaneously controls any imposed asynchrony between converted speech and visual signals may soon benefit listeners with temporal processing deficits, as well as those with peripheral hearing impairment. Similarly, speech processing algorithms that increase the salience of the rapidly changing acoustic elements of speech may offer promise for enhancing comprehension of spoken language among those with CAPD and language impairment (Tallal et al., 1996).

In addition to offering new solutions to processing problems, technological enhancements, especially computer technology, will provide more novel instructional formats, which may elicit greater attention, motivation, and persistence than more traditional formats. The use of CD-ROM and video laser disc technology offers opportunities for interactive applications to support computer-assisted training and adaptive testing. Tallal et al.'s (1996) work with adaptive computerized training demonstrates the potential of this technology in delivering efficacious therapy for CAPD and associated language-related deficits.

Similarly, Miller and Gildea (1987) described a computerized tutorial designed to help children improve their vocabulary skills using the contextual approach described in Chapter 8. Building on children's curiosity and motivation to learn, they are presented with words beyond their current vocabulary level in an interesting context which motivates the child to learn their meanings. They are expected to learn word meaning by requesting information through definitions, sentences, and pictures. Although computer programmed instruction incorporates a technology that would seem to be inherently motivating to most children, the effectiveness of this approach relative to an attentive therapist remains to be ascertained.

Continuing developments in the application of active noise control technology may lead to quieter classrooms and other settings where noise control is desired. Already used in headphones, hearing protection devices, and other enclosed spaces (e.g., exhaust pipes, ducts), active noise control is particularly effective in reducing low frequency noise that cannot be adequately attenuated through traditional passive techniques (Carter, 1984; Eriksson, Allie, Bremigan, & Gilbert, 1989; Landgarten, 1987).

Active noise control relies on sound cancellation by generating a sound field that is an exact mirror image (i.e., *anti-noise*) of the disturbing sound (Hoover & Blazier, 1991). The generated sound cancels the disturbance. Since the destructive interference can selectively cancel unwanted low frequency noise while still allowing a listener to hear the middle and high frequency sounds so important to spoken language recognition, this sound cancellation technique has been investigated for incorporation in wearable hearing aids (Brey, Robinette, Chabries, & Christiansen, 1987; Preves, 1994; Weiss, 1987). Although active noise control is usually limited to low frequency waves, digital signal processing should extend application of the technique to broadband signals (Hoover & Blazier, 1991). It also should reduce the cost of noise control, particularly for the low frequencies which would otherwise require expensive, heavy or bulky passive methods (e.g., absorptive treatments, vibration mounts). Reduced costs should lead to more widespread use of active noise control technology to quiet noisy settings, including classrooms.

CONCLUSIONS

Recent scientific and clinical advances have considerably increased our understanding of CAPD, resulting in improved diagnostic and management services. The neurobiological and technological frontiers reviewed in this chapter promise to further advance clinical practices, perhaps even revolutionizing assessment and treatment procedures. For example, it is conceivable that future pharmacologic treatments may supplant, or more likely complement and potentiate, behavioral management of some types of CAPD (Deberdt, 1994; Klein & Slomkowski, 1993; van Engeland, 1993). Similarly, advances in electrophysiological procedures and neuroimaging techniques will clarify the relationships between neurobiological function and structure and the interdependent processing of stimuli by the peripheral and central auditory systems. No doubt, this knowledge will benefit, if not transform, clinical assessment and managment practices.

While we strive for these dramatic improvements in clinical care, we must remain committed to advancing the more attainable research priorities, which will lead to improved clinical practices in the near term. One of these priorities, developing a more powerful test battery, will improve diagnostic efficiency and advance a second priority, to refine the CAPD classification system. Both developments will lead to greater treatment efficacy by furthering customization of intervention programming. As another priority, we must fully exploit the current opportunities to minimize the impact of CAPD on individuals' lives, including the use of technology (e.g, computer instruction, FM systems) for remediation and compensation. Because computerized programs are tools that can be used in the home, they may be particularly valuable in promoting collaboration and generalization of skills.

Clearly, multidisciplinary collaboration among clinicians, researchers, educators, and families will expedite clinical advances by stimulating new questions and fueling investigation. Understanding neural regeneration, neural reorganization, and the functional consequences of restored neural function, for example, will require the combined undertaking of auditory scientists, audiologists, molecular biologists, and geneticists. This knowledge may generate new rehabilitative or restorative therapies. Even more exciting, this knowledge may signal a new era of prevention as management.

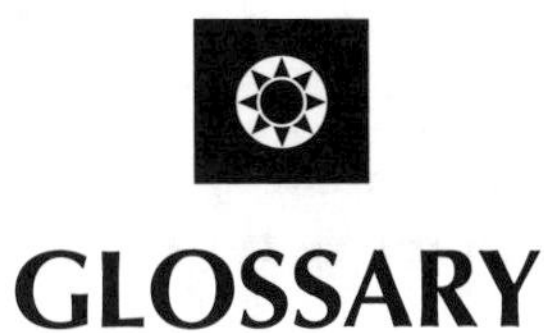

GLOSSARY

Accommodation. Making facilities and programs accessible to and usable by persons with disabilities through appropriate modifications, including policy modifications, task restructuring, modified schedules, equipment acquisition or modification, training, or provision of qualified readers or interpreters, and other similar accommodations.

Acoustic access. Access through the auditory channel, either unaided or aided, to acoustic information.

Analog. Refers to a signal which varies continuously over time.

Assistive Listening System. A device that delivers sound to individuals with peripheral or central auditory deficits to mitigate listening problems (e.g., frequency modulated [FM] systems, personal amplifiers, infrared systems).

Attention. Gateway to conscious experience; maintains primacy of certain information in ongoing information processing.

Selective (focused) attention. Ability to focus on relevant stimuli while ignoring simultaneously presented, but irrelevant stimuli (i.e., distractors).
Divided attention. Ability to attend to multiple stimuli simultaneously.
Sustained attention (vigilance). Ability to inhibit interference; requires sustained focus for a period of time while awaiting the occurrence of a target stimulus.

Attention Deficit Hyperactivity Disorder (ADHD). Persistent pattern of inattention and/or hyperactivity-impulsivity that is more frequent and severe than is typically observed in individuals at a comparable level of development; manifested in at least two settings; interferes with developmentally appropriate social, academic, or occupational functions; and has been present before age 7 years.

Combined type. Attention deficit characterized by hyperactivity-impulsivity and inattention.
Predominantly inattentive type. Presents primary symptoms of inattention.
Predominantly hyperactive-impulsive type. Behavioral regulation disorder.

Binaural interaction. Auditory processing involving the two ears and their neural connections.

Brain imaging. Procedures used to map the structure and metabolic and electrophysiological properties of the brain; includes computed tomography, magnetic resonance imaging, positron emission topography, regional cerebral blood flow, and brain electrical activity mapping.

Bottom-up processing. Information processing that is data driven; properties of the data are primary determinants of higher level representations and constructions.

Central Auditory Nervous System (CANS). The auditory brainstem, subcortical pathways, auditory cortex, and corpus callosum.

Central auditory processes. Auditory system mechanisms and processes responsible for sound localization and lateralization; auditory discrimination; auditory pattern recognition; temporal aspects of audition including, temporal resolution, temporal masking, temporal integration, and temporal ordering; auditory performance with competing acoustic signals; and auditory performance with degraded acoustic signals; these auditory system mechanisms and processes generate electrical brain waves or auditory evoked potentials (i.e., auditory brainstem response, auditory middle-latency response, auditory late-latency response, and auditory event-related response) in response to acoustic stimuli.

Central Auditory Processing Disorder (CAPD). Heterogeneous disorder involving an observed deficit in one or more of the central auditory processes responsible for generating the auditory evoked potentials (i.e., electrocochleography, auditory brainstem response, auditory middle-latency response, auditory late-latency response, and auditory event-related response) and the following behavioral phenomena: sound localization and lateralization; auditory discrimination; auditory pattern recognition; temporal aspects of audition, including temporal resolution, temporal masking, temporal integration, and temporal ordering; auditory performance with competing acoustic signals; and auditory performance with degraded acoustic signals.

Clear speech. Speech produced by a speaker who has been instructed to speak as clearly as possible, as if trying to communicate in a noisy background.

Closure. The ability to subjectively complete and make whole an incomplete form. Listeners use language knowledge and inductive and deductive reasoning, as well as auditory and grammatic closure to derive the meaning of words and messages.

Auditory closure. The ability to recognize a whole word despite the absence of certain elements.

Grammatic closure. The ability to complete phrases or sentences despite missing words or morphemes (e.g., filling in the verb form *are* versus *is* to conjugate with the subject *they*).

Verbal auditory closure. The ability to use spoken contextual information to facilitate speech recognition.

Cognition. Activity of knowing, encompassing the acquisition, organization, and use of knowledge; automatic and unconscious processes that transform, reduce, elaborate, store, recover, and use sensory input; primary phase in the development of knowledge.

Cognitive style. An individual's approach to processing information, problem solving, and cognitive tasks (e.g., bottom-up/top-down, impulsive/reflective, field dependent/field independent).

Commissure. A group of axons of neurons passing from one side of the brain, usually, to a similar structure on the opposite side of the brain.

Compensation. Rehabilitative approach directed toward reducing the negative impact of a disorder or disease not amenable to complete recovery through treatment.

Consonant-Vowel (CV). Nonsense syllable comprised of a consonant followed by a vowel (e.g., ba, da, ga).

Deductive inferencing. Reasoning from the general to the specific.

Dichotic. Simultaneous presentation of two different acoustic events, one to each ear.

Difference Limen (DL). Just noticeable difference or smallest detectable change in a stimulus, usually pertaining to frequency, intensity, or duration.

Dynamic assessment. Approach to evaluation focused on the different ways by which an individual achieves a score rather than the score achieved; approach is characterized by guided learning to determine an individual's potential for change.

Efficacy. Effectiveness, efficiency, and effects of treatments; documenting treatment efficacy requires demonstrating that a particular treatment produces the desired outcomes or behavior change in an efficient manner (e.g., cost effective) as a result of the treatment.

Endogenous. Refers to evoked potentials (e.g., P300) that are relatively invariant to changes in the eliciting physical stimulus, but are highly influenced by subject state and require an internal or mental activity (e.g., perceptual or cognitive process) to generate the potential.

Executive function. Component of metacognition; set of general control processes that coordinate knowledge (i.e., cognition) and metacognitive knowledge, transforming such knowledge into behavioral strategies, which ensure that an individual's behavior is adaptive, consistent with some goal, and beneficial to the individual.

Gyrus (pl. gyri)**.** Bulge on the surface of the cerebral cortex consisting of gray matter with an inner core of white matter.

Induction Learning. Discovery learning; a three-step process through which a learner recognizes a pattern or relationship, explains the pattern or relationship, and hypothesizes the rule governing the pattern or relationship.

Inductive inferencing. Reasoning from the particular facts to a general conclusion.

Inferencing. Reaching a conclusion on the basis of facts or evidence.

Information processing. Assigning meaning to sensory input based on the extraction of cues or constraints through various processes or stages of cognition, including encoding, organizing, storing, retrieving, comparing, and generating or reconstructing information; these stages involve the interaction between sensory (e.g., auditory processes) and central processes (e.g., cognitive and linguistic processes) through feedback and feedforward loops.

Interaural timing. Refers to a behavioral task requiring the subject to determine the order of two acoustic events presented to each ear separately at slightly different times.

Intra-axial. Refers to lesions of the brainstem that evolve from the brainstem tissue itself, as opposed to extra-axial lesions that arise from nonbrainstem tissue. Extra-axial lesions often are in contact with the brainstem.

Isolation point. A real-time word recognition processing event, which occurs at the gate when the listener initially identifies the target word.

Latency. The time between occurrence of a physiologic event, usually a spike or evoked potential, and a stimulus.

Learning disabilities. A heterogeneous group of disorders, presumed to be due to central nervous system dysfunction, manifested by significant difficulties in the acquisition and use of listening, speaking, reading, writing, reasoning, or mathematical abilities.

Learning style. An individual's characteristic cognitive, affective, modality, and physiological behaviors and preferences employed in perceiving, interacting with, and responding to the learning environment.

Lexical access. A spoken language processing event in which a percept comes in contact with various features of stored lexical representations.

Lexical activation. Some change in status of a subset of word candidates contained in the mental lexicon.

Linguistic-contextual information. Anything that influences the a priori probability of an oncoming utterance or the post hoc, retroactive recognition of an ongoing utterance.

Management. Intervention to prevent or remediate a disorder or disease, as well compensatory approaches (e.g., strategies, technologies) to reduce the impact of deficits resistant to remediation.

Memory. Capacity to encode, process, and retrieve events, knowledge, feelings, and decisions of the past.

> **Short-term memory.** Brief storage of limited capacity with minimal processing requirements.
>
> **Working memory.** A component of long-term memory that is at a heightened state of activation for a limited period of time; involves both storage and processing of information (e.g., inference, transformation, executive processing).

Long-term memory. Declarative or explicit memory and procedural or implicit memory; long-term storage of unlimited capacity; involves both storage and processing of information.

Declarative or explicit memory. Conscious awareness or recollection of previously acquired information, retrieved on demand.

Procedural or implicit memory. Use of previous experience or knowledge, in the absence of conscious awareness or recollection, to support learning and guide performance.

Mesencephalic. Referring to the midbrain, just rostral to the pons.

Metacognition. Awareness and appropriate use of knowledge; awareness of the task and strategy variables that affect performance and the use of that knowledge to plan, monitor, and regulate performance, including attention, learning, and the use of language; second phase (following cognition) in the development of knowledge which is active and involves conscious control over knowledge.

Metalinguistics. Aspects of language competence that extend beyond unconscious usage for comprehension and production; involves ability to think about language in its abstract form—to reflect on aspects of language apart from its content, analyze it, and make judgments about it; metalinguistic knowledge underlies performance on a number of tasks, including phonological awareness (e.g., segmentation, rhyming), organization and storage of words (e.g., multiple word meanings), and figurative language (e.g., metaphor, idiom, humor); may be considered a subset of metacognition since using language is one of the goals of metacognitive processes.

Metamemory. Knowledge and awareness of one's own memory systems and strategies.

Mnemonics. Artificial or contrived memory aids for organizing information (e.g., acronyms, rhymes, verbal mediators, visual imagery, drawing).

Myogenic. A response that is generated by muscle contractions.

Neurobiology. Encompasses neuroanatomy, physiology, neurochemistry, and neuropharmacology.

Neuropharmacology. Effects of drugs on neuronal tissue.

Neurotransmitter. Chemical agent released by vesicles of a nerve cell that permits synaptic transmission between neurons.

Otoacoustic emissions. Subaudible sounds generated by the cochlea either spontaneously or evoked by sound stimulation.

Pharmacology. Sources, chemistry, actions, and uses of drugs.

Phonemic analysis. Separating words or syllables into a sequence of phonemes.

Phonemic synthesis. Blending of discrete phonemes into the correctly sequenced, coarticulated sound patterns.

Phonological awareness. Explicit awareness of the sound structure of language, including the recognition that words are comprised of syllables and phonemes.

Plasticity. Malleability of the central nervous system prior to stabilization of neural function; alteration of neurons to conform better to immediate environmental influences, often associated with a change in behavior; neural reorganization may be possible to some extent across the life span, as well as following injury (compensatory plasticity), and in response to learning.

Prevalence. Total number of cases of a specific disease or disorder existing in a given population at a certain time.

Problem solving. Generating a variety of potentially effective responses to a situation and recognizing and implementing the most effective response.

Prosody. Suprasegmental aspects of spoken language; the dynamic melody, timing, rhythm, and amplitude fluctuations of fluent speech.

Real-time speech. The transitory, ephemeral nature of an ongoing speech signal; when speech is presented in a real-time manner, listeners must quickly recognize phonemes, syllables, and words based on preceding linguistic-contextual cues and ongoing acoustic-phonetic information.

Reasoning. Evaluation of arguments, drawing of inferences and conclusions, and generation and testing of hypotheses.

Reciprocal teaching. Alternating roles between the client and clinician, allowing the client to assume the role of teacher as well as learner.

Remediation. Therapy to cure a disorder or disease.

Reverberation. Persistence or prolongation of sound in an enclosed space, resulting from multiple reflections of sound waves off hard surfaces after the source of the sound has ceased. Reverberation time (RT60) refers to the time required for a steady-state sound to decay 60 dB from its initial peak amplitude offset.

Schema. Structured cluster of concepts and expectations; an abstract and generic knowledge structure stored in memory that preserves the relations among constituent concepts and generalized knowledge about a text, event, message, situation, or object.

> **Formal schema.** Linguistic form that organizes, integrates, and predicts relationships across propositions (e.g., additives [*and, furthermore*], adversative [*although, nevertheless, however*], causal [*because, therefore, accordingly*], disjunctive [*but, instead, on the contrary*], and temporal connectives [*before, after, subsequently*], as well as patterns of parallelism and correlative pairs [*not only / but also; neither / nor*]).
>
> **Content or contextual schema.** Provides a generalized interpretation of the content of experience; organizes facts and establishes a framework that imposes certain structures on events, precepts, situations, and objects and facilitates interpretation.

Segmentation. Parsing spoken language into its constituent and successive segments; parsing sentences, words, or syllables into their constituent phonetic units.

Segmentation. The manner in which listeners demarcate the ongoing spoken utterance into units of lexical access.

Semantic network. Construct representing a mental system of nodes and links connecting lexical units; vocabulary building in such a network involves adding new nodes and links, as well as changing activation values of the links between nodes (e.g., building synonymy by strengthening the relationships between nodes).

Signal-to-Noise Ratio. Relationship between the sound levels of the signal and the noise at the listener's ear, commonly reported as the difference in decibels between the intensity of the signal and the intensity of the background noise (e.g., if the speech signal is measured at 70 dB and the noise is 64 dB, the signal-to-noise ratio is +6 dB).

Spoken language processing. An interactive system of peripheral and central functions used to recognize and understand real-world transitory utterances as meaningful speech.

Sulcus. Infoldings on the cerebral surface separating gyri.

Systems theory. Study of systems as an entity rather than a conglomeration of parts; provides a conceptual framework for understanding the organization, interaction, and dynamicity of elements comprising systems.

Temporal processing. Auditory mechanisms and processes responsible for temporal patterning (e.g., phase locking, synchronization) of neural discharges and the following behavioral phenomena: temporal resolution (i.e., detection of changes in durations of auditory stimuli and time intervals between auditory stimuli over time), temporal ordering (i.e., detection of sequence of sounds over time), temporal integration (i.e., summation of power over durations less than 200 milliseconds), and temporal masking (i.e., obscuring of probe by pre- or poststimulatory presentation of masker).

Tonotopic. Organization of auditory neurons in a particular structure according to their responsiveness to specfic frequencies.

Top-down processing. Information processing that is knowledge or concept driven such that higher level constraints guide data processing, leading to data interpretation consistent with these constraints.

TORCH+S complex. A group of perinatal medical problems often linked to hearing loss. T = toxoplasmosis; O = other (e.g., associated ophthalmologic disease); R = rubella; C = cytomegalovirus; H = herpes; S = syphilis.

Total acceptance point. A late event in the real-time word recognition process when a listener recognizes the target word with a high level of confidence.

Treatment. Therapy to prevent or remediate (i.e., cure) a disorder or disease.

Tuning curve. A graph depicting the response of a neuron, plotted as a function of stimulus intensity and frequency. The lowest sound level to which the neuron responds is represented by the tip of the tuning curve (i.e., characteristic frequency).

Word predictability. Amount of fill-in-the blank meaningfulness in a preceding spoken context. In predictability-high (PH) sentences, preceding semantic-contextual information is presented in the form of clue words; no such clue words are available in predictability-low (PL) sentences.

Word recognition. A spoken language processing event marking the conclusion of the word selection phase; also refers to a listener's ability to perceive and correctly identify a set of words usually presented at suprathreshold hearing level.

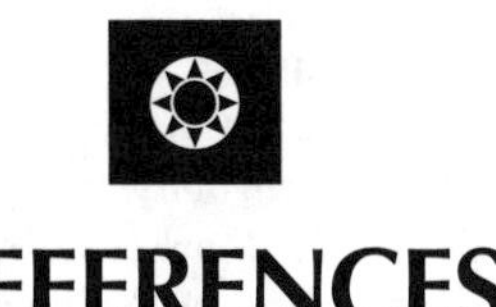

REFERENCES

Abbs, J.H., & Sussman, H.M. (1971). Neurophysiological feature detectors and speech perception: A discussion of theoretical implications. *Journal of Speech and Hearing Research, 14,* 23–36.

Abel, S.M. (1972). Discrimination of temporal gaps. *Journal of the Acoustical Society of America, 52*, 519–524.

Abeles, M., & Goldstein, M. (1972). Responses of a single unit in the primary auditory cortex of the cat to tones and to tone pairs. *Brain Research, 42*, 337–352.

Adams, J., & Wenthold, R. (1987). Immunostaining of GABA-ergic and glycinergic inputs to the anterovental cochlear nucleus. *Neuroscience Abstracts, 13*, 1259.

Adams, M.J. (1990). *Beginning to read: Thinking and learning about print.* Cambridge, MA: MIT Press.

Adelman, H.S., & Taylor, L. (1983). Enhancing motivation for overcoming learning and behavior problems. *Journal of Learning Disabilities, 16,* 384–392.

Adelman, P.B., & Vogel, S.A. (1991). The learning-disabled adult. In B.Y.L. Wong (Ed.), *Learning about learning disabilities* (pp. 564–594). San Diego: Academic Press.

Adesman, A.R., Altshuler, L., Lipkin, P., & Walco, G. (1990). Otitis media in children with learning disabilities and in children with attention deficit disorder with hyperactivity. *Pediatrics, 85*(Suppl.), 442–446.

Adrian, E.D. (1930). The activity of the nervous system of the caterpillar. *Journal of Physiology, 30*, 34–36.

Aitkin, L.M., & Webster, W.R. (1972). Medial geniculate body of the cate: Organization response to tonal stimuli of neurons in the ventral division. *Journal of Neurophysiology, 35*, 365–380.

Aitken, L.M., Webster, W.R., Veale, J.L., & Crosby, D.C. (1975). Inferior colliculus. I. Comparison of response properties of neurons in central, pericentral, and external nuclei of adult cat. *Journal of Neurophysiology, 38*, 1196–1207.

Alberti, R.E., & Emmons, M.L. (1978). *Your perfect right* (3rd ed.). San Luis Obispo, CA: Impact.

Alho, K., Woods, D., Algazi, A., Knight, R., & Naatanen, R. (1994). Lesions of the frontal cortex dimish the auditory mismatch negativity. *Electroencephalography and Clinical Neurophysiology, 91,* 353–362.

Allen, L., & Anderson, K. (1995). Marketing sound-field amplification systems. In C. Crandell, J. Smaldino, & C. Flexer (Eds.), *Sound-field FM amplification* (pp. 201–211). San Diego: Singular Publishing Group.

Allen, P., Wightman, F., Kistler, D., & Dolan, T. (1989). Frequency resolution in children. *Journal of Speech and Hearing Research, 32*, 317–322.

Allen, R.L., Cranford, J.L., & Pay, N. (1996). Central auditory processing in an adult with congenital absence of left temporal lobe. *Journal of the American Academy of Audiology, 7*(4), 282–288.

Allen, W. (1945). Effect of destroying three localized cerebral cortical areas for sound on correct conditioned differential responses of the dog's foreleg. *American Journal of Psychology, 144*, 415–428.

Altschuler, R.A., & Fex, J. (1986). Efferent neurotransmitters. In R.A. Altschuler, D.W. Hoffman, & R.P. Bobbin (Eds.), *Neurobiology of hearing: The cochlea* (pp. 383–396). New York: Raven Press.

Altschuler, R.A., Wenthold, R., Schwartz, A., Haser, W., Curthoys, N., Parakkal, M., & Fex, J. (1984). Immunocytochemical localization of glutaminase-like immunoreactivity in the auditory nerve. *Brain Research, 29*, 173–178.

American Psychiatric Association. (1994). *Diagnostic and statistical manual of mental disorders: DSM-IV* (4th ed.). Washington, DC: American Psychiatric Association.

American Speech-Language-Hearing Association. (1990). Audiological assessment of central auditory processing: An annotated bibliography. *Asha, 32*(Suppl. 1), 13–30.

American Speech-Language-Hearing Association. (1991). Amplification as a remediation technique for children with normal peripheral hearing. *Asha, 33*(Suppl. 3), 22–24.

American Speech-Language-Hearing Association. (1992). Issues in central auditory processing disorders: A report from the ASHA Ad Hoc Committee on Central Auditory Processing. Rockville, MD: American Speech-Language-Hearing Association.

American Speech-Language-Hearing Association. (1994). Guidelines for fitting and monitoring FM systems. *Asha, 36*(Suppl. 12), 1–9.

American Speech-Language-Hearing Association. (1995). Position statement and guidelines for acoustics in educational settings. *Asha, 37*(Suppl. 14), 15–19.

American Speech-Language-Hearing Association Task Force on Central Auditory Processing Consensus Development. (1996). Central auditory processing: Current status of research and implications for clinical practice. *American Journal of Audiology, 5*(2), 41–54.

Ames, C., & Ames, R. (1984). Systems of student and teacher motivation: Toward a qualitative definition. *Journal of Educational Psychology, 76,* 535–556.

Ames, C., & Felker, D. W. (1979). An examination of children's attributions and achievement-related evaluations in competitive, cooperative, and individualistic reward structures. *Journal of Educational Psychology, 71,* 413–420.

Anderson, J. (1988, January). *Cognitive styles and multicultural populations.* Paper presented at the American Speech-Language-Hearing Association Sea Island Multicultural Institute, Sea Island, GA.

Anderson, K.L. (1989). *S.I.F.T.E.R.: Screening instrument for targeting educational risk*. Austin, TX: Pro-Ed.

Anderson, K.L. (1991). Speech perception in children. *Educational Audiology Monograph, 1,*(1), 15–29.

Anderson, N.B. (1991). Understanding cultural diversity. *American Journal of Speech-Language Pathology, 1*(1), 9–10.

Anderson, P.P., & Fenichel, E.S. (1989). Serving culturally diverse families of infants and toddlers with disabilities. Washington, DC: National Center for Clinical Infant Programs.

Aoki, C., & Siekevitz, P. (1988). Plasticity in brain development. *Scientific American, 259*(6), 56–64.

Arehole, S., Augustine, L., & Simhadri, R. (1995). Middle latency response in children with learning disabilities: Preliminary findings. *Journal of Communications Disorders, 28*, 21–38.

Art, J.J., & Fettiplace, R. (1984) Efferent desensitization of auditory nerve fibre responses in the cochlea of the turtle pseudemys scripta elegans. *Journal of Physiology, 356,* 507–523.

Auerbach, S., Allard, T., Naeser, M., Alexander, M., & Albert, M. (1982). Pure word deafness. Analysis of a case with bilateral lesions and a defect at the prephonemic level. *Brain, 105*, 271–300.

August, G., & Garfinkel, B. (1990). Comorbidity of ADHD and reading disability among clinic-refereed children. *Journal of Abnormal Child Psychology, 18*, 29–45.

Augustine, L.E., & Damico, J.S. (1995). Attention deficit hyperactivity disorder: The scope of the problem. *Seminars in Speech and Language, 16*(4), 243–258.

Ausubel, D.P., & Robinson, F.C. (1969). *School learning*. New York: Holt, Rinehart, and Winston.

Bacon, S.E. (1992). Speech-language management of central auditory processing disorders. In J. Katz, N.A. Stecker, & D. Henderson (Eds.), *Central auditory processing: A transdisciplinary view* (pp. 199–204). St. Louis: Mosby Year Book.

Bailey, C.H., & Chen, M. (1988). Long-term memory in Aplysia modulates the total number of varicosities of single identified sensory neurons. *Proceedings of the National Academy of Sciences of the United States of America, 85,* 2373–2377.

Bain, B., & Dollaghan, C. (1991). Treatment efficacy: The notion of clinically significant change. *Language, Speech, and Hearing Services in Schools, 22*, 264–270.

Ball, E.W., & Blachman, B.A. (1991). Does phoneme segmentation training in kindergarten make a difference in early word recognition and developmental spelling. *Reading Research Quarterly, 26,* 49–66.

Banay-Schwartz, M., Laztha, A., & Palkovits, M. (1989). Changes with aging in the levels of amino acids in rat CNS structural elements: I. Glutamate and related amino acids. *Neurochemical Research, 14,* 555–562.

Barajas, J. (1990). The effects of age on human P3 latency. *Acta Otolaryngologica, 476*(Suppl.), 157–160.

Baran, J.A., & Musiek, F.E. (1991). Behavioral assessment of the central auditory nervous system. In W.F. Rintelmann (Ed.), *Hearing assessment* (pp. 549–602). Austin, TX: Pro-Ed.

Baran, J.A., & Musiek, F.E. (1994). Evaluation of the adult with hearing complaints and normal audiograms. *Audiology Today, 6*, 9–11.

Baran, J.A., Musiek, F.E., & Reeves, A.G. (1986). Central auditory function following anterior sectioning of the corpus callosum. *Ear and Hearing, 7*(6), 359–362.

Baran, J.A., Verkest, S., Gollegly, K., Kibbe-Michal, K., & Rintelmann, W. (1985). Use of time-compressed speech in the assessment of central nervous system disorders. *Journal of the Acoustical Society of America, 78* (Suppl. 1), S41.

Bard, E. G., Schillcock, R. C., & Altmann, G.T.M. (1988). The recognition of words after their acoustic offsets in spontaneous speech: Effects of subsequent context. *Perception and Psychophysics, 44*(5), 395–408.

Barkley, R.A. (1990). *Attention-deficit hyperactivity disorder: A handbook for diagnosis and treatment.* New York: Guilford Press.

Barkley, R.A. (1994). Delayed responding and response inhibition: Toward a unified theory of attention deficit hyperactivity disorder. In D.K. Routh (Ed.), *Disruptive behavior disorders in children: Essays in honor of Herbert Quay* (pp. 11–57). New York: Plenum.

Barkley, R.A. (1996). Linkages between attention and executive functions. In G.R. Lyon & N.A. Krasnegor (Eds.), *Attention, memory, and executive function* (pp. 307–326). Baltimore, MD.: Paul H. Brookes.

Barnes, W., Magon, H., & Ranson, S. (1943). The ascending auditory pathway in the brain stem of the monkey. *Journal of Comparative Neurology, 79*, 129–152.

Barr, D.F. (1976). *Auditory perceptual disorders* (2nd ed.). Springfield: Charles C. Thomas.

Bartoli, J., & Botel, M. (1988). *Reading / learning disability: An ecological approach.* New York: Teachers College Press.

Bashford, J.A., Reiner, K.R., & Warren, R.M. (1992). Increasing the intelligibility of speech through multiple phonemic restorations. *Perception and Psychophysics, 51*, 211–217.

Bashford, J.A., & Warren, R.M. (1987). Multiple phonemic restoration follows the rules for auditory induction. *Perception and Psychophysics, 42*(2), 114–121.

Bashir, A.S., & Scavuzzo, A. (1992). Children with learning disabilities: Natural history and academic success. *Journal of Learning Disabilities, 25*, 53–65.

Battle, D.E. (1993). Introduction. In D.E. Battle (Ed.), *Communication disorders in multicultural populations* (pp. xv–xxiv). Boston: Andover Medical Publishers.

Bauer, R.H., & Emhert, J. (1984). Information processing in reading disabled and nondisabled children. *Journal of Experimental Child Psychology, 37*, 271–281.

Baumann, S., Rogers, R., Papanicolaou, A., & Saydjari, C. (1990). Intersession replicability of dipole parameters in three components of the auditory evoked magnetic field. *Brain Topography, 3*, 311–319.

Bear, M.F., Kleinschmidt, A., Gu, Q., & Singer, W. (1990). Disruption of experience-dependent synaptic modifications in striate cortex by infusion of an NMDA receptor antagonist. *Journal of Neuroscience, 10*(3), 909–925.

Beasley, D., Forman, B., & Rintelmann, W. (1972). Intelligibility of time compressed CNC monosyllables by normal listeners. *Journal of Auditory Research, 12,* 71–75.

Bellis, T. (1996). *Assessment and management of central auditory processing disorders in the educational setting: From science to practice*. San Diego: Singular Publishing Group.

Benerento, L., & Coleman, P. (1970). Responses of single cells in cat inferior colliculus to binaural click stimuli: Combinations of intensity levels, time differences, and intensity differences. *Brain Research, 17*, 387–405.

Benson, D., & Teas, D. (1976). Single unit study of binaural interaction in the auditory cortex of the chinchilla. *Brain Research, 103*, 313–338.

Beranek, L. (1986). *Acoustics*. Woodbury, NY: Acoustical Society of America.

Berg, F.S. (1987). FM equipment. *Facilitating classroom listening: A handbook for teachers of normal and hard of hearing children*. Boston: College-Hill Press.

Berg, F.S. (1993). *Acoustics and sound systems in schools.* San Diego: Singular Publishing Group.

Bergenske, M. D. (1987). The missing link in narrative story mapping. *The Reading Teacher, 41*, 333–335.

Bergman, M. (1980). *Aging and the perception of speech*. Baltimore: University Park Press.

Berlin, C., Hood, L., Secola, P., Jackson, D., & Szabo, P. (1993). Does Type I afferent neuron dysfunction reveal itself through lack of efferent suppression? *Hearing Research, 65*, 40–50.

Berlin, C.L., Lowe-Bell, S.S., Jannetta, P.J., & Kline, D.G. (1972). Central auditory deficits after temporal lobectomy. *Archives of Otolaryngology, 96*, 4–10.

Berrick, J.M., Shubow, G.F., Schultz, M.C., Freed, H., Fournier, S.R., & Hughes, J.P. (1984). Auditory processing tests for children: Normative and clinical results on the SSW Test. *Journal of Speech and Hearing Disorders, 49*, 318–325.

Bess, F. (1985). The minimally hearing-impaired child. *Ear and Hearing, 6*, 43–47.

Bess, F., Sinclair, J., & Riggs, D. (1984). Group amplification in schools for the hearing impaired. *Ear and Hearing, 5*, 138–144.

Bickford, R., Jacobson, J., & Cody, D. (1964). Nature of averaged evoked potentials to sound and other stimuli in man. *Annals of the New York Academy of Science, 112*, 204–223.

Bilger, R.C., Neutzel, J.M., Rabinowitz, W.M., & Rzeczkowski, C. (1984). Standardization of a test of speech perception in noise. *Journal of Speech and Hearing Research, 27*, 32–48.

Bindman, L.J., Murphy, K.P.S.J., & Pockett, S. (1988). Postsynaptic control of the induction of long-term changes in efficacy of transmission at neurocortical synapses in slices of rat brain. *Journal of Neurophysiology, 60*, 1053–1065.

Blaettner, U., Scherg, M., & Von Cramen, D. (1989). Diagnosis of unilateral telenecephalic hearing disorders: Evaluation of a simple psychoacoustic pattern discrimination test. *Brain, 112*, 177–195.

Blair, J., Myrup, C., & Viehweg, S. (1989). Comparison of the listening effectiveness of hard-of-hearing children using three types of amplification. *Educational Audiology Monograph, 1*, 48–55.

Blake, R., Field, B., Foster, C., Platt, F., & Wertz, P. (1991). Effect of FM auditory trainers on attending behaviors of learning-disabled children. *Language, Speech, and Hearing Services in Schools, 22*, 111–114.

Blank, M., & Foss, D. J. (1978). Semantic facilitation and lexical access during sentence processing. *Memory and Cognition, 6*, 644–652.

Blashfield, R.K. (1993). Models of classification as related to a taxonomy of learning disabilities. In G.R. Lyon, D.B. Gray, J.F. Kavanaugh, & N.A. Krasnegor (Eds.), *Better understanding learning disabilities* (pp. 17–26). Baltimore: Paul H. Brookes.

Bledsoe, S., Bobbin, R., & Puel, J. (1988). Neurotransmission in the inner ear. In A. Jahn & J. Santo-Sacchi (Eds.), *Physiology of the ear* (pp. 385–406). New York: Raven Press.

Bleitchman, J.H., Hood, J., & Inglis, A. (1990). Psychiatric risk in children with speech and language disorders. *Journal of Abnormal Child Psychology, 18*, 283–296.

Bliss, T., & Lomo, T. (1973). Long-lasting potentiation of synaptic transmission in the dentate area of the anaesthetized rabbit following stimulation of the perforant path. *Journal of Physiology, 232*(2), 331–356.

Bloom, B. (1956). *Taxonomy of educational objectives handbook I: Cognitive domain.* New York: McKay.

Blumstein, S., & Cooper, W. (1974). Hemisphere processing of intonation contours. *Cortex, 10*, 146–158.

Blumstein, S.E., Katz, B., Goodglass, H., Shrier, R., & Dworetsky, B. (1985). The effects of slowed speech on auditory comprehension in aphasia. *Brain and Language, 24,* 246–265.

Bobbin, R.P., & Konishi, T. (1971). Acetylcholine mimics crossed olivocochlear bundle stimulation. *Nature, 231,* 222–224.

Bocca, E. (1958). Clinical aspects of cortical deafness. *Laryngoscope, 68,* 301–309.

Bocca, E., Calearo, C., & Cassinari, V. (1954). A new method for testing hearing in temporal lobe tumor. *Acta Otolaryngologica, 44*, 219–221.

Bocca, E., Calearo, C., Cassinari, V., & Migliavacca, F. (1955). Testing "cortical" hearing in temporal lobe tumors. *Acta Otolaryngologica, 42*, 289–304.

Bohne, B., & Harding, G. (1992). Neuronal regeneration in the noise damaged chinchilla cochlea. *Laryngoscope, 102*, 693–703.

Bolshakov, V.Y., & Siegelbaum, S.A. (1995). Regulation of hippocampal transmitter release during development and long-term potentiation. *Science, 269,* 1730–1733.

Bolt R., & MacDonald, A. (1949). Theory of speech masking by reverberation. *Journal of the Acoustical Society of America, 21*, 577–580.

Boothroyd, A., & Nittrouer, S. (1988). Mathematical treatment of context effects in phoneme and word recognition. *Journal of the Acoustical Society of America, 84*(1), 101–114.

Borg, E. (1973). On the organization of the acoustic middle ear reflex: A physiologic and anatomic study. *Brain Research, 100,* 113–116.

Borkowski, J.G., & Burke, J.E. (1996). Theories, models, and measurement of executive functioning: An information processing perspective. In G.R. Lyon & N.A. Krasnegor (Eds.), *Attention, memory, and executive function* (pp. 235–261). Baltimore: Paul H. Brookes.

Borkowski, J.G., Estrada, M.T., Milstead, M., & Hale, C. (1989). General problem-solving skills: Relations between metacognition and strategic processing. *Learning Disability Quarterly, 12*, 57–70.

Borkowski, J.G., Johnston, M.B., & Reid, M.K. (1987). Metacognition, motivation, and controlled performance. In S.J. Ceci (Ed.), *Handbook of cognitive, social, and neuropsychological aspects of learning disabilities* (Vol. 2, pp. 147–174). Hillsdale, NJ: Lawrence Erlbaum.

Borkowski, J.G., Milstead, M., & Hale, C. (1988). Components of children's metamemory: Implications for strategy generalization. In F. Weinert & M. Perlumutter (Eds.), *Memory development: Individual differences and universal changes* (pp. 73–100). Hillsdale, NJ: Lawrence Erlbaum.

Borkowski, J.G., Weyhing, R.S., & Carr, M. (1988). Effects of attributional retraining on strategy-based reading comprehension in learning-disabled students. *Journal of Education Psychology, 80*, 46–53.

Born, D., & Rubel, E. (1985). Afferent influences on brainstem auditory nuclei of the chicken: Neuron number and size following cochlear removal. *Journal of Comparative Neurology, 231*, 435–445.

Bornstein, M.R., Bellack, A.S., & Hersen, M. (1977). Social-skills training for unassertive children. A multiple-baseline analysis. *Journal of Applied Behavior Analysis, 10,* 183–195.

Bornstein, S.P., & Musiek, F.E. (1984). Implication of temporal processing for children with learning and language problems. In D. Beasley (Ed.), *Contemporary issues in audition* (pp. 25–65). San Diego: College-Hill Press.

Bornstein, S. P., & Musiek, F.E. (1992). Recognition of distorted speech in children with and without learning problems. *Journal of the American Academy of Audiology, 3,* 22–32.

Bos, C., & Filip, D. (1982). Comprehension monitoring skills in learning disabled and average students. *Topics in Learning Disabilities, 2*, 79–85.

Boudreau, J.C., & Tsuchitani, C. (1970). Cat superior olive S-segment cell discharge to tonal stimulation. In W.D. Neff (Ed.), *Contributions to sensory physiology* (Vol. 4, pp. 143–213). New York: Academic Press.

Bradley, J. (1986). Speech intelligibility studies in classrooms. *Journal of the Acoustical Society of America, 80*(3), 846–854.

Bradley, L., & Bryant, P. (1985). *Rhyme and reason in reading and spelling.* [International Academy for Research in Learning Disabilities Monograph Series, No. 1.] Ann Arbor: University of Michigan Press.

Brainard, M.S., & Knudsen, E.I. (1993). Experience-dependent plasticity in the inferior colliculus: A site for visual calibration of the neural representation of auditory space in the barn owl. *Journal of Neuroscience, 13*(11), 4589–4608.

Brainard, M.S., & Knudsen, E.I. (1995). Dynamics of visually guided auditory plasticity in the optic tectum of the barn owl. *Journal of Neurophysiology, 73*(2), 595–614.

Breedin, S.D., Martin, R.C., & Jerger, S. (1989). Distinguishing auditory and speech-specific perceptual deficits. *Ear and Hearing, 10*(5), 311–316.

Bremer, F., Brihaye, J., & Andre-Balisaux, G. (1956). Physologie et pathologie du corps calleux. *Archives Suisses de Neurologie et de Psychiatrie, 78,* 31–32.

Brey, R.H., Robinette, S., Chabries, D.M., & Christiansen, R.W. (1987). Improvement in speech intelligibility in noise employing an adaptive filter with normal and hearing-impaired subjects. *Journal of Rehabilitation Research and Development, 24*(4),75–86.

Brody, J.A., Overfield, T., & McAllister, R. (1965). Draining ears and deafness among Alaskan Eskimos. *Archives of Otolaryngology, 81*, 29.

Brophy, J.E. (1981). Teacher praise: A functional analysis. *Review of Educational Research, 51*, 5–32.

Brophy, J.E. (1983). Research on the self-fulfilling prophecy and teacher expectations. *Journal of Educational Psychology, 75,* 631–661.

Brown, A.L., Bransford, J., Ferrara, R.A., & Campione, J.C. (1983). Learning, remembering, and understanding. In J. Flavell & E.M. Markman (Eds.),

Carmichael's manual of child psychology (Vol. 1, pp. 77–166). New York: John Wiley & Sons.

Brown, A.L., Campione, J., & Barclay, C.R. (1979). Training self-checking routines for estimating test readiness: Generalization for list learning to prose recall. *Child Development, 50*, 501–512.

Brown, A.L., Campione, J.C., & Day, J.D. (1981). Learning to learn: On training students to learn from texts. *Educational Researcher, 10*, 14–21.

Brown, A.L., & French, L. (1979). The zone of potential development: Implications for intelligence testing in the year 2000. *Intelligence, 2,* 46–53.

Brown, D.P. (1994). Speech recognition in recurrent otitis media: Results in a set of identical twins. *Journal of the American Academy of Audiology, 5*, 1–6.

Brown, T.H., Chapman, P.F.E., Kairiss, W., & Keenan, C.L. (1988). Long-term synaptic potentiation. *Science, 242*, 724–728.

Bruder, G.E. (1983). Cerebral laterality and psychopathology: Dichotic listening studies in schizophrenia and affective disorders. *Schizophrenia Bulletin, 9,* 134–151.

Brugge, I.F, & Geisler, C.E. (1978). Auditory mechanisms of the lower brain stem. *American Review of Neuroscience, 1,* 363–394.

Bruner, J.S. (1957). On perceptual readiness. *Psychological Review, 64,* 123–152.

Bryan, T. (1991). Social problems and learning disabilities. In B.Y.L. Wong (Ed.), *Learning about learning disabilities* (pp. 195–229). San Diego: Academic Press.

Buchanan, L. H., Moore, E.J., & Counter, S.A. (1993). Hearing disorders and auditory assessment. In D. Battle (Ed.), *Communication disorders in multicultural populations* (pp. 256–279). Boston: Andover Medical Publishers.

Buchwald, J. (1990). Animal models of event-related potentials. In J. Rohrbaugh, R. Parasuraman, & R. Johnson (Eds.), *Event related potentials of the brain* (pp. 57–75). New York: Oxford Press.

Bunch, C.C. (1929). Age variations in auditory acuity. *Archives of Otolaryngology, 9*, 625–626.

Bunch, C.C. (1931). Further observations on age variations in auditory acuity. *Archives of Otolaryngology, 13*, 170–180.

Burd, L., & Fisher, W. (1986). Central auditory processing disorder or attention deficit disorder? *Journal of Developmental and Behavioral Pediatrics, 7*, 215–216.

Bush, P.J., & Rabin, D.L. (1980). Racial differences in encounter rates for otitis media. *Pediatric Research, 14*, 1115–1117.

Butkowski, I.S., & Willows, D.M. (1980). Cognitive-motivational characteristics of children varying in reading ability: Evidence for learned helplessness in poor readers. *Journal of Educational Psychology, 72*, 408–422.

Butler, K.G. (1983). Language processing-selective attention and mnemonic strategies. In E.Z. Lasky & J. Katz (Eds.), *Central auditory processing disorders* (pp. 297–315). Baltimore: University Park Press.

Butler, R., Keidel, W., & Spreng, M. (1969). An investigation of the human cortical evoked potential under conditions of monaural and binaural stimulation. *Acta Otolaryngologica, 68*, 317–326.

Butterfield, E.C., & Albertson, L.R. (1995). On making cognitive theory more general and developmentally pertinent. In F. Weinert & W. Schneider (Eds.), *Research on memory development* (pp. 73–99). Hillsdale, NJ: Lawrence Erlbaum.

Buttrill, J., Niizawa, J., Biemer, C., Takahashi, C., & Hearn, S. (1989). Serving the language learning disabled adolescent: A strategies-based model. *Language, Speech, and Hearing Services in Schools, 20,* 185–203.

Cacace, A., & McFarland, D. (1995). Modality specificity as a criterion for diagnosing central auditory processing disorders. *The American Journal of Audiology, 4*, 36–48.

Cairns, H.S., & Hsu, J.R. (1980). Effects of prior context upon lexical access during sentence comprehension: A replication and reinterpretation. *Journal of Psycholinguistic Research, 9,* 319–326.

Calearo, C., & Lazzaroni A. (1957). Speech intelligibility in relation to the speech of the message. *Laryngoscope, 67,* 410–419.

Campain, R., & Minckler, J. (1976). A note in gross configurations of the human auditory cortex. *Brain and Language, 3*, 318–323.

Campbell, M., & Cueva, J.E. (1995). Psychopharmacology in child and adolescent psychiatry: A review of the past seven years. Part I. *Journal of the American Academy of Child and Adolescent Psychiatry, 34*(9), 1124–1132.

Campbell, T., & McNeil, M. (1985). Effects of presentation rate and divided attention on auditory comprehension in children with acquired language disorder. *Journal of Speech and Hearing Research, 28*, 513–520.

Campione, J., & Brown, A. (1987). Linking dynamic assessment with school achievement. In C. Lidz (Ed.), *Dynamic assessment* (pp. 82–115). New York: Guilford Press.

Campo, P., Subramaniam, M., & Henderson, D. (1991). The effect of "conditioning" exposures on hearing loss from traumatic exposure. *Hearing Research, 55,* 195–200.

Canlon, B., Borg, E., & Flock, A. (1988). Protection against noise trauma by pre-exposure to a low level acoustic stimulus. *Hearing Research, 34,* 197–200.

Canlon, B., Borg, E., & Lofstrand, P. (1991). Physiological and morphological aspects to low level acoustic stimulation. In A.L. Dancer, D. Henderson, R.J. Salvi, & R.P. Hamernik (Eds.), *Noise-induced hearing loss* (pp. 489–499). St. Louis: Mosby.

Canterbury, D. (1990). Changes in hearing status of Alaskan natives. *Annals of Otology, Rhinology, and Laryngology, 99*(Suppl. 149), 23–29.

Cantwell, D.P., & Baker, L. (1985). Psychiatric and learning disorders in children with speech and language disorders: A descriptive analysis. In K.D. Gadow (Ed.), *Advances in learning and behavioral disabilities* (Vol. 4). Greenwich, CT: JAL.

Cantwell, D.P., Baker, L., & Mattison, R.E. (1979). The prevalence of psychiatric disorder in children with speech and language disorder: A epidemiological study. *Journal of the American Academy of Child Psychiatry, 18,* 450–459.

Carmon, A., & Nachshon, I. (1971). Effect of unilateral brain damage on perception of temporal order. *Cortex, 7,* 410–418.

Carney, L.J., & Chermak, G.D. (1991). Performance of Native American children with fetal alcohol syndrome on the Test of Language Development. *Journal of Communication Disorders, 24*(2),123–134.

Carpenter, M., & Sutin, J. (1983). *Human neuroanatomy*. Baltimore: Williams & Wilkins.

Carter, J. (1984). *Active noise reduction.* [Report No. MRL-TR-84-003.] Dayton, OH: Wright-Patterson Air Force Base.

Casanova, U. (1989). Being the teacher helps students learn. Instructor, 98(9), 12-13.

Caspary, D.M., Milbrandt, J.C., & Helfert, R.H. (1995). Central auditory aging: GABA changes in the inferior colliculus. *Experimental Gerontology, 30*, 349–360.

Caspary, D.M., Raza, A., Lawhorn-Armour, B., Pippin, J., & Arneric, S. (1990). Immunocytochemical and neurochemical evidence for age-related loss of GABA in the inferior colliclus: Implications for neural presbycusis. *Journal of Neuroscience, 10*(7), 2363–2372.

Casterline, C., Flexer, C., & DePompei, R. (1989, November). *Use of assistive listening devices with head injured survivors.* Paper presented at the annual convention of the American Speech-Language-Hearing Association, St. Louis, MO.

Catts, H.W. (1991). Facilitating phonological awareness: Role of speech-language pathologists. *Language, Speech, and Hearing Services in Schools, 22*, 196–203.

Cavanaugh, J.C., & Perlmutter, M. (1982). Metamemory: A critical examination. *Child Development, 53*, 11–28.

Celebisoy, N., Aydogdu, I., Ekmekci, O., & Akurekli, O. (1996). Middle latency auditory evoked potentials (MLAEPs) in MS. *Acta Neurologica Scandinavica, 93*, 318–321.

Celesia, G. (1976). Organization of auditory cortical areas in man. *Brain, 99*, 403–414.

Chalfant, J.C., & Scheffelin, M.A. (1969). *Central processing dysfunction in children: A review of research.* [NINDS Monograph NO. 9.] Washington, DC: U.S. Department of Health, Education, and Welfare.

Chambers, R., & Griffiths, S. (1991). Effects of age on the adult auditory middle latency resonse. *Hearing Research, 51*, 1–10.

Chang, H.T. (1953). Cortical response to activity of callosal neurons. *Journal of Neurophysiology, 16,* 1409–1410.

Chapin, M., & Dyck, D.G. (1976). Persistence in children's reading behavior as a function of N length and attribution retraining. *Journal of Abnormal Psychology, 85,* 511–515.

Chappell, P.B., Riddle, M.A., Scahill, L., Lynch, K.A., Schultz, R., Arnsten, A., Leckman, J.F., & Cohen, D.J. (1995). Guanfacine treatment of comorbid attention-deficit hyperactivity disorder and Tourette's syndrome: Preliminary clinical experience. *Journal of the American Academy of Child and Adolescent Psychiatry, 34*(9), 1140–1146.

Chedru, F., Bastard, V., & Efron, R. (1978). Auditory micropattern discrimination in brain damaged subjects. *Neuropsychologia, 16,* 141–149.

Cheng, L.L. (1987). Cross-cultural and linguistic considerations in working with Asian populations. *Asha, 29*(6), 33–38.

Chermak, G.D. (1981). *Handbook of audiological rehabilitation.* Springfield, IL: Charles C. Thomas.

Chermak, G.D. (1993). Dynamics of collaborative consultation with families. *American Journal of Audiology, 2*(3),38–43.

Chermak, G.D. (1996). Central testing. In S.A. Gerber (Ed.), *Handbook of pediatric audiology* (pp. 206–253). Washington, DC: Gallaudet University Press.

Chermak, G.D., Curtis, L., & Seikel, J.A. (1996). The effectiveness of an interactive hearing conservation program for elementary school children. *Language, Speech, and Hearing Services in Schools, 27*(1), 29–39.

Chermak, G.D., & Montgomery, M. (1992) Form equivalency of the selective auditory attention task administered to six-year-old children. *Journal of Speech and Hearing Research, 35,* 661–665.

Chermak, G.D., & Musiek, F.E. (1992). Managing central auditory processing disorders in children and youth. *American Journal of Audiology, 1*(3), 61–65.

Chermak, G.D., Vonhof, M., & Bendel, R.B. (1989). Word identification performance in the presence of competing speech and noise in learning disabled adults. *Ear and Hearing, 10,* 90–93.

Cherry, R.S. (1980). Selective Auditory Attention Test. St. Louis: Auditec.

Chiappa, K. (1983). *Evoked potentials in clinical medicine.* New York: Raven Press.

Chmiel, R., & Jerger, J. (1996). Hearing aid use, central auditory disorder, and hearing handicap in elderly persons. *Journal of the American Academy of Audiology, 7,* 190–202.

Churchland, P.S., & Sejnowski, T.J. (1988). Perspectives on cognitive neuroscience. *Science, 242,* 741–746.

Clark, D.H. (1967). *The psychology of education.* New York: Cambridge University Press.

Clark, W.W., Bohne, B.A., & Boettcher, F.A. (1987). Effect of periodic rest on hearing loss and cochlear damage following exposure to noise. *Journal of the Acoustical Society of America, 82,* 1253–1264.

Clarke, J., MacPherson, B., Holmes, D., & Jones, R. (1986). Reducing adolescent smoking: A comparison of peer-led, teacher-led, and expert interventions. *Journal of School Health, 98*(2), 92–96.

Clifford, M.M. (1978). Have we underestimated the facilitative effects of failure? *Canadian Journal of Behavioral Science, 10,* 308–316.

Clopton, B., & Silverman, M. (1978). Changes in latency and duration of neural responding following developmental auditory deprivation. *Experimental Brain Research, 32,* 39–47.

Codding, K.G., & Gardner, M.F. (1988). *Auditory-perceptual development.* Burlington, CA: Psychological and Educational Publications.

Cody, A.R., & Johnstone, B.M. (1982). Temporary threshold shift modified by binaural acoustic stimulation. *Hearing Research, 6*, 199–205.

Cohen, G. (1987). Speech comprehension in the elderly: The effects of cognitive changes. *British Journal of Audiology, 21*, 221–226.

Cokely, C.G., & Humes, L.E. (1992). Reliability of two measures of speech recognition in elderly people. *Journal of Speech and Hearing Research, 35*, 654–660.

Colavita, F. (1972). Auditory cortical lesions and visual patterns discrimination in cats. *Brain Research, 39*, 437–447.

Colavita, F. (1974). Insular-temporal lesions and vibrotactile temporal pattern discrimination in cats. *Psychological Behavior, 12*, 215–218.

Colclasure, J., & Graham, S. (1981). Intracranial aneurysm occurring as a sensorineural hearing loss. *Otolaryngology—Head and Neck Surgery, 89*, 283–287.

Cole, L. (1989). Multicultural imperatives. *Asha, 9*, 66–70.

Cole, L., & Anderson, N.B. (1985). The economically disadvantaged. In L. Cole (Ed.), *National colloquium on underserved populations* (pp. 60–94). Rockville, MD: American Speech-Language-Hearing Association.

Cole, R., & Jakimik, J. (1980). A model of speech perception. In R. Cole (Ed.), *Perception and prediction of fluent speech* (pp. 133–160). Engelwood Cliffs, NJ: Lawrence Erlbaum.

Cole, R.A., & Rudnicky, A.I. (1983). What's new in speech perception? The research ideas of William Chandler Bagley, 1874–1946. *Psychological Review, 90,* 94–104.

Coleman, J., & O'Connor, P. (1979). Effects of monaural and binaural sound deprivation on cell development in the anteroventral cochlear nucleus of rats. *Experimental Neurology, 64*, 553–566.

Collard, M. (1984). Central auditory tests in patients with intractable seizures. *Seminars in Hearing, 5*, 277–296.

Collet, L., Veuillet, E., Bene, J., & Morgan, A. (1992). Effects of contralateral white noise on click evoked emissions in normal and sensorineural ears: Towards an explanation of the medial olivocochleaer system. *Audiology, 31*, 1–7.

Colson, K., Robin, D., & Luschei, E. (1991). Auditory processing and sequential pitch and timing changes following frontal opercular damage. *Clinical Aphasiology, 20,* 317–325.

Comis, S., & Whitfield, I. (1968). Influence of centrifugal pathways on unit activity in the coclear nucleus. *Journal of Neurophysiology, 31*, 62–68.

Committee on Hearing, Bioacoustics, and Biomechanics (CHABA) Working Group on Speech Understanding and Aging. (1988). Speech understanding and aging. *Journal of the Acoustical Society of America, 83*, 859–893.

Connell, P.J. (1988). Induction, generalization, and deduction: Models for defining language generalization. *Language, Speech, and Hearing Services in Schools, 19*(3), 282–291.

Connell, P.J. (1989). Facilitating generalization through induction teaching. In L.V. McReynolds & J.E. Spradlin (Eds.), *Generalization strategies in the treatment of communication disorders* (pp. 44–62). Philadelphia: B.C. Decker.

Cook, J.R., Mausbach, T., Burd, L., Gascon, G.G., Slotnick, H.B., Patterson, B., Johnson, R.D., Hankey, B., & Reynolds, B.W. (1993). A preliminary study of the relationship between central auditory processing disorder and attention deficit disorder. *Journal of Psychiatry and Neuroscience, 18*(3), 130–137.

Cooper, J., & Cutts, B. (1971). Speech discrimination in noise. *Journal of Speech and Hearing Research, 14,* 332–337.

Cooper, J.C., Jr., & Gates, G.A. (1991). Hearing in the elderly—The Framingham Cohort, 1983–1985: Part II. Prevalence of central auditory processing disorders. *Ear & Hearing, 12*, 304–311.

Correa, V.I. (1989). Involving culturally diverse families in the educational process. In S.H. Fradd & M.J. Weismatel (Eds.), *Meeting the needs of culturally diverse and linguistically different students: A handbook for educators* (pp. 130–144). Boston: Little, Brown.

Corwin, J.T., & Cotanche, D.A. (1988). Regeneration of sensory hair cells after acoustic trauma. *Science, 240,* 1772–1774.

Cotanche, D.A. (1987). Regeneration of hair cell stereociliary bundles in the chick cochlea following severe acoustic trauma. *Hearing Research, 30,* 181–194.

Cotton, S., & Grosjean, F. (1984). The gating paradigm: A comparison of successive and individual presentation formats. *Perception and Psychophysics, 35*, 41–48.

Coufal, K.L., Hixson, P.K., & Stick, S.L. (1990, November). *Collaborative consultation—an alternative treatment: Efficacy data and policy issues.* Paper presented at the annual Convention of the American Speech-Language-Hearing Assocation, Seattle, WA.

Cousillas, H., Cole, K.S., & Johnstone, B.M. (1988). Effect of spider venom on cochlear nerve activity consistent with glutamatergic transmission at hair cell-afferent dendrite synapse. *Hearing Research, 36*, 213–220.

Cowan, N. (1993). Activation, attention, and short-term memory. *Memory and Cognition, 21*, 162–167.

Cowan, W.M., Fawcett, J.W., O'Leary, D.M., & Stanfield, B. (1984). Regressive events in neurogenesis. *Science, 255,* 1258–1265.

Craig, C.H. (1988). Effects of three conditions of predictability on word-recognition performance. *Journal of Speech and Hearing Research, 31,* 588–592.

Craig, C.H. (1992) Effects of time-gating and word length on isolated word-recognition performance. *Journal of Speech and Hearing Research, 35,* 234–238.

Craig, C.H., & Kim, B. (1990). Effects of time-gating on isolated-word recognition performance. *Journal of Speech and Hearing Research, 33,* 808–815.

Craig, C.H., Kim, B.W., Rhyner, P.M.P., & Chirillo, T.K.B. (1993). Effects of word predictability, child development, and aging on time-gated speech recognition performance. *Journal of Speech and Hearing Research, 36,* 832–841.

Craig, C.H., Warren, R.M., Bashford, J.A., & Chirillo, T. (1994). The influence of context on spoken language perception and processing among elderly and hearing impaired listeners. *Proceedings of the ICSLP '94, 4,* 2047–2051.

Craighead, W.E., Wilcoxon-Craighead, L., & Meyers, A. (1978). New directions in behavior modification with children. In M. Hersen, R. Eisler, & P. Miller (Eds.), *Progress in behavior modification* (Vol. 6, pp. 159–201). New York: Academic Press.

Crais, E.R. (1991). Moving from "parent involvement" to family-centered services. *American Journal of Speech-Language Pathology, 1*(1), 5–8.

Crandell, C. (1991). Classroom acoustics for normal-hearing children: Implications for rehabilitation. *Educational Audiology Monograph, 2*(1), 18–38.

Crandell, C. (1992). Classroom acoustics for hearing-impaired children. *Journal of the Acoustical Society of America, 92*(4), 2470.

Crandell, C. (1993a). A comparison of commercially available frequency modulation and field amplification systems. *Educational Audiology Monograph, 3,* 15–20.

Crandell, C. (1993b). Speech recognition in noise by children with minimal degrees of sensorineural hearing loss. *Ear & Hearing, 14*(3), 210–216.

Crandell, C., & Bess, F. (1986, November). Speech recognition of children in a "typical" classroom setting. Paper presented at the annual convention of the American Speech-Language-Hearing Association, Detroit, MI.

Crandell, C., & Smaldino, J. (1994). An update of classroom acoustics for children with hearing impairment. *Volta Review, 96,* 291–306.

Crandell, C., & Smaldino, J. (1995a). Acoustical modifications in classrooms. In C. Crandell, J. Smaldino, & C. Flexer, *Sound-field FM amplification* (pp. 83–92). San Diego: Singular Publishing Group.

Crandell, C., & Smaldino, J. (1995b). The importance of room acoustics. In R.S. Tyler & D.J. Schum (Eds.), *Assistive devices for persons with hearing impairment* (pp. 142–164). Boston: Allyn and Bacon.

Crandell, C., Smaldino, J., & Flexer, C. (1995). *Sound-field FM amplification.* San Diego: Singular Publishing Group.

Cranford, J. (1979). Detection versus discrimination of brief tones by cats with auditory cortex lesions. *Journal of the Acoustical Society of America, 65,* 1573–1575.

Cranford, J. (1984). Brief tone detection and discimination tests in clinical audiology with emphasis on their use in central nervous system lesions. *Seminars in Hearing, 5,* 263–275.

Cranford, J., Boose, M., & Moore, C. (1990). Tests of the precedence effect in sound localization reveal abnormalities in multiple sclerosis. *Ear & Hearing, 11*, 282–288.

Cranford, J., Igarashi, M., & Stramler, J. (1976). Effect of auditory neocortical ablation on pitch perception in the cat. *Journal of Neurophysiology, 39*, 143–152.

Cranford, J.L., Kennalley, T., Svoboda, W., & Hipp, K. (1996). Changes in central auditory processing following temporal lobectomies in children. *Journal of the American Academy of Audiology, 7*(4), 289–295.

Cranford, J., Stream, R., Rye, C., & Slade, T. (1982). Detection versus discrimination of brief duration tones: Findings in patients with temporal lobe damage. *Archives of Otolaryngology, 108*, 350–356.

Crelin, E. (1973). *Functional anatomy in the newborn*. New Haven: Yale University Press.

Cronbach, L.J., & Snow, R. (1981). *Aptitudes and instructional methods* (2nd ed.). New York: Irvington.

Crowder, R.G. (1982). The demise of short-term memory. *Acta Psychologica, 50,* 291–293.

Crum, M., & Matkin, N. (1976). Room acoustics: The forgotten variable? *Language, Speech, and Hearing Services in Schools, 7,* 106–110.

Cruz, R.M., Lambert, P.R., & Rubel, E.W. (1987). Light microscopic evidence of hair cell regeneration after gentamicin toxicity in chick cochlea. *Archives of Otolaryngology—Head and Neck Surgery, 113*(10), 1058–1062.

Cullen, J., & Thompson, C. (1974). Masking release for speech in subjects with temporal lobe resections. *Archives of Otolaryngology, 100,* 113–116.

Cutler, A., & Foder, J.A. (1979). Semantic focus and sentence comprehension. *Cognition, 7,* 49–59.

Cutler, A., & Foss, D.J. (1977). On the role of sentence stress in sentence processing. *Language and Speech, 20*, 1–10.

Cutler, A., & Norris, D. (1988). The role of strong syllables in segmentation for lexical access. *Journal of Experimental Psychology: Human Perception and Performance, 14*, 113–121.

Damasio, H., & Damasio, A. (1979). Paradoxic ear extension in dichotic listening: Possible anatomic significance. *Neurology, 25*(4), 644–653.

Damasio, H., & Damasio, A. (1989). *Lesion analysis in neuropsychology*. New York: Oxford Press.

Damico, J.S., Augustine, L.E., & Hayes, P.A. (1996). Formulating a functional model of attention deficit hyperactivity disorder for the practicing speech-language pathologist. *Seminars in Speech and Language, 17*(1), 5–20.

Damico, J.S., & Simon, C.A. (1993). Assessing language abilities in school-age children. In A. Gerber (Ed.), *Language-related learning disabilities* (pp. 279–299). Baltimore: Paul H. Brookes.

Danks, J.H., & End, L.J. (1987). Processing strategies for reading and listening. In R. Horowitz & S.J. Samuels (Eds.), *Comprehending oral and written language* (pp. 271–294). San Diego, CA: Academic Press.

Davis, P. (1939) Effects of acoustic stimuli on the waking human brain. *Journal of Neurophysiology, 2,* 494–499.

Deberdt, W. (1994). Interaction between psychological and pharmacological treatment in cognitive impairment. *Life Sciences, 55*(25–26), 2057–2066.

DeConde, C. (1984). Children with central processing disorders. In R.H. Hull & K.I. Dilka (Eds.), *The hearing impaired child in school* (pp. 141–161). New York: Grune & Stratton.

DeMarco, S., Harbour, A., Hume, W., & Givens, G. (1989). Perception of time-altered monosyllables in a specific group of phonologically disordered children. *Neuropsychologia, 27,* 753–757.

Denckla, M.B. (1989). Executive function, the overlap zone between attention deficit hyperactivity disorder and learning disabilities. *International Pediatrics, 4,* 155–160.

Denckla, M.B. (1996). A theory and model of executive function: A neuropsychological perspective. In G.R. Lyon & N.A. Krasnegor (Eds.), *Attention, memory, and executive function* (pp. 263–278). Baltimore: Paul H. Brookes.

Denckla, M.B., & Reader, M. (1993). Education and psychosocial interventions: Executive dysfunction and its consequences. In R. Kurlan (Ed.), *Handbook of Tourette's syndrome and related tic and behavioral disorders* (pp. 431–451). New York: Marcel Dekker.

Denes, P.B., & Pinson, E.N. (1993). *The speech chain: The physics and biology of spoken language.* New York: W.H. Freeman.

Desmedt, J. (1975). Physiological studies of the efferent recurrent auditory system. In W. Keidel & W. Neff (Eds.), *Handbook of sensory physiology* (pp. 219–246). Berlin: Springer-Verlag.

Devor, M., & Wall, P.D. (1978). Reorganization of spinal cord sensory map after peripheral nerve injury. *Nature, 276,* 75–76.

Dewson, J.H. (1968). Efferent olivocochlear bundle: Some relationship to stimulus discrimination in noise. *Journal of Neurophysiology, 31,* 122–130.

Diamond, I., & Neff, W. (1957). Ablation of temporal cortex and discrimination of auditory patterns. *Journal of Neurophysiology, 20,* 300–315.

Dillon, G.L. (1981). *Constructing texts.* Bloomington: Indiana University Press.

DiSimoni, F. (1978). *The Token Test for Children.* Hingham, MA: Teaching Resources Corporation.

Divenyi, P.L., & Robinson, A.J. (1989). Nonlinguistic auditory capabilities in aphasia. *Brain and Language, 37,* 290–326.

Dodd, B. (1977). The role of vision in the perception of speech. *Perception, 6,* 31–40.

Dodd, B. (1980). Interaction of auditory and visual information in speech perception. *British Journal of Psychology, 71,* 541–549.

Dolan, D.F., & Nuttall, A.L. (1988). Masked cochlear whole-nerve response intensity functions altered by electrical stimulation of the crossed olivocochlear bundle. *Journal of the Acoustical Society of America, 83,* 1081–1086.

Donchin, E., Kutas, M., & McCarthy, G. (1976). Electrocortical indices of hemispheric utilization. In S. Harnad & R. Doty (Eds.), *Lateralization in the nervous system* (pp. 339–384). New York: Academic Press.

Dooling, R.J., Manabe, K., & Ryals, B.M. (1996, February). *Effect of masking and hearing loss on vocal production and vocal learning in budgerigars.* Paper presented at the Association for Research in Otolaryngology Nineteenth Midwinter Research Meeting, St. Petersburg Beach, FL.

Doris, J.L. (1993). Defining learning disabilities: A history of the search for consensus. In G.R. Lyon, D.B. Gray, J.F. Kavanagh, & N.A. Krasnegor (Eds.), *Better understanding learning disabilities: New views from research and their implications for education and public policies* (pp. 95–115). Baltimore: Paul H. Brookes.

Downs, D.W., & Crum, M.A. (1978). Processing demands during auditory learning under degraded listening conditions. *Journal of Speech and Hearing Research, 21*, 702–714.

Dublin, W. (1976). *Fundamentals of sensorineural auditory pathology.* Springfield: Charles C. Thomas.

Dublin, W. (1985). The cochlear nuclei-pathology. *Otolaryngology—Head and Neck Surgery, 93,* 448–463.

Dublin, W. (1986). Central auditory pathology. *Otolaryngology—Head and Neck Surgery, 95*(3) (Suppl. Pt. II), 365–420.

Duffy, F.H. (1986). Topographic mapping of evoked potentials in learning-disabled children. In R.Q. Cracco & I. Bodis-Wollner (Eds.), *Evoked potentials* (pp. 485–496). New York: Alan R. Liss.

Duffy, F.H., Deckla, M.B., Bartell, R.H., & Sandini, G. (1980). Regional differences in brain electrical activity by topographic mapping. *Annals of Neurology, 5,* 412–420.

Duquesnoy, A.J., & Plomp, R. (1980). Effect of reverberation and noise on the intelligibility of sentences in cases of presbycusis. *Journal of the Acoustical Society of America, 68,* 537–544.

Duranti, A., & Goodwin, C. (1990). *Rethinking context: Language as an interactive phenomenon.* Cambridge, UK: Cambridge University Press.

Duyk, G., Gastier, J.M., & Mueller, R.F. (1992). Traces of her workings. *Nature Genetics,* 2, 5–8.

Dweck, C.S. (1975). The role of expectations and attributions in the alleviation of learned helplessness. *Journal of Personality and Social Psychology, 31*, 674–685.

Dweck, C.S. (1977). Learned helplessness and negative evaluation. *The Educator, 14,* 44–49.

D'Zurilla, T.J. (1986). *Problem-solving therapy: A social competence approach to clinical intervention.* New York: Springer.

Ebner, A., Haas, J., Lucking, C., Schily, M., Wallesh, C., Zimmerman, P., Goldstein, L., Jaynes, J., & Krauthamer, G. (1986). Event-related brain potentials (P300) and neuropsychological deficit in patients with focal brain lesions. *Neuroscience Letters, 64*, 330–334.

Edeline, J.M., & Weinberger, N.M. (1991). Thalamic short-term plasticity in the auditory system: Associative retuning of receptive fields in the ventral medial geniculate body. *Behavioral Neuroscience, 105*, 618–639.

Edwards, C. (1995). Listening strategies for the classroom teacher. In C. Crandell, J. Smaldino, & C. Flexer, *Sound-field FM amplification* (pp. 83–92). San Diego: Singular Publishing Group.

Efron, R. (1963). Temporal perception, aphasia, and deja vu. *Brain, 86*, 403–424.

Efron, R., Yund, E.W., Nichols, D., & Crandall, P.H. (1985). An ear asymmetry for gap detection following anterior temporal lobectomy. *Neuropsychologia, 23*, 43–50.

Egan, J. (1948). Articulation testing methods. *Laryngoscope, 58*, 955–991.

Eggermont, J. (1991). Rate and synchronization measures of periodicity coding in cat primary auditory cortex. *Hearing Research, 56,* 153–167.

Eisenmann, L. (1974). Neurocoding of sound localizations: An electrophysiological study in auditory cortex of the cat using free field stimuli. *Brain Research, 75*, 203–214.

Eitan, S., Solomon, A. Lavie, V., Yoles, E., Hirschberg, D.L., Belkin, M., & Schwartz, M. (1994). Recovery of visual response of injured adult rat optic nerves treated with transglutaminase. *Science, 264*, 1764–1768.

Elbert, T., Pantev, C., Wienbruch, C., Rockstroh, B. & Taub, E. (1995). Increased cortical representation of the fingers of the left hand in string players. *Science, 270*, 305–306.

Elkonin, D.B. (1973). USSR. In J. Downing (Ed.), *Comparative reading: Cross-national studies of behavior and processes in reading and writing* (pp. 551–579). New York: Macmillan.

Elliott, L.L. (1979). Performance of children aged 9 to 17 years on a test of speech intelligibility in noise using sentence material with controlled word predictability. *Journal of the Acoustical Society of America, 66*, 651–653.

Elliott, L.L. (1982). Effects of noise on perception of speech by children and certain handicapped individuals. *Sound and Vibration, 16*, 10–14.

Elliott, L.L. (1986). Discrimination and response bias for CV syllables differing in voice onset time among children and adults. *Journal of the Acoustical Society of America, 80,* 1250–1255.

Elliott, L.L. (1995). Verbal auditory closure and the Speech Perception in Noise (SPIN) test. *Journal of Speech and Hearing Research, 38*, 1363–1376.

Elliott, L.L., & Busse, L.A. (1987). Auditory processing by learning disabled young adults. In D.J. Johnson & J.W. Blalock (Eds.), *Adults with learning disabilities* (pp. 107–129). Orlando, FL: Grune and Stratton.

Elliott, L.L., Connors, S., Kille, E., Levin, S., Ball, K., & Katz, D. (1979). Children's understanding of monosyllabic nouns in quiet and in noise. *Journal of the Acoustical Society of America, 66,* 12–21.

Elliott, L.L., & Hammer, M. (1988). Longitudinal changes in auditory discrimination in normal children and children with language-learning problems. *Journal of Speech and Hearing Disorders, 53*, 467–474.

Elliott, L.L., Hammer, M., & Evan, K. (1987). Perception of gated highly familiar spoken monosyllabic nouns by children, teenagers and older adults. *Perception and Psychophysics, 42*(2), 150–157.

Elliott, L.L., & Katz, D.R. (1980). *Development of a new children's speech discrimination test.* St. Louis: Auditec.

Ellis, E.S., & Friend, P. (1991). Adolescents with learning disabilities. In B.Y.L. Wong (Ed.), *Learning about learning disabilities* (pp. 506–561). San Diego: Academic Press.

Ellis, E.S., Lenz, B.K., & Sabornie, E.J. (1987). Generalization and adaptation of learning strategies to natural environments—Part 2: Research into practice. *Remedial and Special Education, 8*(2), 6–23.

Ellis Weismer, S., & Hesketh, L. (1993). The influence of prosodic and gestural cues on novel word acquisition by children with specific language impairment. *Journal of Speech and Hearing Research, 36,* 1013–1026.

Elman, J.L. (1989). Connectionist approaches to acoustic/phonetic processing. In W.D. Marslen-Wilson (Ed.), *Lexical representation and process* (pp. 227–260). Cambridge, MA: MIT Press.

Elman, J.L. (1993). Learning and development in neural networks: The importance of starting small. *Cognition, 48*, 71–99.

Elman, J.L., & McClelland, J.L. (1984). Speech perception as a cognitive process: The interactive activation model. In N. Lass (Ed.), *Speech and Language,* Vol. *10.* New York: Academic Press.

Elman, J.L., & McClelland, J.L. (1986). Exploring lawful variability in the speech waveform. In J.S. Perkell & D.H. Klatt (Eds.), *Invariance and variablity in speech processing* (pp. 360–385). Hillsdale, NJ: Lawrence Erlbaum.

Erber, N. (1969). An interaction of audition and vision in recognition of oral speech stimuli. *Journal of Speech and Hearing Research, 12*(2), 423–425.

Erickson, J., & Inglesias, A. (1986). Assessment of communication disorders in non-English proficient children. In O.L. Taylor (Ed.), *Nature of communication disorders in culturally and linguistically diverse populations* (pp. 181–217). San Diego: College-Hill Press.

Eriksson, L., Allie, M., Bremigan, C., & Gilbert, J. (1989). Active noise control on systems with time-varying sources and parameters. *Sound and Vibration, 23,* 16–21.

Eshel, Y., & Klein, Z. (1981). Development of academic self-concept of lower-class and middle-class primary school children. *Journal of Educational Psychology, 73,* 287–293.

Eslinger, P.J. (1996). Conceptualizing, describing, and measuring components of executive function: A summary. In G.R. Lyon & N.A. Krasnegor (Eds.), *Attention, memory, and executive function* (pp. 367–398). Baltimore, MD: Paul H. Brookes.

Eslinger, P.J., & Grattan, L.M. (1993). Frontal lobe and frontal-striatal substrates for different forms of human cognitive flexibility. *Neuropsychologia, 31*, 17–28.

Evans, E. (1968). Cortical representation. In A. de Reuck & J. Knight (Eds.), *Hearing mechanisms in vertebrates* (pp. 227–287). London: Churchill Livingstone.

Evans, W., Webster, D., & Cullen, J. (1983). Auditory brainstem responses in neonatally sound deprived CBA/J mice. *Hearing Research, 10*, 269–277.

Fabricius, W.V., & Hagen, J.W. (1984). Use of causal attributions about recall performance to assess metamemory and predict strategic memory behavior in young children. *Developmental Psychology, 20*, 975–987.

Faingold, C.L., Hoffmann, W.E., & Caspary. D.M. (1989). Effects of excitant amino acids on acoustic responses of inferior colliculus neurons. *Hearing Research, 40*, 127–136.

Fant, G. (1967). Auditory patterns of speech. In W. Wathen-Dunn (Ed.), *Models for the perception of speech and visual form* (pp. 111–125). Cambridge, MA: MIT Press.

Farkas, C. (1986). Ethno-specific communication patterns: Implications for nutrition education. *Journal of Nutrition Education, 18*(3), 99–103.

Feagans, L.V., Sanyal, M., Henderson, F., Collier, A., & Appelbaum, M. (1987). Relationship of middle ear disease in early childhood to later narrative and attentional skills. *Journal of Pediatric Psychology, 12*, 581–594.

Feldman, D.E., Brainard, M.S., & Knudsen, E.I. (1996). Newly learned auditory responses mediated by NMDA receptors in the owl inferior colliculus. *Science, 271,* 525–528.

Feng, A., & Rogowski, B. (1980). Effects of monaural and binaural occlusion on morphology of neurons in the medial superior olivary nucleus of the rat. *Brain Research, 189*, 530–534.

Ferraro, J., & Minckler, J. (1977). The human lateral lemniscus and its nuclei. The human auditory pathways. A quantitative study. *Brain and Language, 4*, 277–294.

Ferre, J.M., & Wilber, L.A. (1986). Normal and learning disabled children's central auditory processing skills: An experimental test battery. *Ear & Hearing, 7,* 336–343.

Finitzo, T., Gunnarson, A., & Clark, J. (1990). Auditory deprivation and early conductive hearing loss from otitis media. *Topics in Language Disorders, 11*, 29–42.

Finitzo, T., & Pool, K.D. (1987). Brain electrical activity mapping. *Asha, 29*, 21–25.

Finitzo-Hieber, T. (1988). Classroom acoustics. In R. Roeser (Ed.), *Auditory disorders in school children* (2nd ed., pp. 221–223). New York: Thieme-Stratton.

Finitzo-Hieber, T., & Tillman, T. (1978). Room acoustics effects monosyllabic word discrimination ability for normal and hearing-impaired children. *Journal of Speech and Hearing Research, 21*, 440–458.

Fire, K.M., Lesner, S.A., & Newman, C. (1991). Hearing handicap as a function of central auditory abilities in the elderly. *American Journal of Otolaryngology, 122*, 105–108.

Fisher, L. (1976). *Fisher's auditory problems checklist.* Bemidji, MN: Life Products.

Fitzgibbons, P.J., & Gordon-Salant, S. (1996). Auditory temporal processing in elderly listeners. *Journal of the American Academy of Audiology, 7,* 183–189.

Flavell, J.H. (1981). Cognitive monitoring. In W.P. Dickson (Ed.), *Children's oral communication skills* (pp. 35–60). New York: Academic Press.

Flavell, J.H., & Wellman, H.M. (1977). Metamemory. In R.V. Kail & J.W. Hagan (Eds.), *Perspectives on the development of memory and cognition* (pp. 3–33). Hillsdale, NJ: Lawrence Erlbaum.

Fletcher, H. (1929). *Speech and hearing.* New York: Van Nostrand.

Fletcher, H. (1953). *Speech and hearing in communication.* New York: Von Nostrand.

Fletcher, H., & Galt, R.H. (1950). The perception of speech and its relation to telephony. *Journal of the Acoustical Society of America, 22*, 89–151.

Fletcher, H., & Steinberg, H.J.M. (1947). Factors governing the intelligibility of speech sounds. *Journal of the Acoustical Society of America, 19*, 90–119.

Fletcher, J.M., Taylor, H.G., Levin, H.S., & Satz, P. (1995). Neuropsychological and intellectual assessment of children. In H.I. Kaplan & B.J. Sadock (Eds.), *Comprehensive textbook of psychiatry / VI* (pp. 581–601). Baltimore: Williams & Wilkins.

Flexer, C. (1989). Turn on sound: An odyssey of sound field amplification. *Educational Audiology Association Newsletter, 5,* 6.

Flexer, C. (1992). FM classroom public address systems. In M. Ross (Ed.), *FM auditory training systems: Characteristics, selection and use* (pp. 189–210). Timonium, MD: York Press.

Flexer, C. (1994). *Facilitating hearing and listening in young children.* San Diego: Singular Publishing Group.

Flexer, C., Millin, J., & Brown, L. (1990). Children with developmental disabilities: The effects of sound field amplification in word identification. *Language, Speech, and Hearing Services in Schools, 21,* 177–182.

Florentine, M., Fastl, H., & Buss, S. (1988). Temporal integration in normal hearing, cochlear impairment, and impairment simulated by masking. *Journal of the Acoustical Society of America, 84*, 195–203.

Flowers, A., Costello, M., & Small, V. (1973). *Flowers-Costello tests of central auditory abilities.* Deerborn, MI: Perceptual Learning Systems.

Folsum, R., Weber, B., & Thompson, G. (1983). Auditory brainstem responses in children with early recurrent middle ear disease. *Annals of Otolology, Rhinology, and Otolaryngology, 92*, 249–253.

Forge, A., Li, L., Corwin, J.T., & Nevill, G. (1993). Ultrastructural evidence for hair cell regeneration in the mammalian inner ear. *Science, 29,* 1616–1619.

Forman-Franco, B., Karayalin, G., Mandel, D., & Abramson, A. (1982). The evaluation of auditory function in homozygous sickle cell disease. *Otolaryngology, Head and Neck Surgery, 89*, 850–856.

Forster, K.I. (1976). Accessing the mental lexicon. In R.J. Wales, & E. Walker (Eds.), *New approaches to language mechanisms* (pp. 257–287). Amsterdam: North-Holland.

Forster, K.I. (1981). Priming and the effects of sentence and lexical contexts on naming time: Evidence for autonomous lexical processing. *Quarterly Journal of Experimental Psychology, 33,* 465–495.

Forster, K.I., & Bednall, E.S. (1976). Terminating an exhaustive search in lexical access. *Memory and Cognition, 4*(1), 53–61.

Fowler, R., Hart, J., & Sheehan, M. (1972). A prosthetic memory: An application of the prosthetic environment concept. *Rehabilitation Counseling Bulletin, 15*, 80–85.

Fowler, S.M., & Baer, D.M. (1981). "Do I have to be good all day?" The timing delayed reinforcement as a factor in generalization. *Journal of Applied Behavior Analysis, 14*, 12–24.

Fox, R.A., Wall, L.G., & Gokcen, J. (1992). Age-related differences in processing dynamic information to identify vowel quality. *Journal of Speech and Hearing Research, 35*, 892–902.

French, J. (1957). The reticular formation. *Science America, 66*, 1–8.

French, L., & Nelson, K. (1985). *Young children's knowledge of relational terms.* New York: Springer-Verlag.

French, N., & Steinberg, J. (1947). Factors governing the intelligibility of speech sounds. *Journal of the Acoustical Society of America, 19,* 90–119.

Friedman, E., Luban, N., Herer, G., & Williams I. (1980). Sickle cell anemia and hearing. *Annals of Otolaryngology, Rhinolaryngology, and Laryngology, 89,* 342–347.

Friel-Patti, S. (1994a). Auditory linguistic processing and language learning. In G.P. Wallach & K.G. Butler (Eds.), *Language learning disabilities in school-age children and adolescents* (pp. 373–392). New York: Merrill.

Friel-Patti, S. (1994b). Commitment to theory. *American Journal of Speech-Language Pathology, 3*, 30–34.

Frumkin, N.L., Potchen, E.J., Aniskiewicz, A.S., Moore, J.B., & Cooke, P.A. (1989). Potential impact of magnetic resonance imaging on the field of communication disorders. *Asha, 31,* 95–99.

Gajar, A. (1985). American Indian personnel preparation in special education: Needs, program components, programs. *Journal of American Indian Education, 24*(2), 7–15.

Gajar, A.H. (1989). A computer analysis of written language variables and a comparison of compositions written by university students with and without learning disabilities. *Journal of Learning Disabilities, 22*, 125–130.

Galaburda, A.M. (1989). Ordinary and extraordinary brain development: Anatomical variation in developmental dyslexia. *Annals of Dyslexia, 39*, 67–80.

Galaburda, A.M., & Eidelberg, D. (1982). Symmetry and asymmetry in the human posterior thalamus: II. Thalamic lesions in a case of developmental dyslexia. *Archives of Neurology, 39*, 333–336.

Galaburda, A.M., & Kemper T. (1978). Cytoarchitectonic abnormalities in developmental dyslexia: A case study. *Annals of Neurology, 6*, 94–101.

Galaburda, A., & Sanides, F. (1980). Cytoarchitectonic organization of the human auditory cortex. *Journal of Comparative Neurology, 190*, 597–610.

Galaburda, A., Sherman, G., Rosen G., Aboitz, F., & Geschwind, N. (1971). Cytoarchitectonic organization of the human auditory cortex. *Journal of Comparative Neurology, 190*, 597–610.

Galaburda, A.M., Sherman, G.F., Rosen, G.D., Aboitz, F., & Geshwind, N. (1985). Developmental dyslexia: Four consecutive patients with cortical anomalies. *Annals of Neurology, 18*, 222–233.

Galambos, R. (1956). Suppression of auditory nerve activity by stimulation of efferent fibers to cochlea. *Journal of Neurophysiology, 19*, 424–437.

Gascon, G.G., Johnson, R., & Burd, L. (1986). Central auditory processing in attention deficit disorders. *Journal of Child Neurology, 1*, 27–33.

Gazzaniga, M., & Sperry, R. (1962). Some functional effects of sectioning the cerebral commissure in man. *Procedures of the National Academy of Science, USA, 48*, 1765–1769.

Geisler, C., Frishkopf, L., & Rosenblith, W. (1958). Extra cranial responses to acoustic clicks in man. *Science, 128*, 1210–1211.

Gengel, R.W. (1972). Auditory temporal integration at relatively high masked-threshold levels. *Journal of the Acoustical Society of America, 51*, 1849–1851.

Gerber, A. (1981). Remediation of language processing problems of the school-age child. In A. Gerber & D.N. Bryen (Eds.), *Language and learning disabilities* (pp. 159–215). Baltimore: University Park Press.

Gerber, A. (1993a). Interdisciplinary language intervention in education. In A. Gerber (Ed.), *Language-related learning disabilities: Their nature and treatment* (pp. 301–322). Baltimore: Paul H. Brookes.

Gerber, A. (1993b). Intervention: Preventing or reversing the failure cycle. In A. Gerber (Ed.), *Language-related learning disabilities: Their nature and treatment* (pp. 323–393). Baltimore: Paul H. Brookes.

Gerber, A. (Ed.). (1993c). *Language-related learning disabilities: Their nature and treatment.* Baltimore: Paul H. Brookes.

Gershuni, J., Baru, A., & Karaseva, T. (1967). Role of auditory cortex and discrimination of acoustic stimuli. *Neurology Science Transactions, 1*, 370–372.

Geschwind, N., & Levitsky, W. (1968). Human brain: Left-right asymmetries in temporal speech region. *Science, 161*, 186–187.

Giacobini, E., & Becker, R. (1989). Present progress and future development in the therapy of Alzheimer's disease. *Progress in Neuropsychopharmacology and Biological Psychiatry, 13*, 1121–1154.

Gibson, J.J. (1966). *The senses considered as perceptual systems*. Boston: Houghton Mifflin.

Gibson, J.J. (1979). *The ecological approach to visual perception*. Boston: Houghton Mifflin.

Gilbert, C.D., & Wiesel, T.N. (1992). Receptive field dynamics in adult primary visual cortex. *Nature, 356,* 150–152.

Gillet, P. (1993). *Auditory processes.* Novato, CA: Academic Therapy Publications.

Giolas, T.C., Cooker, H., & Duffy, J.R. (1970). Predictability of words in sentences. *Journal of Auditory Research, 10,* 328–334.

Godfrey, D., Carter, J., Berger, S., Lowry, D., & Matschinsky, F. (1977). Quantitative histochemical mapping of candidate transmitter amino acids in the cat cochlear nucleus. *Journal of Histochemistry and Cytochemistry, 25,* 417–431.

Godfrey, D., Park, J., Dunn, J., & Ross, C. (1985). Cholinergic neurotransmission in the cochlear nucleus. In D. Frecher (Ed.), *Auditory neurochemistry* (pp. 163–183). Springfield, IL: Charles C. Thomas.

Goetzinger, C.P., Proud, G.O., & Emery, J. (1961). A study of hearing in advanced age. *Archives of Otolaryngology, 73,* 662–674.

Goldberg, J.M., & Moore, R.Y. (1967). Ascending projections of the lateral lemniscus in the cat and the monkey. *Journal of Comparative Neurology, 129,* 143–155.

Goldenberg, G., Oder, W., Spatt, J., & Podreka, I. (1992). Cerebral correlates of disturbed executive function and memory in survivors of severe closed head injury: A SPECT study. *Journal of Neurology, Neurosurgery and Psychiatry, 55,* 362–368.

Goldfried, M.R., & Davison, G.C. (1976). *Clinical behavior therapy*. New York: Holt, Rinehart & Winston.

Goldinger, S.D., Pisoni, D.B., & Luce, P.A. (1996). Speech perception and spoken word recognition: Research and theory. In N.J. Lass (Ed.), *Principles of experimental phonetics* (pp. 277–327). St. Louis: Mosby.

Goldstein, H. (1990). Assessing clinical significance. In L.B. Olswang, C.K. Thompson, S.F. Warren, & N.J. Minghetti (Eds.), *Treatment efficacy research in communication disorders* (pp. 91–98). Rockville, MD: American Speech-Language-Hearing Foundation.

Goldstein, M., DeRibaupierre, R., & Yeni-Komshian, G. (1971). Cortical coding of periodicity pitch. In M. Sachs (Ed.), *Physiology of the auditory system* (pp. 299–306). Baltimore, MD: National Education Consultants, Inc.

Goldstein, S., & Goldstein, M. (1990). *Managing attention disorder in children*. New York: John Wiley.

Goodin, D., Aminoff, M., Chernoff, D., & Hollander, H. (1990). Long latency event-related potentials in patients infected with human immunodeficiency virus. *Annals of Neurology, 27*, 414–420.

Goodman, G., & Poillion, M.J. (1992). ADD: Acronym for any dysfunction or difficulty. *Journal of Special Education, 26*, 37–56.

Goodwin, E.H., Shaw, J., & Feldman, C.M. (1980). Distribution of otitis media among four Indian populations in Arizona. *Public Health Reports, 95*(6), 589–594.

Goodyear, P., & Hynd, G.W. (1992). Attention-deficit disorder with (ADD/H) and without (ADD/WO) hyperactivity: Behavioral and neuropsychological differentiation. *Journal of Clinical Child Psychology, 21*, 273–305.

Gordon, B. (1972). The inferior colliculus of the brain. *Scientific American, 227*, 72–82.

Gordon, C.J. (1989). Teaching narrative text structure: A process approach to reading and writing. In K.D. Muth (Ed.), *Children's comprehension of text* (pp. 79–102). Newark, DE: International Reading Association.

Gordon, C.J., & Rennie, B.J. (1986). Restructuring content schemata: An intervention study. *Reading Reseach and Instruction, 26*, 162–188.

Gordon, M. (1991). *ADHD/hyperactivity: A consumer's guide*. Dewitt, NY: GSI Publications.

Gordon-Salant, S., & Fitzgibbons, P. J. (1993). Temporal factors and speech recognition performance in elderly listeners. *Journal of Auditory Research, 36*, 1276–1285.

Gould, H.J., Crawford, M.R., Smith, W.R., Beckford, N., Gibson, W.R., Pettit, L., & Bobo, L. (1991). Hearing disorders in sickle cell disease: Cochlear and retrocochlear findings. *Ear & Hearing, 12*(5), 352–354.

Graham, S., & Harris, K. R. (1996). Addressing problems in attention, memory, and executive functioning: An example from self-regulated strategy development. In G.R. Lyon & N.A. Krasnegor (Eds.), *Attention, memory, and executive function* (pp. 349–365). Baltimore: Paul H. Brookes.

Grattan, L.M., Bloomer, R., Archambault, F.X., & Eslinger, P.J. (1994). Cognitive flexibility and empathy after frontal lobe lesion. *Neuropsychiatry, Neurophyschology and Behavioral Neurology, 7*, 251–259.

Grattan, L.M., & Eslinger, P.J. (1992). Long-term psychological consequences of childhood frontal lobe lesion in patient DT. *Brain and Cognition, 20*, 185–195.

Gravel, J.S., & Wallace, I.F. (1992). Listening and language at four years of age: Effects of early otitis media. *Journal of Speech and Hearing Research, 35*, 588–595.

Gravel, J.S., & Wallace, I.F. (1995). Early otitis media, auditory abilities, and educational risk. *American Journal of Speech-Language Pathology, 4*(3), 89–94.

Green, D.M., Birdsall, T.G., & Tanner, W.P. (1957). Signal detection as a function of signal intensity and duration. *Journal of the Acoustical Society of America, 29*, 523–531.

Greenberg, S. (1996). Auditory processing of speech. In N.J. Lass (Ed.), *Principles of experimental phonetics* (pp. 362–407). St. Louis: Mosby.

Greenough, W., & Bailey, C. (1988). Anatomy of memory: Convergence of results across a diversity of tests. *Trends in Neuroscience, 11*, 142–146.

Griffiths, H., & Craighead, E.W. (1972). Generalization in operant speech therapy for misarticulation. *Journal of Speech and Hearing Disorders, 37*, 485–492.

Grimes, A.M., Grady, C.L., Foster, N.L., Sunderland, T., & Patronas, N.J. (1985). Central auditory function in Alzheimer's disease. *Neurology, 35*, 352–358.

Groen, J. (1969). Diagnostic value of lateralization ability for dichotic time differences. *Acta Otolaryngology, 67*, 326–332.

Grose, J.H. (1996). Binaural performance and aging. *Journal of the Academy of Audiology, 7,* 168–174.

Grose, J.H., Hall, J.W., & Gibbs, C. (1993). Temporal analysis in children. *Journal of Speech and Hearing Research, 36*, 351–356.

Grosjean, F. (1980). Spoken word-recognition processes and the gating paradigm. *Perception and Psychophysics, 28,* 267–283.

Grosjean, F. (1985). The recognition of words after acoustic offset: Evidence and implications. *Perception and Psychophysics, 38*, 299–310.

Grosjean, F., & Hirt, C. (1996). Using prosody to predict the end of sentences in English and French: Normal and brain-damaged subjects. *Language and Cognitive Processes, 11,* 107–134.

Guevremont, D. (1990). Social skills and peer relationship training. In R.A. Barkley (Ed.), *Attention-deficit hyperactivity disorder: A handbook for diagnosis and treatment* (pp. 540–572). New York: Guilford Press.

Guilford, P., Ayadi, H., Blanchard, S., Chaib, H., Le Pasier, D., Weissenbach, J., Drira, M., & Petit, C. (1994). A human gene responsible for neurosensory, non-syndromic recessive deafness is a candidate homologue of the mouse *sh-1* gene. *Human Molecular Genetics, 3*, 989–993.

Guilford, P., Ben, A.S., Blanchard, S., Levilliers, J., Weissenbach, J., Belkahia, A., & Petit, C. (1994). A non-syndromic form of neurosensory, recessive deafness maps to the pericentromeric region of chromosome 13q. *Nature Genetics, 6*, 24–28.

Gulya, J. (1991). Structural and physiological changes of the auditory and vestibular mechanisms with aging. In D. Ripich (Ed.), *Handbook of geriatric communication disorders* (pp. 39–54). Austin, TX: Pro-Ed.

Gunnerson, A., & Finitzo, T. (1991). Conductive hearing loss during infancy: Effects on later auditory brainstem electrophysiology. *Journal of Speech and Hearing Research, 34*, 1207–1215.

Gustafsson, B., & Wigstrom, H. (1988). Physiologic mechanisms underlying long term potentiation. *Trends in Neuroscience, 11*(4), 156–162.

Guth, P., & Melamed, B. (1982). Neurotransmission in the auditory system: A primer for pharmacologists. *Annual Review of Pharmacology and Toxicology, 22,* 383–412.

Haaga, D.A., & Davison, G.C. (1986). Cognitive change methods. In F.H. Kanfer & A.P. Goldstein (Eds.), *Helping people change: A textbook of methods* (pp. 236–282). New York: Pergamon Press.

Haenlein, M., & Caul, W.F. (1987). Attention deficit disorder with hyperactivity: A specific hypothesis of reward dysfunction. *Journal of the American Academy of Child and Adolescent Psychiatry, 26*, 356–362.

Hall, J.G. (1976). The cochlear nuclei in monkeys after dihydrostreptomycin or noise exposure. *Acta Otolaryngologica, 81,* 344–352.

Hall, J.W. III (1985). The acoustic reflex in central auditory dysfunction. In M.L. Pinheiro & F.E. Musiek (Eds.), *Assessment of central auditory dysfunction: Foundations and clinical correlates* (pp. 103–130). Baltimore: Williams & Wilkins.

Hall, J.W. III (1992). *Handbook of auditory evoked responses*. Boston: Allyn & Bacon.

Hall, J.W. III, & Grose, J.H. (1990). The masking-level difference in children. *Journal of the American Academy of Audiology, 1*, 81–88.

Hall, J.W. III, & Grose, J.H. (1991). Notched-noise measures of frequency selectivity in adults and children using fixed-masker-level and fixed-signal-level presentation. *Journal of Speech and Hearing Research, 34*, 651–660.

Hall, J.W., & Grose, J.H. (1993). The effect of otitis media with effusion on the masking level difference and the auditory brainstem response. *Journal of Speech and Hearing Research, 36,* 210–217.

Hall, J.W., & Grose, J.H. (1994). The effect of otitis media with effusion on comodulation masking release in children. *Journal of Speech and Hearing Research, 37,* 1441–1449.

Hall, J.W., Grose, J.H., & Pillsbury, H.C. (1994). Long-term effects of chronic otitis media on binaural hearing in children. *Archives of Otolaryngology-Head and Neck Surgery, 37,* 1441–1449.

Hall, J.W., Grose, J.H., & Pillsbury, H.C. (1995). Long-term effects of chronic otitis media on binaural hearing in children. *Archives of Otolaryngology-Head and Neck Surgery, 121,* 847–852.

Hallahan, D.P., & Kneedler, R.D. (1979). *Strategy deficits in the information processing of learning-disabled children.* (Technical Report No. 6). Charlottesville: University of Virginia Learning Disabilities Research Institute.

Halliday, M.A.K., & Hasan, R. (1976). *Cohesion in English*. London: Longman.

Halpern, D.F. (1984). *Thought and knowledge: An introduction to critical thinking.* Hillsdale, NJ: Lawrence Erlbaum.

Hamernik, R.P., Ahroon, W.A., Davis, R.I., & Lei, S.F. (1994). Hearing threshold shifts from repeated 6-h daily exposure to impact noise. *Journal of the Acoustical Society of America, 95*, 444–453.

Handel, S. (1989). *Listening: An introduction to the perception of auditory events.* Cambridge, MA: The MIT Press.

Handrock, M., & Zeisberg, J. (1982). The influence of the efferent system on adaptation, temporary and permanent threshold shift. *Archives of Otolaryngology, 234*, 191–195.

Hari, R., Aittonieme, K., Jarvinen, M., Katila, T., & Varpula, T. (1980). Auditory evoked transient and sustained magnetic fields of the human brain. *Experimental Brain Reserach, 40*, 237–240.

Harley, R., & Lawrence, G. (1977). *Visual impairment in the schools*. Springfield, IL: Charles C. Thomas.

Harrell, M., Parente, F., Bellingrath, E.G., & Lisicia, K.A. (1992). *Cognitive rehabilitation of memory: A practical guide.* Gaithersburg, MD: Aspen.

Harris, A.J., & Sipay, E.R. (1990). *How to increase reading ability* (9th ed.). New York: Longman.

Harris, G.A. (1993). American Indian cultures: A lesson in diversity. In D.E. Battle (Ed.), *Communication disorders in multicultural populations* (pp. 78–113). Boston: Andover Medical Publishers.

Harris, J.D. (1960). Combinations of distortion in speech: The twenty-five percent factor by multiple-cueing. *Archives of Otolaryngology, 72,* 227–232.

Harris, J.E. (1992). Ways to help memory. In B. Wilson & N. Moffat (Eds.), *Clinical management of memory problems* (pp. 56–82). San Diego: Singular Publishing Group.

Harris, K.R., & Graham, S. (1985). Improving learning disabled students' composition skills: Self-control strategy training. *Learning Disability Quarterly, 8,* 27–36.

Harris, P.L. (1978). Developmental aspects of memory: A review. In M.M. Gruneberg, P.E. Morris, & R.N. Sykes (Eds.), *Practical aspects of memory* (pp. 369–377). London: Academic Press.

Harris, P.L., & Terwogt, M.M. (1978). How does memory write a synnopsis. In M.M. Gruneberg, P.E. Morris, & R.N. Sykes (Eds.), *Practical aspects of memory.* (pp. 385–392). London: Academic Press.

Harris, R.W., & Reitz, M.L. (1985). Effects of room reverberation and noise on speech discrimination by the elderly. *Audiology, 24,* 319–324.

Harrison, J., & Howe, M. (1974). Anatomy of the descending auditory system (mammalian). In W. Keidel & W. Neff (Eds.), *Handbook of sensory physiology* (pp. 363–368). Berlin: Springer-Verlag.

Hart, K.J., & Morgan, J.R. (1993). Cognitive-behavioral procedures with children: Historical context and current status. In A.J. Finch, W.M. Nelson, & E.S. Ott (Eds.), *Cognitive-behavioral procedures with children and adolescents* (pp. 1–24). Boston: Allyn & Bacon.

Harter, S. (1982). A developmental perspective on some parameters of self-regulation in children. In P. Karoly & F.H. Kanfer (Eds.), *Self-management and behavior change: From theory to practice* (pp. 165–204). New York: Pergamon Press.

Hassamannova, J., Myslivecek, J., & Novakova, V. (1981). Effects of early auditory stimulation on cortical areas. In J. Syka & L. Aitkin (Eds.), *Neuronal mechanisms of hearing* (pp. 355–359). New York: Plenum Press.

Hausler, R., & Levine, R. (1980). Brainstem auditory evoked potentials are related to interaural time discrimination in patients with multiple sclerosis. *Brain Research, 91,* 589–594.

Hawkins, D. (1984). Comparisons of speech recognition in noise by mildly-to-moderately hearing-impaired children using hearing aids and FM systems. *Journal of Speech and Hearing Disorders, 49*(4), 409–418.

Hayes, S.C., Gifford, E.V., & Ruckstuhl, L.E. (1996). Relational frame theory and executive function: A behavioral approach. In G.R. Lyon & N.A. Krasnegor (Eds.), *Attention, memory, and executive function* (pp. 279–326). Baltimore: Paul H. Brookes.

Heasley, B.E. (1980). *Auditory processing disorders and remediation.* Springfield, IL: Charles C. Thomas.

Heaton, R.K. (1981). *A manual for the Wisconsin Card Sorting Test.* Odessa, FL: Psychological Assessment Resources.

Heffner, H., & Heffner, R. (1986). Hearing loss in Japanese Macaques following bilateral auditory cortex lesions. *Journal of Neurophysiology, 55,* 256–271.

Heffner, H., Heffner, R., & Porter, W. (1985, October). Effects of auditory cortex lesion on absolute thresholds in Macaques. *Proceedings of the Society for Neuroscience*, Annual Meeting, Dallas, TX.

Hegde, M.N. (1993). *Treatment procedures in communicative disorders.* Austin, TX: Pro-Ed.

Helfert, R., Altschuler, R., & Wenthold, R. (1987). GABA and glycine immunoreactivity in the guinea pig superior olivary complex. *Neuroscience Abstracts, 13,* 544.

Helman, C. (1984). *Culture, health and illness*. Bristol: John Wright and Sons.

Henderson, D., Campo, P. Subramaniam, M., & Fiorino, F. (1992). Development of resistance to noise. In A.L. Dancer, D. Henderson, R.J. Salvi, & R.P. Hamernik (Eds.), *Noise-induced hearing loss* (pp. 476–488). St. Louis: Mosby.

Henderson, D., Subramaniam, M., Spongr, V., & Attansaio, G. (1996). Biological mechanisms of the "toughening" phenomenon. In R.J. Salvi, D. Henderson, F. Fiorino, & V. Colletti (Eds.), *Auditory system plasticity and regeneration* (pp. 143–154). New York: Thieme.

Henselman, L.W., Henderson, D., Subramaniam, M., & Sallustio, V. (1994). The effect of "conditioning" exposures on hearing loss from impulse noise. *Hearing Research, 78,* 1–10.

Henri, B.P. (1994). Graduate student preparation: Tomorrow's challenge. *Asha, 36*, 43–46.

Heshusius, L. (1989). The Newtonian mechanistic paradigm, special education, and contours of alternatives: An overview. *Journal of Learning Disabilities, 22*(7), 403–415.

Heyer, J. (1995). The responsibilities of speech-language pathologists toward children with ADHD. *Seminars in Speech and Language, 16*(4), 275–288.

Hirsh, I.J. (1959). Auditory perception of temporal order. *Journal of the Acoustical Society of America, 31*, 759–767.

Hirsh, I.J., Reynolds, E.G., & Joseph, M. (1954). Intelligibility of different speech materials. *The Journal of the Acoustical Society of America, 35*(2), 200–206.

Hirsh, L., Davis, H., Silverman, S., Reynolds, E. Eldert, E., & Benson, R. (1952). Development of materials for speech audiometry. *Journal of Speech and Hearing Disorders, 17*, 321–337.

Hock, F.J. (1995). Therapeutic approaches for memory impairments. *Behavioral Brain Research, 66*, 143–150.

Hodgson, W. (1967). Audiological report of a patient with left hemispherectomy. *Journal of Speech and Hearing Disorders, 32,* 39–45.

Hodson, B., & Paden, E. (1983) *Targeting intelligible speech.* San Diego: College-Hill Press.

Hoffman, D.W. (1986). Opioid mechanisms in the inner ear. In R.A. Altschuler, D.W. Hoffman, & R.P. Bobbin (Eds.), *Neurobiology of hearing: The cochlea* (pp. 371–382). New York: Raven Press.

Holborow, P.L., & Berry, P.S. (1986). Hyperactivity and learning difficulties. *Journal of Learning Disabilities, 19*, 426–431.

Hooks, K., Milich, R., & Lorch, E. P. (1994). Sustained and selective attention in boys with attention deficit hyperactivity disorder. *Journal of Clinical Child Psychology, 23,* 69–77.

Hoover, R.M., & Blazier, W.E. (1991). Noise control in heating, ventilating, and air-conditioning systems. In C.M. Harris (Ed.), *Handbook of acoustical measurements and noise control* (pp. 42.1–42.31). New York: McGraw-Hill.

Horton, D.L., & Mills, C.B. (1984). Human learning and memory. *Annual Review of Psychology, 35*, 361–394.

Hoskins, B. (1983). Semantics. In C. Wren (Ed.), *Language learning disabilities* (pp. 85–111). Rockville, MD: Aspen Systems.

Houck, C.K., & Billingsley, B.S. (1989). Written expression of students with and without learning disabilities: Differences across the grades. *Journal of Learning Disabilities, 22*, 561–572.

Houtgast, T. (1981). The effect of ambient noise on speech intelligibility in classrooms. *Applied Acoustics, 14*, 15–25.

Houtgast, T., & Steeneken, H.J.M. (1985). Review of the MTF concept for estimating speech intelligibility in auditoria. *Journal of the Acoustical Society of America, 72*, 1069–1077.

Howe, M.J.A., & Ceci, S.J. (1978). Why older children remember more: Contributions of strategies and existing knowledge of developmental changes in memory. In M.M. Gruneberg, P.E. Morris, & R.N. Sykes (Eds.), *Practical aspects of memory* (pp. 393–400). London: Academic Press.

Howes, D. (1952). The intelligibility of spoken messages. *American Journal of Psychology, 65,* 460–465.

Huber, M., Kittner, B., Hojer, C., Fink, G.R., Neveling, M., & Heiss, W.D. (1993). Effect of propentofylline on regional cerebral glucose metabolism in acute ischemic stroke. *Journal of Cerebral Blood Flow and Metabolism, 13*(3), 526–530.

Hughes, G.B. (1985). *Texbook of clinical otology*. New York: Thieme-Stratton.

Hughes, L.F., Tobey, E.A., & Miller, C.J. (1983). Temporal aspects of dichotic listening in brain-damaged subjects. *Ear & Hearing, 4*(6), 306–310.

Humes, L.E. (1996). Speech understanding in the elderly. *Journal of the American Academy of Audiology, 7*, 161–167.

Humes, L.E., & Christopherson, L. (1991). Speech identification difficulties of hearing-impaired elderly persons: The contributions of auditory processing deficits. *Journal of Speech and Hearing Research, 34*, 686–693.

Humes, L.E., Dirks, D.D., Bell, T.S., Ahlstrom, C., & Cincaid, G.E. (1986). Application of the articulation index and the speech transmission index to the recognition of speech by normal-hearing and hearing-impaired listeners. *Journal of Speech and Hearing Research, 29*, 447–462.

Humes, L.E., & Roberts, L. (1990). Speech-recognition difficulties of the hearing-impaired elderly: The contributions of audibility. *Journal of Speech and Hearing Research, 33*, 726–735.

Humes, L.E., Watson, B.U., Christensen, L.A., Cokely, C.G., Haling, D.C., & Lee, L. (1994). Factors associated with individual differences in clinical measures of speech recognition among the elderly. *Journal of Speech and Hearing Research, 37*, 465–474.

Hunt, R.D., Arnsten, A.F., & Asbell, M.D. (1995). An open trial of guanfacine in the treatment of attention-deficit hyperactivity disorder. *Journal of the American Academy of Child and Adolescent Psychiatry, 34*(1), 50–54.

Hunt, R.D., Minderaa, R., & Cohen, D.J. (1985). Clonidine benefits children with attention deficit disorder and hyperactivity: Report of a double-blind placebo crossover therapeutic trial. *Journal of the American Academy of Child and Adolescent Psychiatry, 24*, 617–629.

Hutchings, M.E., Meyer, S.E., & Moore, D.R. (1992). Binaural masking level differences in infants with and without otitis media with effusion. *Hearing Research, 63,* 71–78.

Hynd, G.W., & Semrud-Clikeman, M. (1989). Dyslexia and neurodevelopmental pathology: Relationships to cognition, intelligence, and reading acquisition. *Journal of Learning Disabilities, 22*, 204–216.

Hynd, G.W., Semrud-Clikeman, M., Lorys, A.R., Novey, E.S., & Eliopulos, D. (1990). Brain morphology in developmental dyslexia and attention deficit disorder/hyperactivity. *Archives of Neurology, 47,* 916–919.

Hynd, G.W., Semrud-Clikeman, M., Lorys, A.R., Novey, E.S., Eliopulos, D., & Lyytinen, H. (1991). Corpus callosum morphology in attention deficit-hyeractivity disorder: Morphometric analysis of MRI. *Journal of Learning Disabilities, 24,* 141–146.

Hynd, G.W., Semrud-Clikeman, M., & Lyytinen, H. (1991). Brain imaging in learning disabilities. In J.E. Obrzut & G.W. Hynd (Eds.), *Neuropsychological foundations of learning disabilities* (pp. 475–511). San Diego: Academic Press.

Ibanez, V., Deiber, P., & Fischer, C. (1989). Middle latency auditory evoked potentials and cortical lesions: Criteria of interhemispheric asymmetry. *Archives of Neurology, 46,* 1325–1332.

Idol, L. (1987). Group story mapping: A comprehension strategy for both skilled and unskilled readers. *Journal of Learning Disabilities, 20,* 196–205.

Iler Kirk, K., Pisoni, D.B., & Osberger, M.J. (1995). Lexical effects on spoken word recognition by pediatric cochlear implant users. *Ear & Hearing, 16*(5), 470-481.

Ikeda, T., Yamamoto, K., Takahashi, K., Kahu, Y., Uchiyama, M., Sugiyama, K., & Yamada, M. (1992). Treatment of Alzheimer-type dementia with intravenous mecobalamin. *Clinical Therapeutics, 14*(3), 426–427.

Interagency Committee on Learning Disabilities. (1987). *Learning disabilities: A report to the U.S. Congress*. Washington, DC: Government Printing Office.

Irvine, D.R.F., Rajan, R., & Robertson, D. (1992). Plasticity in auditory cortex of adult mammals with restricted cochlear lesions. In R. Naresh Singh (Ed.), *Nervous systems: Principles of design and function* (pp. 319–350). New Delhi: Wiley-Eastern Ltd.

Irwin, R.J., Ball, A.K., Kay, N., Stillman, J.A., & Bosser, J. (1985). The development of auditory temporal acuity in children. *Child Development, 56*, 614–620.

Jacob, J.E., & Paris, S.G. (1987). Children's metacognition about reading: Issues in definition, measurement and instruction. *Educational Psychology, 22*(3/4), 255–278.

Jacobsen, M. (1991). *Developmental neurobiology*. New York: Plenum.

Jacobson, J.T., Deppe, U., & Murray, T.J. (1983). Dichotic paradigms in multiple sclerosis. *Ear & Hearing, 4*(6), 311–317.

Jean-Baptiste, M., & Morest D. (1975). Transneuronal changes of synaptic endings and nuclear chromatic in the trapezoid body following cochlear ablations in cats. *Journal of Comparative Neurology, 162,* 111–134.

Jeffress, L., & McFadden, D. (1971). Differences of interaural phase and level of detection and lateralization. *Journal of the Acoustical Society of America, 49*, 1169–1179.

Jeffries, J.H., & Jeffries, R.D. 1991). *Auditory processing activities.* Phoenix: ECL Publications.

Jenkins, W.M., Merzenich, M.M., Ochs, M.T., Allard, T., & Guic-Robles, E. (1990). Functional reorganization of primary somatosensory cortex in adult owl monkeys after behaviorally controlled tactile stimulation. *Journal of Neurophysiology, 63,* 82–104.

Jenkins, W.M., Merzenich, M.M., & Recanzone, G.H. (1990). Neocortica representational dynamics in adult primates: Implications for neuropsychology. *Neuropsychologia, 28*(6), 573–584.

Jensen, J., & Neff, D. (1989, April). *Discrimination of intensity, frequency and duration differences in preschool children: Age effects and longitudinal data*. Presented at the SRCH Biennial Meeting, Kansas City, MO.

Jensen, J.K., & Neff, D.L. (1993). Development of basic auditory discrimination in preschool children. *Pyschological Science, 4*(2), 104–107.

Jerger, J. (1973). Audiological findings in aging. *Advances in Otology, Rhinology and Laryngology, 20*, 115–124.

Jerger, J. (1992). Can age-related decline in speech understanding be explained by peripheral hearing loss? *Journal of the American Academy of Audiology, 3*, 33–38.

Jerger, J. (1996). ALD use in the elderly: A speech test that can help us predict success. *The Hearing Journal, 49*(10), 72–75.

Jerger, J., & Jerger, S. (1971). Diagnostic significance of PB word functions. *Archives of Otolaryngology, 93*, 573–580.

Jerger, J., & Jerger, S. (1974). Auditory findings in brain stem disorders. *Archives of Otolaryngology, 99,* 342–350.

Jerger, J., Jerger, S., Oliver, T., & Pirozzolo, F. (1989). Speech understanding in the elderly. *Ear & Hearing, 10*(2), 79–89.

Jerger, J., Jerger, S., & Pirozzolo, F. (1991). Correlational analysis of speech audiometric scores, hearing loss, age, and cognitive abilities in the elderly. *Ear & Hearing, 12*(2), 103–109.

Jerger, J., Johnson, K., Jerger, S., Coker, N., Pirozzolo, F., & Gray, L. (1991). Central auditory processing disorder: A case study. *Journal of the American Academy of Audiology, 2*(1), 36–54.

Jerger, J., Oliver, T., Chmiel, R., & Rivera, V. (1986). Patterns of auditory abnormality in multiple sclerosis. *Audiology, 25,* 193–209.

Jerger, J., Silman, S., Lew, H., & Chmiel, R. (1993). Case studies in binaural interference: Converging evidence from behavioral and electrophysiological measures. *Journal of the American Academy of Audiology, 4,* 122–131.

Jerger, J., Stach, B., Pruitt, J., Harper, R., & Kirby, H. (1989). Comments on "Speech understanding and aging." *Journal of the Acoustical Society of America, 85*(3), 1352–1354.

Jerger, J., Weikers, N., Sharbrough, F., & Jerger, S. (1969). Bilateral lesions of the temporal lobe. A case study. *Acta Otolaryngologica, 258*(Suppl.), 1–51.

Jerger, S., Elizondo, R., Dinh, T., Sanchez, P., & Chavira, E. (1994). Linguistic influences on the auditory processing of speech by children with normal hearing or hearing impairment. *Ear & Hearing, 15*(2), 138–159.

Jerger, S., Grimes, A., Tran, T., Chen, C., & Martin, R. (1996). Childhood hearing impairment: Processing dependencies in multi-dimensional speech perception for auditory level of analysis. Unpublished manuscript.

Jerger, S., & Jerger, J. (1984). *Pediatric Speech Intelligibility Test: Manual for administration.* St. Louis: Auditech.

Jerger, S., & Jerger, J. (1985). Audiological applications of early, middle and late auditory evoked potentials. *The Hearing Journal, 38*, 31–36.

Jerger, S., Jerger, J., & Abrams, S. (1983). Speech audiometry in the young child. *Ear & Hearing, 4*, 56–66.

Jerger, S., Jerger, J., Alford, B.R., & Abrams, S. (1983). Development of speech intelligibility in children with recurrent otitis media. *Ear & Hearing, 4,* 138–145.

Jerger, S., Johnson, K., & Loiselle, L. (1988). Pediatric central auditory dysfunction: Comparison of children with a confirmed lesion versus suspected processing disorders. *American Journal of Otology, 9*, 63–71.

Jerger, S., Martin, R.C., & Jerger, J. (1987). Specific auditory perceptual dysfunction in a learning disabled child. *Ear & Hearing, 8*(2), 78–86.

Jerger, S., Stout, G., Kent, M., Albritton, E., Loiselle, L., Blondeau, R., & Jorgenson, S. (1993). Auditory stroop effects in children with hearing impairment. *Journal of Speech and Hearing Research, 36*, 1083–1096.

Jirsa, R.E. (1992). The clinical utility of the P3 AERP in children with auditory processing disorders. *Journal of Speech and Hearing Research, 35,* 903–912.

Jirsa, R.E., & Clontz, K.B. (1990). Long latency auditory event–related potentials from children with auditory processing disorders. *Ear & Hearing, 11*, 222–232.

Johnson, D.J., & Myklebust, H.R. (1967). *Learning disabilities: Educational principles and practices*. New York: Grune & Stratton.

Jones, E., & Powell, T. (1970). An anatomical study of converging sensory pathways within the cerebral cortex of the monkey. *Brain, 93*, 793–820.

Jungert, S. (1958). Auditory pathways in the brain stem. A neurophysiologic study. *Acta Otolaryngology*, Suppl. 138.

Kail, R.V. (1990). *The development of memory in children*. New York: W.H. Freeman.

Kalikow, D.N., Stevens, K.N., & Elliott, L.L. (1977). Development of a test of speech intelligibility in noise using sentence materials with controlled word predictability. *Journal of Acoustical Society of America, 61*(5), 1337–1351.

Kalil, R.E. (1989). Synapse formation in the developing brain. *Scientific American, 261*(6), 76–85.

Kamhi, A.G. (1991). Clinical forum: Treatment efficacy, an introduction. *Language, Speech, and Hearing Services in Schools, 22*(4), 254.

Kane, E.C. (1974). Patterns of degeneration in the caudal cochlear nucleus of the cat after cochlear ablation. *Anatomy Record, 179*, 67–91.

Kanfer, F.H., & Gaelick, L. (1991). Self–management methods. In F.H. Kanfer & A.P. Goldstein (Eds.), *Helping people change: A textbook of methods* (4th ed., pp. 305–360). Needham Heights, MA: Allyn & Bacon.

Karlsson, A., & Rosenhall, U. (1995). Clinical application of distorted speech audiometry. *Scandinavian Audiology, 24*, 155–160.

Kass, C., & Myklebust, H. (1969). Learning disability: An educational definition. *Journal of Learning Disabilities, 2*, 38–40.

Kass, J.H. (1991). Plasticity of sensory and motor maps in adult mammals. *Annual Review of Neuroscience, 14*, 137–167.

Katz, J. (1962). The use of staggered spondaic words for assessing the integrity of the central auditory system. *Journal of Auditory Research, 2*, 327–337.

Katz, J. (1983). Phonemic synthesis. In E.Z. Lasky & J. Katz (Eds.), *Central auditory processing disorders: Problems of speech, language and learning* (pp. 269–296). Baltimore: University Park Press.

Katz, J. (1992). Classification of auditory processing disorders. In J. Katz, N.A. Stecker, & D. Henderson (Eds.), *Central auditory processing: A transdisciplinary view* (pp. 81–92). St. Louis: Mosby Year Book.

Katz, J., & Harmon, C. (1982). *Phonemic synthesis*. Allen, TX: Developmental Learning Materials.

Katz, J., & Illmer, R. (1972). Auditory perception in children with learning disabilities. In J. Katz (Ed.), *Handbook of clinical audiology* (pp. 540–563). Baltimore: Williams & Wilkins.

Katz, J., & Smith, P. (1991). The Staggered Spondaic Word Test: A ten minute look at the CNS through the ears. In R. Zapulla, F.F. LeFever, J. Jaeger, & R. Bilder (Eds.), *Windows on the brain: Neuropsychology's technical frontiers* (pp. 1–19). *Annals of the New York Academy of Sciences, 620*, 233–251.

Katz, J., Stecker N.A., & Henderson, D. (1992). *Central auditory processing: A transdisciplinary view*. St. Louis: Mosby Year Book.

Katz, J., & Wilde, L. (1994). Auditory processing disorders. In J. Katz (Ed.), *Handbook of clinical audiology* (4th ed., pp. 490–502). Baltimore: Williams & Wilkins.

Kaufman, W., & Galaburda, A. (1989). Cerebrocortical microdysgenesis in neurologically normal subjects: A histopathological study. *Neurology, 39*, 238–243.

Kavanagh, G., & Kelly, J. (1988). Hearing in the ferret (Mustela putorius): Effects of primary auditory cortical lesions on thresholds for pure tone detection. *Journal of Neurophysiology, 60*, 879–888.

Keefe, J.W. (1987). *Learning style theory and practice.* Reston, VA: National Assocation of Secondary School Principals.

Keidel, W., Kallert, S., Korth, M., & Humes, L. (1983). *The physiological basis of hearing.* New York: Thieme–Stratton.

Keith, R.W. (Ed.). (1977). *Central auditory dysfunction.* New York: Grune & Stratton.

Keith, R.W. (1981a). Audiological and auditory-language tests of central auditory function. In R.W. Keith (Ed.), *Central auditory and language disorders in children* (pp. 61–76). Houston, TX: College-Hill Press.

Keith, R. W. (Ed.). (1981b). *Central auditory and language disorders in children.* San Diego: College-Hill Press.

Keith, R.W. (1981c). Tests of central auditory function. In R.J. Roeser & M.P. Downs (Eds.), *Auditory disorders in school children* (pp. 159–173). New York: Thieme-Stratton.

Keith, R.W. (1983). Interpretation of the staggered spondaic word (SSW) test. *Ear & Hearing, 4*(6), 297–292.

Keith, R.W. (1986). *SCAN: A screening test for auditory processing disorders.* San Antonio, TX: Psychological Corporation.

Keith, R.W. (1994a). *SCAN-A: A test for auditory processing disorders in adolescence and adults*. San Antonio, TX: The Psychological Corporation.

Keith, R.W. (1994b). *ACPT: Auditory continuous performance test.* San Antonio, TX: Psychological Corporation.

Keith, R.W., & Engineer, P. (1991). Effects of methylphenidate on the auditory processing abilities of children with attention deficit-hyperactivity disorder. *Journal of Learning Disabilities, 24*, 630–636.

Keith, R.W., & Jerger, S. (1991). Central auditory disorders. In J.T. Jacobson & J.L. Northern (Eds.), *Diagnostic audiology* (pp. 235–250). Austin, TX: Pro-Ed.

Keith, R.W., & Novak, K.K. (1984). Relationships between tests of central auditory function and receptive language. *Seminars in Hearing, 5*(3), 243–250.

Keith, R.W., Rudy, J., Donahue, P.A., & Katbamna, B. (1989). Comparison of SCAN results with other auditory and language measures in a clinical population. *Ear & Hearing, 10*(6), 382–386.

Keller, W.D. (1992). Auditory processing disorder or attention-deficit disorder? In J. Katz, N.A. Stecker, & D. Henderson (Eds.), *Central auditory processing: A transdisciplinary view* (pp. 107–114). St. Louis: Mosby Year Book.

Kelley, C. (1979). *Assertion training: A facilitator's guide*. San Diego: University Associates.

Kelly, D.A. (1995). *Central auditory processing disorder: Strategies for use with children and adolescents.* San Antonio, TX: Communication Skill Builders.

Kelly, T., Lee, W., Charrette, L., & Musiek, F. (1996, April). *Middle latency evoked response sensitivity and specificity.* Paper presented at the Annual Meeting of the American Auditory Society, Salt Lake City, UT.

Kendall, P.C. (1992). *Anxiety disorders in youth.* Boston: Allyn and Bacon.

Kendall, P.C., & Braswell, L. (1982). Cognitive-behavioral self-control therapy for children. A components analysis. *Journal of Consulting and Clinical Psychology, 50*, 672–689.

Kennedy, B.A., & Miller, D.J. (1976). Persistent use of verbal rehearsal as a function of information about its value. *Child Development, 47*, 566–569.

Kiang, N.Y.S. (1975). Stimulus representation in the discharge patterns of auditory neurons. In D.B. Tower (Ed.), *The nervous system: Human communication and its disorders* (pp. 8l–96). New York: Raven Press.

Kilb, L. (1993). Title II—Public Services, Subtitle A: State and local governments' role. In L.O. Gostin, & H.A. Beyer (Eds.), *Implementing the Americans With Disabilities Act* (pp. 87–108). Baltimore: Paul H. Brookes.

Kileny, P., & Kripal, J. (1987). Test/retest variablity of auditory event–related potentials. *Ear & Hearing, 8*, 110–114.

Kileny, P., Paccioretti, D., & Wilson, A. (1987). Effects of cortical lesions on middle latency auditory evoked respones (MLR). *Electroencephalography and Clinical Neurophysiology, 66*, 108–120.

Kimelman, M.D.Z. (1991). The role of target word stress in auditory comprehension by aphasic listeners. *Journal of Speech and Hearing Research, 34,* 334–339.

Kimura, D. (1961a). Cerebral dominance and the perception of verbal stimuli. *Canadian Journal of Psychology, 15*, 166–171.

Kimura, D. (1961b). Some effects of temporal lobe damage on auditory perception. *Canadian Journal of Psychology, 15*, 157–165.

Kinney, S.E., Hughes, G.B., & Hardy, R.W. (1985). Acoustic tumors. In G.B. Hughes (Ed.), *Textbook of clinical otology* (pp. 404–415). New York: Thieme-Stratton.

Kintsch, W. (1977). On comprehending stories. In M.A. Just & P.A. Carpenter (Eds.), *Cognitive processes in comprehension* (pp. 33–62). Hillsdale, NJ: Lawrence Erlbaum.

Kintsch, W. (1988). The role of knowledge in discourse comprehension: A construction-integration model. *Psychological Review, 95*, 163–182.

Kistner, J.A., Osborne, M., & LeVerrier, L. (1988). Causal attributions of learning-disabled children: Developmental patterns and relation to academic progress. *Journal of Education Psychology, 80*, 82–89.

Klatt, D.H. (1976). Linguistic uses of segmental duration in English: Acoustic and perceptual evidence. *Journal of the Acoustical Society of America, 59,* 1208–1221.

Klatt, D.H. (1979). A model of acoustic-phonetic analysis and lexical access. *Journal of Phonetics, 7*, 279–312.

Klein, R.G., & Slomkowski, C. (1993). Treatment of psychiatric disorders in children and adolescents. *Psychopharmacology Bulletin, 29*(4), 525–535.

Knight, R. (1990). Neuromechanisms of event-related potentials: Evidence from human lesion studies. In J. Roharabaugh, R. Parasuraman, & R. Johnson (Eds.), *Event related potentials: Basic issues in applications* (pp. 3–18). New York: Oxford University Press.

Knight, R., Hillyard, S., Woods, D., & Neville, H. (1980). The effects of frontal and temporal-parietal lesions on the auditory evoked potential in man. *Electroencephalography and Clinical Neurophysiology, 50*, 112–124.

Knight, R., Scabini, D., Woods, D., & Clayworth, C. (1988). The effects of lesions of the superior temporal gyrus and inferior parietal lobe on temporal and vertex components of the human AEP. *Electroencephalography and Clinical Neurophysiology, 70*, 499–509.

Knox, C., & Roeser, R. (1980). Cerebral dominance in auditory perceptual asymmetries in normal and dyslexic children. *Seminars in Speech, Language, and Hearing, 1*, 181–194.

Knudsen, E.I. (1987). Early auditory experience shapes auditory localization behavior and the spatial tuning of auditory units in the barn owl. In J. Rauschecker & P. Marler (Eds.), *Imprinting and cortical plasticity* (pp. 7–23). New York: John Wiley.

Knudsen, E.I. (1988). Experience shapes sound localization and auditory unit properties during development in the barn owl. In G. Edelman, W. Gall, & W. Kowan (Eds.), *Auditory function: Neurobiological basis of hearing* (pp. 137–152). New York: John Wiley.

Knudsen, E.I. (1994). Supervised learning in the brain. *Journal of Neuroscience, 14*(7), 3985–3997.

Knudsen, E.I., Esterly, S.D., & du Lac, S. (1991). Stretched and upside-down maps of auditory space in the optic tectum of blind-reared owls: Acoustic basis and behavioral correlates. *Journal of Neuroscience, 11*(6), 1727–1747.

Knudsen, E.I., Esterly, S.D., & Olsen, J.F. (1994). Adaptive plasticity of the auditory space map in the optic tectum of adult and baby barn owls in response to external ear modification. *Journal of Neurophysiology, 71*(1), 79–94.

Knudsen, E.I., & Konishi, M. (1978). Space and frequency are represented separately in auditory midbrain of the owl. *Journal of Neurophysiology, 41*, 870–884.

Knudsen, E.I., & Konishi, M. (1980). Monaural occlusion shifts receptive-field locations of auditory midbrain of the owl. *Journal of Neurophysiology, 41*, 870–884.

Knudsen, V., & Harris, C. (1978). *Acoustical designing in architecture*. Washington, DC: The American Institute of Physics for the Acoustical Society of America.

Kodaras, M. (1960). Reverberation times of typical elementary school settings. *Noise Control, 6*, 17–19.

Koegel, L.K., Koegel, R.L., & Ingham, J.C. (1986). Programming rapid generalization of correct articulation through self-monitoring procedures. *Journal of Speech and Hearing Disorders, 51*, 24–32.

Kolb, B. (1995). *Brain plasticity and behavior*. Mahwah, NJ: Lawrence Erlbaum.

Konkle, D.F., Beasley, D.S., & Bess, F.G. (1977). Intelligibility of time-altered speech in relation to chronological aging. *Journal of Speech and Hearing Research, 20*, 108–115.

Korber, C., Pfeiffer, R., Warr, B., & Kiang, N. (1966). Spontaneous spike discharges some single units in the cochlear nucleus after destruction of the cochlea. *Experimental Neurology, 16*, 199–130.

Kotsonis, M.E., & Patterson, C.J. (1980). Comprehension monitoring skills in learning disabled children. *Developmental Psychology, 16,* 541–542.

Kraus, N., Kileny, P., & McGee, T.J. (1994). Middle latency auditory evoked potentials. In J. Katz (Ed.), *Handbook of clinical audiology* (4th ed., pp. 387–405). Baltimore: Williams & Wilkins.

Kraus, N., & McGee, T.J. (1994). Mismatch negativity in the assessment of central auditory function. *American Journal of Audiology, 3*(2), 39–51.

Kraus, N., McGee, T.J., Carrell, T.D., Zecker, S.G., Nicol, T.G., & Koch, D.B. (1996). Auditory neurophysiologic responses and discrimination deficits in children with learning problems. *Science, 273*, 971–973.

Kraus, N., McGee, T.J., & Comperatore, C. (1989). MLR's in children are consistently present during wakefulness, Stage I and REM sleep. *Ear & Hearing, 10*, 339–345.

Kraus, N., McGee, T.J., Ferre, J., Hoeppner, J., Carrell, T., Sharma, A., & Nicol, T. (1993). Mismatch negativity in the neurophysiologic/behavioral evaluation of auditory processing deficits: A case study. *Ear & Hearing, 14*(4), 223–234.

Kraus, N., McGee, T., Micco, A., Sharma, A., Carrell, T., & Nicol, T. (1993). Mismatch negativity in school-age children to speech stimuli that are just perceptibly different. *Electroencephalography and Clinical Neurophysiology, 88*, 123–130.

Kraus, N., McGee, T.J., & Naatanen, R. (1992). *Attention and brain function.* Hillsdale, NJ: Lawrence Erlbaum.

Kraus, N., Ozdamar, O., Hier, D., & Stein, L. (1982). Auditory middle latency response in patients with cortical lesions. *Electroencephalography and Clinical Neurophysiology, 5*, 247–287.

Kraus, N., Smith, D., Reed, N. Stein, L., & Cartee, C. (1985). Auditory middle latency responses in children: Effects of age and diagnostic category. *Electroencephalography and Clinical Neurophysiology, 62*, 343–351.

Kreitler, S., & Kreitler, H. (1978). Plans and planning: Their motivational and cognitive antecedents. In S.L. Friedman, E.K. Scholnick, & R.R. Cocking (Eds.), *Blueprints for thinking* (pp. 110–178). New York: Cambridge University.

Kreutzer, M.A., Leonard, C., & Flavell, J.H. (1975). An interview study of children's knowledge about memory. *Monographs of the Society for Research in Child Development, 40*(Serial No. 159), 1–58.

Krueger, W.C.F. (1929). The effect of overlearning on retention. *Journal of Experimental Psychology, 12*, 71–78.

Kryter, K., & Ades, H. (1943). Studies on the function of the higher acoustic center in the cat. *American Journal of Psychology, 56*, 501–536.

Kudo, M. (1981). Projections of the nuclei of the lateral lemniscus in the cat. An autoradiograhic study. *Brain Research, 221*, 57–69.

Kurdziel, S., Noffsinger, D., & Olsen, W. (1976). Performance by cortical lesion patients on 40% and 60% time-compressed materials. *Journal of the American Audiological Society, 2*, 3–7.

Kutus, M., Hillyard, S., & Volpe, B. (1990). Late positive event-related potentials after commissural section in humans. *Journal of Cognitive and Neuroscience, 2*, 258–271.

Lackner, J.R. (1982). Alterations and resolution of temporal order after cerebral injury in man. *Experimental Neurology, 75*, 501–509.

Lackner, J.R., & Teuber, H.L. (1973). Alterations in auditory fusion thresholds after cerebral injury in man. *Neuropsychologia, 11*, 408–415.

Lahey, B., Schaughency, E., Hynd, G., Carlson, C., & Nieves, N. (1987). Attention deficit disorder with and without hyperactivity: Comparison of behavioral characteristics of clinic-referred children. *Journal of the American Academy of Child and Adolescent Psychiatry, 26*, 718–723.

Lambert, P.R. (1994). Inner ear hair cell regeneration in a mammal: Identification of a triggering factor. *Laryngoscope, 104*, 701–718.

Landgarten, H. (1987). The cancellation of repetitive noise and vibration by active methods. *Sound and Vibration, 21*, 6–10.

Lasky, E.Z., & Cox, L.C. (1983). Auditory processing and language interaction: Evaluation and intervention strategies. In E.Z. Lasky & J. Katz (Eds.), *Central auditory processing* (pp. 243–268). Baltimore: University Park Press.

Lasky, E.Z., & Tobin, H. (1973). Linguistic and nonlinguistic competing message effects. *Journal of Learning Disabilities, 6*, 243–250.

Lasky, E.Z., Weidner W.E., & Johnson, J.P. (1976). Influence of linguistic complexity, rate of presentation and interphrase pause time on auditory–verbal comprehension of adult aphasic patients. *Brain and Language, 3*, 386–395.

Lauter, J., Herscovitch, P., Formby, C., & Raichle, M. (1985). Tonotopic organization of human auditory cortex revealed by position emission tomography. *Hearing Research, 20*, 199–205.

Lawrence, A. (1970). *Architectural acoustics*. Amsterdam: Elsevier Publishing Company.

Lazzari, A.M., & Peters, P.M. (1994). *Handbook of exercises for language processing*. East Moline, IL: Linguisystems.

Leavitt, R. (1991). Group amplification systems for students with hearing impairment. *Seminars in Hearing, 12*, 380–387.

LeDoux, J., Sakaguchi, A., & Reis, D. (1983). Subcortical efferent projections of the medial geniculate nucleus mediate emotional responses conditioned to acoustic stimuli. *Journal of Neuroscience, 4*, 683–698.

Lee, L.W., & Humes, L.E. (1992). Factors associated with speech-recognition ability of the hearing-impaired elderly. *Asha, 34*(10), 212.

Lefebvre, P.P., Malgrange, B., Staecker, H., Moonen, G., & Van De Water, T.R. (1993). Retinoic acid stimulates regeneration of mammalian auditory hair cells. *Science, 260*, 692–695.

Lehiste, I., Olive, J., & Streeter, L. (1976). Role of duration in syntactic disambiguation. *Journal of the Acoustical Society of America, 60*, 1199–1202.

Lehiste, I., & Peterson, G.E. (1959). Linguistic considerations in the study of speech intelligibility. *Journal of the Acoustical Society of America, 31*(4), 280–286.

Lenhart, M., Shaia, F., & Abedi, E. (1985). Brainstem evoked responses waveform variation associated with recurrent otitis media. *Archives of Otolaryngology, 111*, 315–316.

Lenz, B.K. (1984). *The effect of advance organizers on the learning and retention of learning disabled adolescents within the context of a cooperative planning model*. Final research report submitted to the U.S. Department of Education, Special Education Services. Lawrence: University of Kansas.

Leonard, L., Sabbadini, L., Volterra, V., & Leonard, J.S. (1988). Some influences on the grammar of English- and Italian-speaking children with specific language impairment. *Applied Psycholinguistics, 9*, 39–57.

Levin, J.R. (1976). What have we learned about maximizing what children learn? In J.R. Levin & V.L. Allen (Eds.), *Cognitive learning in children* (pp. 105–134). New York: Academic Press.

Levine, R., Gardner, J., Stufflebeam, S., Fullterton, B., Carlisle, E., Furst, N., Rosen, B., & Kiang, M. (1993). Effects of multiple sclerosis brainstem lesions on sound lateralization and brainstem auditory evoked potentials. *Hearing Research, 68*, 73–88.

Lewis, D.E. (1994). Assistive devices for classroom listening: FM systems. *American Journal of Audiology, 3*, 70–83.

Lewis, D.E. (1995). Orientation to the use of frequency modulated systems. In R.S. Tyler & D.J. Schum (Eds.), *Assistive devices for persons with hearing impairment* (pp. 165–184). Boston: Allyn and Bacon.

Lewkowitz, N. (1980). Phonemic awareness training: What to teach and how to teach it. *Journal of Educational Psychology, 72*, 686–700.

Liberman, A.M. (1970). The grammars of speech and language. *Cognitive Psychology, 1*, 301–323.

Liberman, A.M., Cooper, F.S., Shankweiler, D., & Studdert-Kennedy, M. (1967). Perception of the speech code. *Psychological Review, 74*, 431–461.

Liberman, I., Shankweiler, D., Blachman, B., Camp, L., & Werfelman, M. (1980). Steps toward literacy. In P. Levinson, & C. Sloan (Eds.), *Auditory processing and language: Clinical and research perspectives* (pp. 189–215). New York: Grune & Stratton.

Licht, B., & Kistner, J.A. (1986). Motivational problems of learning-disabled children: Individual differences and their implications for treatment. In J.K. Torgesen & B.Y.L. Wong (Eds.), *Psychological and educational perspectives on learning disabilities* (pp. 225–255). San Diego: Academic Press.

Licht, B., Kistner, J., Ozkaragoz, T., Shapiro, S., & Clausen, L. (1985). Causal attributions of learning disabled children: Individual differences and their implications for persistence. *Journal of Educational Psychology, 77*, 208–216.

Liden, G., & Rosenthal, V. (1981). New developments in diagnostic auditory neurological problems. In M. Paparella & W. Meyerhoff (Eds.), *Sensorineural hearing loss* (pp. 273–294). Baltimore: Williams & Wilkins.

Lieske, M. (1994). Infrared systems. In M. Ross (Ed.), *Communication access for persons with hearing loss* (pp. 42–50). Baltimore: York Press.

Liles, B.Z. (1985). Cohesion in the narratives of normal and language disordered children. *Journal of Speech and Hearing Research, 28*, 123–133.

Liles, B.Z. (1987). Episode organization and cohesive conjunctions in narratives of children with and without language disorders. *Journal of Speech and Hearing Research, 30*, 185–196.

Lim, H.H., Jenkins, O.H., Myers, M.W., Miller, J.M., & Altschuler, R.A. (1993). Detection of HSP 72 synthesis after acoustic overstimulation in rat cochlea. *Hearing Research, 69*, 146–150.

Lincoln, A., Courchesne, E., Kilman, B., & Galambos, R. (1985). Neuropsychological correlates of information processing by children with Down's syndrome. *American Journal of Mental Deficiency, 89*, 403–414.

Lindamood, C., & Lindamood, P. (1971). *The Lindamood Auditory Test of Conceptualization* (LAC). Boston: Teaching Resources Corporation.

Lindamood, C., & Lindamood, P. (1975). *Auditory discrimination in depth* (rev. ed.). Austin, TX: Pro–Ed.

Lindgren, S.D., & Lyons, D.A. (1984). *Pediatric Assessment of Cognitive Efficiency* (PACE). Iowa City: University of Iowa, Department of Pediatrics.

Lloyd, J. (1980). Academic instruction and cognitive behavior modification: The need for attack strategy training. *Exceptional Education Quarterly, 1*, 53–64.

Lodico, M.G., Ghatala, E.S., Levin, J.R., Pressley, M., & Bell, J.A. (1983). The effects of strategy-monitoring training on children's selection of effective memory strategies. *Journal of Experimental Child Psychology, 35*, 263–277.

Loftus, G.F., & Loftus, E.F. (1976). *Human memory: The processing of information*. Hillsdale, NJ: Lawrence Erlbaum.

Loiselle, D., Stamm, J., Maitinsky, S., & Whipple, S. (1980). Evoked potential and behavioral signs of attention dysfunction in hyperactive boys. *Psychophysiology, 17*, 193–201.

Loose, F. (1984). *Learning disabled students use FM wireless systems.* Rochester, MN: Telex Communications.

Lou, H.C., Henriksen, L., & Bruhn, P. (1984). Focal cerebral hypoperfusion in children with dysphasia and/or attention deficit disorder. *Archives of Neurology, 41*, 825–829.

Lou, H.C., Henriksen, L., Bruhn, P., Borner, H., & Nielsen, J.B. (1989). Striatal dysfunction in attention deficit and hyperkinetic disorder. *Archives of Neurology, 46*, 48–52.

Lubert, N. (1981). Auditory perceptual impairment in children with specific language disorders. *Journal of Speech and Hearing Disorders, 46*, 3–9.

Lubinsky, J. (1986). Choosing aural rehabilitative directions: Suggestions from a model of information processing. *Journal of the Academy of Aural Rehabilitative Audiologists, 19*, 27–41.

Luce, P. (1986). *Neighborhoods of words in the mental lexicon* (Research on Speech Perception Technical Report No. 6). Bloomington, IN: Department of Psychology, Speech Research Laboratory, Indiana University.

Luce, P.A., Pisoni, D.B., & Goldinger, S.D. (1990). Similarity neighborhoods of words. In G. Altmann (Ed.), *Cognitive models of speech processing* (pp. 122–147). Cambridge, MA: MIT Press.

Ludlow, C. (1980). Impaired language development: Hypotheses for research. *Bulletin of the Orton Society, 130*, 153–169.

Ludlow, C., Cudahy, E., Bassich, C., & Brown, G. (1983). Auditory processing of hyperactive, language-impaired and reading disabled boys. In E. Lasky & J. Katz (Eds.), *Central auditory processing disorders* (pp. 163–184). Baltimore: University Park Press.

Lund, R. (1978). *Development and plasticity of the brain: An introduction.* New York: Oxford University Press.

Luterman, D.M. (1990). Audiological counseling and the diagnostic process. *American Speech-Language-Hearing Association, 32*(4), 35–37.

Lynn, G.E., Cullis, P., & Gilroy, J. (1983). Olivopontocerebellar degeneration: Effects of auditory brainstem responses. *Seminars in Hearing, 4*, 375–384.

Lynn, G.E., & Gilroy, J. (1977). Evaluation of central auditory dysfunction in patients with neurological disorders. In R.W. Keith (Ed.), *Central auditory dysfunction* (pp. 177–221). New York: Grune & Stratton.

Lynn, G.E., Gilroy, J., Taylor, P.C., & Leiser, R.P. (1981). Binaural masking level differences in neurological disorders. *Archives of Otolaryngology, 107*, 357–362.

Maag, J.W., & Reid, R. (1994). Attention-deficit hyperactivity disorder: A functional approach to assessment and treatment. *Behavioral Disorders, 20*, 5–23.

Maag, J.W., & Reid, R. (1996). Treatment of attention deficit hyperactivity disorder: A multi-modal model for schools. *Seminars in Speech and Language, 17*(1), 37–58.

Mandler, J.M. (1984). *Stories, scripts, and scenes: Aspects of schema theory.* Hillsdale, NJ: Lawrence Erlbaum.

Mann, C.A., Lubar, J.F., Zimmerman, A.W., Miller, C.A., & Muenchen, R.A. (1992). Quantitative analysis of EEG in boys with attention-deficit-hyperactivity disorder: Controlled study with clinical implications. *Pediatric Neurology, 8*, 30–36.

Mann, V. (1991). Language problems: A key to early reading problems. In B.Y.L. Wong (Ed.), *Learning about learning disabilities* (pp. 130–162). San Diego: Academic Press.

Manning, W., Johnson, K., & Beasley, D. (1977). The performance of children with auditory perceptual disorders on a time-compressed speech discrimination measure. *Journal of Speech and Hearing Disorders, 42*, 77–84.

Margulies, N. (1991). *Mapping inner space.* Tucson, AZ: Zephyr Press.

Markides, A. (1986). Speech levels and speech-to-noise ratios. *British Journal of Audiology, 20*, 115–120.

Marlowe, W. (1992). The impact of right prefrontal lesion on the developing brain. *Brain and Cognition, 20*, 205–213.

Marosi, E., Harmony, T., & Becker, J. (1990). Brainstem evoked potentials in learning-disabled children. *International Journal of Neuroscience, 50*, 233–342.

Marshall, L. (1981). Auditory processing in aging listeners. *Journal of Speech and Hearing Disorders, 46*, 226–240.

Marslen-Wilson, W.D. (1987). Functional parallelism in spoken word-recognition. *Cognition, 25*, 71–102.

Marslen-Wilson, W.D., & Tyler, L.K. (1980). The temporal structure of spoken language understanding. *Cognition, 8*, 1–71.

Marslen-Wilson, W.D., & Welsh, A. (1978). Processing interactions during word-recognition in continuous speech. *Cognitive Psychology, 10*, 29–63.

Martin, F., & Clark, J. (1977). Audiologic detection of auditory processing disorders in children. *Journal of the American Audiological Society, 3*, 140–146.

Mason, S., & Mellor, D. (1984). Brainstem, middle latency and late cortical potentials in children with speech and language disorders. *Electroencephalography and Clinical Neurophysiology, 59*, 297–309.

Massaro, D.W. (1975a). Language and information processing. In D.W. Massaro (Ed.), *Understanding language: An information-processing analysis of speech perception, reading, and psycholinguistics* (pp. 3–28). New York: Academic Press.

Massaro, D.W. (1975b). *Understanding language: An information-processing analysis of speech perception, reading, and psycholinguistics.* New York: Academic Press.

Massaro, D.W. (1976). Auditory information processing. In W.K.W. Estes (Ed.), *Handbook of learning and cognitive processes: Vol. 4: Attention and memory* (pp. 275–320). Hillsdale, NJ: Lawrence Erlbaum.

Massaro, D.W. (1987). *Speech perception by ear and eye: A paradigm for psychological inquiry.* Hillsdale, NJ: Lawrence Erlbaum.

Masterson, B., Thompson, G.C., Bechtold, J.K., & Robards, M.J. (1975). Neuroanatomical basis of binaural phase difference analysis for sound localization: A comparative study. *Journal of Comparative Physiology and Psychology, 89*, 379–386.

Masterton, R.B. (1992). Role of the central auditory system in hearing: The new direction. *Trends in Neuroscience, 15*, 280–285.

Matathias, O., Sohmer, H., & Biton, V. (1985). Central auditory tests and auditory nerve brainstem evoked respones in multiple sclerosis. *Acta Otolaryngology, 99*, 369–376.

Matkin, N., & Carhart, R. (1966). Auditory profiles associated with Rh incompatibility. *Archives of Otolaryngology, 84*, 502–513.

Matkin, N., & Hook, P. (1983). A multidisciplinary approach to central auditory evaluations. In E. Lasky & J. Katz (Eds.), *Central auditory processing disorders* (pp. 223–342). Baltimore: University Park Press.

Mattingly, I.G. (1972). Reading, the linguistic process, and linguistic awareness. In J.F. Kavanaugh & I.G. Mattingly (Eds.), *Language by ear and by eye: The relationship between speech and reading* (pp. 133–148). Cambridge: MIT Press.

Matzker, J. (1959). Two methods for the assessment of central auditory function in cases of brain disease. *Annals of Otology, Rhinology and Laryngology, 68*, 1155–1197.

Mavrogenes, N.A. (1983). Teaching implications of the schemata theory of comprehension. *Reading World, 22*, 295–305.

Maxon, A.B., & Hochberg, I. (1982). Development of psychoacoustic behavior: Sensitivity and discrimination. *Ear & Hearing, 3*(6), 301–308.

McClelland, J.L., & Elman, J.L. (1986). The TRACE model of speech perception. *Cognitive Psychology, 18*, 1–86.

McCroskey, F., & Devens, J. (1975, April). Acoustic characteristics of public school classrooms constructed between 1980 and 1960. *NOISEXPO Proceedings*, 101–103.

McCroskey, R., & Thompson, N. (1973). Comprehension of rate-controlled speech by children with learning problems. *Journal of Learning Disorders, 6*, 621–627.

McFarland, D.J., & Cacace, A.T. (1995). Modality specificity as a criterion for diagnosing central auditory processing disorders. *American Journal of Audiology, 4*(3), 36–48.

McIntyre, T. (1989). *A resource book for remediating common behaviors and learning Problems*. Boston: Allyn and Bacon.

McKenna, T., Ashe, J., Hui, G., & Weinberger, N. (1988). Muscarinic agonists modulate spontaneous and evoked unit discharge in auditory cortex of the cat. *Synapse, 2*, 54–68.

McKenzie, G.G., Neilson, A.R., & Braun, C. (1981). The effects of linguistic connectives and prior knowledge on comprehension of good and poor readers. In M. Kamil (Ed.), *Directions in reading: Research and instruction* (pp. 215–218). Washington, DC: National Reading Conference

McNeil, M.R. (1995, July). *The notion and importance of modularity.* Paper presented at the American Speech-Language-Hearing Association Workshop on Practical Approaches to Treating Central Auditory Processing Disorders, Snowbird, UT.

McNeil, M.R., & Prescott, T.E. (1978). *Revised Token Test.* Baltimore, MD: University Park Press.

McPherson, D. (1996). *Late potentials of the auditory system*. San Diego: Singular Publishing Group.

McReynolds, L.V. (1989). Generalization issues in the treatment of communication disorders. In L. V. McReynolds & J.E. Spradlin (Eds.), *Generalization strategies in the treatment of communication disorders* (pp. 1–12). Philadephia: B.C. Decker.

McShane, D. (1982). Otitis media and American Indians: Prevalence, etiology, psychoeducational consequences, prevention and intervention. In S.M. Manson (Ed.), *New directions in prevention among American Indian and Alaska Native communities* (pp. 265–295). Portland: Oregon Health Sciences University.

Medway, F.J., & Venino, G.R. (1982). The effects of effort feedback and performance patterns on children's attributions and task persistence. *Contemporary Educational Psychology, 7*, 26–34.

Medwetsky, L. (1994). Educational audiology. In J. Katz (Ed.), *Handbook of clinical audiology* (4th ed., pp. 503–520). Baltimore: Williams & Wilkins.

Mehler, J. (1981). The role of syllables in speech processing: Infants and adult data. *Philosophical Transactions of the Royal Society, B*(295), 333–352.

Meichenbaum, D. (1976). Cognitive factors as determinants of learning disabilities: A cognitive functional approach. In R. Knights & D. Bakker (Eds.), *The neuropsychology of learning disorders: Theoretical approaches* (pp. 423–442). Baltimore: University Park Press.

Meichenbaum, D. (1986). Cognitive-behavior management. In F.H. Kanfer & A.P. Goldstein (Eds.), *Helping people change: A textbook of methods* (3rd ed., pp. 346–380). New York: Pergamon Press.

Meichenbaum, D., & Goodman, J. (1971). Training impulsive children to talk to themselves: A means of developing self-control. *Journal of Abnormal Psychology, 77*, 115–126.

Merzenich, M., & Brugge, J. (1973). Representation of the cochlear partition on the superior temporal plane of the Macaque monkey. *Brain Research, 50*, 275–296.

Merzenich, M.M., Jenkins, W.M., Johnston, P., Schreiner, C., Miller, S.L., & Tallal, P. (1996). Temporal processing deficits of language-learning impaired children ameliorated by training. *Science, 271*, 77–80.

Merzenich, M.M., Nelson, R.J., Stryker, M.P., Cynader, M.S., Schoppmann, A., & Zook, J.M. (1984). Somatosensory cortical map changes following digit amputation in adult monkeys. *Journal of Comparative Neurology, 224*(4), 591–605.

Merzenich, M.M., & Reid, M.D. (1974). Representation of the cochlea within the inferior colliculus of the cat. *Brain Research, 77*, 397–415.

Meyer, D., & Woolsey, C. (1952). Effects of localized cortical destruction on auditory discriminative conditioning in the cat. *Journal of Neurophysiology, 15*, 149–162.

Meyers, S.C., Hughes, L.F., & Schoeny, Z.G. (1989). Temporal-phonemic processing skills in adult stutterers and nonstutterers. *Journal of Speech and Hearing Research, 32*, 274–280.

Miller, G.A. (1988). The challenge of universal literacy. *Science, 241*, 1293–1299.

Miller, G.A., & Gildea, P.M. (1987). How children learn words. *Scientific American, 257*, 94–99.
Miller, G.A., Heise, G., & Lichten, W. (1951). The intelligibility of speech as a function of the context of the test materials. *Journal of Experimental Psychology, 41*, 329–335.
Miller, G.A., & Licklider, J.C.R. (1950). The intelligibility of interrupted speech. *Journal of the Acoustical Society of America, 22*, 167–173.
Miller, G.A., & Nicely, P. (1955). An analysis of perceptual confusions among some English consonants. *Journal of the Acoustical Society of America, 27*, 338–352.
Miller, J.D. (1974). Effects of noise on people. *Journal of the Acoustical Society of America, 56*, 724–764.
Miller, R.L., Brickman, P., & Bolen, D. (1975). Attribution versus persuasion as a means for modifying behavior. *Journal of Personality and Social Psychology, 31*, 430–441.
Milner, B. (1962). Laterality effects in audition. In V.B. Mountcastle (Ed.), *Interhemispheric relations and cerebral dominance* (pp. 177–195). Baltimore: Johns Hopkins Press.
Milner, B., Kimura, D., & Taylor, L. B. (1965, April). *Nonverbal auditory learning after frontal or temporal lobectomy in man*. Paper presented at the annual meeting of the Eastern Psychological Association, Boston.
Milner, B., Taylor, S., & Sperry, R. (1968). Lateralized suppression of dichoticly presented digits after commissural section in man. *Science, 161,* 184–185.
Mishkin, M., & Appenzeller, T. (1987). The anatomy of memory. *Scientific American, 256,* 421–446.
Miyakita, T., Hellstrom, P.A., Frimanson, E., & Axelsson, A. (1992). Effect of low level acoustic stimulation on temporary threshold shift in young humans. *Hearing Research, 60*, 149–155.
Miyaska, E., Nakamura, A., Seiyama, A., Imai, A., & Takagi, T. (1994, September). A new approach to compensate degeneration of speech intelligibility for elderly: Development of a real-time speech rate conversion system. *Proceedings of the Second International Symposium on Speech and Hearing Sciences,* 1–8.
Mogdans, J., & Knudsen, E.I. (1992). Adaptive adjustment of unit tuning to sound localization cues in response to monaural occlusion in developing owl optic tectum. *Journal of Neuroscience, 12*(9), 3473–3484.
Mogdans, J., & Knudsen, E.I. (1993). Early monaural occlusion alters the neural map of interaural level differences in the inferior colliculus of the barn owl. *Brain Research, 619*, 29–38.
Mogdans, J., & Knudsen, E.I. (1994). Site of auditory plasticity in the brain stem (VLVp) of the owl revealed by early monaural occlusion. *Journal of Neurophysiology, 72*(6), 2875–2891.
Mohr, E., Cox, C., Williams, J., Chase, T.N., & Fedio, P. (1990). Impairment of central auditory function in Alzheimer's disease. *Journal of Clinical and Experimental Neuropsychology, 12*, 235–246.

Moller, A.R. (1983). *Auditory physiology*. New York: Academic Press.

Moller, A.R. (1985). Physiology of the ascending auditory pathway with special reference to the auditory brain stem response (ABR). In M.L. Pinheiro & F.E. Musiek (Eds.), *Assessment of central auditory dysfunction: Foundations and clinical correlates* (pp. 23–41). Baltimore: Williams & Wilkins.

Moller, H.J., Maurer, I., & Saletu, B. (1994). Placebo controlled trial of the xanthine derivative propentofylline in dementia. *Psychopharmacology, 101*(2), 147–159.

Moller, M., & Moller, A. (1985). Auditory brain stem evoked responses (ABR) in diagnosis of eighth nerve and brain stem lesions. In M.L. Pinheiro & F.E. Musiek (Eds.), *Assessment of central auditory dysfunction: Foundations and clinical correlates* (pp. 43–65). Baltimore: Williams & Wilkins.

Moore, B.C.J. (1973). Frequency difference limens for short-duration tones. *Journal of the Acoustical Society of America, 54*, 610–619.

Moore, C., Cranford, J., & Rahn, A. (1990). Tracking a "moving" fused auditory image under conditions that elicit the precedence effect. *Journal of Speech and Hearing Research, 33*, 141–148.

Moore, D.R. (1983). Development of the inferior colliculus and binaural audition. In R. Romand (Ed.), *Development of auditory and vestibular system* (pp. 121–159). New York: Academic Press.

Moore, D.R. (1993). Plasticity of binaural hearing and some possible mechanisms following late-onset deprivation. *Journal of the American Academy of Audiology, 4*(5), 227–283.

Moore, D.R., Hutchings, M.E., & Meyer, S.E. (1991). Binaural masking level differences in children with a history of otitis media. *Audiology, 30,* 91–101.

Moore, J.K. (1987). The human auditory brainstem: A comparative view. *Hearing Research, 29*, 1–32.

Morales-Garcia, C., & Poole, J.O. (1972). Masked speech audiometry in central deafness. *Acta Otolaryngologica, 74*, 307–316.

Morest, D.K. (1964). The neuronal architecture of medial geniculate body of the cat. *Journal of Anatomy, 98*, 611–630.

Morest, K. (1983). Degeneration in the brain following exposure to noise. In R.P. Hamernik, D. Henderson, & R.J. Salvi (Eds.), *New perspectives on noise-induced hearing loss* (pp. 87–94). New York: Raven Press.

Morton, J. (1969). Interaction of information in word recognition. *Psychological Review, 76*(2), 165–178.

Mountcastle, V. (1962). *Interhemispheric relations and cerebral dominance.* Baltimore: Johns Hopkins Press.

Mountcastle, V. (1968). Central neural mechanisms in hearing. In V. Mountcastle (Ed.), *Medical physiology* (Vol. 2, pp. 1296–1355). St. Louis: C.V. Mosby.

Moynahan, E.D. (1978). Assessment and selection of paired associate strategies: A developmental study. *Journal of Experimental Child Psychology, 26*, 257–266.

Mueller, H., Beck, W., & Sedge, R. (1987). Comparison of efficiency of cortical level speech tests. *Seminars in Hearing, 8*, 279–298.

Mueller, H.G., & Killion, M.C. (1990). An easy method for calculating the articulation index. *The Hearing Journal, 43*(9), 1–4.

Murdock, J.Y., Garcia, E.E., & Hardman, M.L. (1977). Generalizing articulation training with trainable mentally retarded subjects. *Journal of Applied Behavior Analysis, 10*, 717–733.

Musiek, F.E. (1983a). Assessment of central auditory dysfunction: The Dichotic Digit Test revisited. *Ear and Hearing, 4*, 79–83.

Musiek, F.E. (1983b). The evaluation of brainstem disorders using ABR and central auditory test. *Monographs in Contemporary Audiology, 4*, 1–24.

Musiek, F.E. (1985). Application of central auditory tests: An overview. In J. Katz (Ed.), *Handbook of clinical audiology* (3rd ed., pp. 321–336). Baltimore: Williams & Wilkins.

Musiek, F.E. (1986a). Neuroanatomy, neurophysiology and central auditory assessment. Part II: The cerebrum. *Ear & Hearing, 7*, 283–294.

Musiek, F.E. (1986b). Neuroanatomy, neurophysiology, and central auditory assessment: Part III: Corpus callosum and efferent pathways. *Ear & Hearing, 7*(6), 349–358.

Musiek, F.E. (1991). Auditory evoked respones in site of lesion assessment. In W. Rintelmann (Ed.) *Hearing assessment* (pp. 383–428). Boston: Allyn & Bacon.

Musiek, F.E. (1992). Otoacoustic emissions and the olivocochlear bundle. *The Hearing Journal, 45*, 12–15.

Musiek, F.E. (1994). Frequency (pitch) and duration pattern tests. *Journal of the American Academy of Audiology, 5*, 265–268.

Musiek, F.E., & Baran, J.A. (1984). Neuroaudiological results from split-brain patients. *Seminars in Hearing, 5*, 219–229.

Musiek, F.E., & Baran, J.A. (1986). Neuroanatomy, neurophysiology, and central auditory assessment. Part 1: Brain stem. *Ear and Hearing, 7*, 207–219.

Musiek, F.E., & Baran, J.A. (1987). Central auditory assessment: Thirty years of change and challenge. *Ear and Hearing, 8*(Suppl.), 22–35.

Musiek, F.E., & Baran, J.A. (1991). Assessment of the human auditory system. In R. Altschuler, R. Bobbin, B. Clopton, & D. Hoffman (Eds.), *Neurobiology of hearing: The central auditory system* (pp. 411–438). New York: Raven Press.

Musiek, F.E., & Baran, J.A. (1996). Amplification and the central auditory nervous system. In M. Valente (Ed.), *Hearing aids: Standards, options and limitations* (pp. 407–437). New York: Thieme.

Musiek, F., & Baran, J.A. (1997). Central auditory assessment: Thirty years of change and challenge. *Ear and Hearing, 8*(Suppl.), 22–35.

Musiek, F.E., Baran, J.A., & Pinheiro, M.L. (1990). Duration pattern recognition in normal subjects and patients with cerebral and cochlear lesions. *Audiology, 29*, 304–313.

Musiek, F.E., Baran, J.A., & Pinheiro, M.L. (1992). P300 results in patients with lesions of the auditory areas of the cerebrum. *Journal of the American Academy of Audiology, 3*, 5–15.

Musiek, F.E., Baran, J.A., & Pinheiro, M.L. (1994). *Neuroaudiology case studies*. San Diego: Singular Publishing Group.

Musiek, F.E., Bornstein, S., & Rintelmann, W. (1995). Transient evoked otoacoustic emissions and pseudohypacusis. *Journal of the American Academy of Audiology, 6*, 293–301.

Musiek, F.E., & Chermak, G.D. (1994). Three commonly asked questions about central auditory processing disorders: Assessment. *American Journal of Audiology: A Journal of Clinical Practice, 3*(3), 23–27.

Musiek, F.E., & Chermak, G.D. (1995). Three commonly asked questions about central auditory processing disorders: Management. *American Journal of Audiology, 4*(1), 15–18.

Musiek, F.E., & Geurkink, N.A. (1980). Auditory perceptual problems in children: Considerations for the otolaryngologist and audiologist. *Laryngoscope, 90*, 962–971.

Musiek, F.E., & Geurkink, N.A. (1981). Auditory brainstem and middle latency evoked response sensitivity near threshold. *Annals of Otology, Rhinology, and Laryngology, 90*, 236–240.

Musiek, F.E., & Geurkink, N. (1982). Auditory brain stem response and central auditory test findings for patients with brain stem lesions. *Laryngoscope, 92*, 891–900.

Musiek, F.E., Geurkink, N.A., & Keitel, S. (1982). Test battery assessment of auditory perceptual dysfunction in children. *Laryngoscope, 92*, 251–257.

Musiek, F.E., Geurkink, N.A., Weider, D., & Donnelly, K. (1984). Past, present and future applications of the auditory middle latency response. *Laryngoscope, 94*, 1545–1552.

Musiek, F.E., & Gollegly, K.M. (1985). ABR in eighth nerve and low brain stem lesions. In J.T. Jacobson (Ed.), *The auditory brain stem response* (pp. 181–202). San Diego: College-Hill Press.

Musiek, F.E., & Gollegly, K. (1988). Maturational considerations in the neuroauditory evaluation of children. In F. Bess (Ed.), *Hearing impairment in children* (pp. 231–252). Parkton, MD: York Press.

Musiek, F.E., Gollegly, K., & Baran, J. (1984). Myelination of the corpus callosum and auditory processing problems in children: Theoretical and clinical correlates. *Seminars in Hearing, 5*, 231–242.

Musiek, F.E., Gollegly, K., Kibbe, K., & Reeves, A. (1989). Electrophysiologic and behavioral auditory findings in multiple sclerosis. *American Journal of Otology, 10*, 343–350.

Musiek, F.E., Gollegly, K., Kibbe, K., & Verkest, S. (1988). Current concepts on the use of ABR and auditory psychophysical tests in the evaluation of brain stem lesions. *American Journal of Otology, 9*(Suppl.), 25–35.

Musiek, F.E., Gollegly, K., Kibbe, K., & Verkest-Lenz, S. (1991). Proposed screening tests for central auditory disorders: Follow-up on the Dichotic Digits Test. *American Journal of Otology, 12*, 109–113.

Musiek, F.E., Gollegly, K., Lamb, L., & Lamb, P. (1990). Selected issues in screening for central auditory processing of dysfunction. *Seminars in Hearing, 11*, 372–384.

Musiek, F.E, Gollegly, K., & Ross, M. (1985). Profiles of types of central auditory processing disorder in children with learning disabilities. *Journal of Childhood Communication Disorders, 9*, 43–63.

Musiek, F.E., & Hoffman, D.W. (1990). An introduction to the functional neurochemistry of the auditory system. *Ear and Hearing, 11*(6), 395–402.

Musiek, F.E., Josey, A., & Glasscock, M. (1986). Auditory brainstem response interwave measurements in acoustic neuromas. *Ear & Hearing, 7,* 100–105.

Musiek, F.E., Kibbe, K., & Baran, J.A. (1984). Neuroaudiological results from split-brain patients. *Seminars in Hearing, 5*, 219–230.

Musiek, F.E., Kibbe, K., Rackliffe, L., & Weider, D. (1984). The auditory brainstem response I–V amplitude ratio in normal, cochlear and retrocochlear ears. *Ear & Hearing, 5*, 52–55.

Musiek, F.E., & Kibbe-Michael, K. (1986). The ABR wave IV–V abnormalities from the ear opposite large CPE tumors. *American Journal of Otolaryngology, 7*, 253–257.

Musiek, F.E, Kibbe-Michael, K., Geurkink, N., Josey, A., & Glasscock, M. (1986). ABR results in patients with posterior fossa tumors and normal pure tone hearing. *Otolaryngology—Head and Neck Surgery, 94*, 568–573.

Musiek, F.E., & Lee, W. (1995). Auditory brainstem response in patients with cochlear pathology. *Ear & Hearing, 16*, 631–636.

Musiek, F.E., & Lee, W. (in press). Conventional and maximum length sequences middle latency response in patients with central nervous system lesions. *Journal of the American Academy of Audiology.*

Musiek, F.E., Lenz, S., & Gollegly, K.M. (1991). Neuroaudiologic correlates to anatomical changes of the brain. *American Journal of Audiology, 1*(1), 19–24.

Musiek, F.E., McCormick, C., & Hurley, R. (1996). Hit and false alarm rates of selected ABR indices in differentiating cochlear disorders from acoustic tumors. *American Journal of Audiology, 5*, 90–96.

Musiek, F.E., & Pinheiro, M.L. (1985). Dichotic speech tests in the detection of central auditory dysfunction. In M.L. Pinheiro & F.E. Musiek (Eds.), *Assessment of central auditory dysfunction: Foundations and clinical correlates* (pp. 201–217). Baltimore: Williams & Wilkins.

Musiek, F.E., & Pinheiro, M. L. (1987). Frequency patterns in cochlear, brainstem, and cerebral lesions. *Audiology, 26*, 79–88.

Musiek, F.E., Pinheiro, M.L., & Wilson, D. (1980). Auditory pattern perception in split-brain patients. *Archives of Otolaryngology, 106*, 610–612.

Musiek, F.E., & Reeves, A.G. (1990). Asymmetries of the auditory areas of the cerebrum. *Journal of the American Academy of Audiology, 1*, 240–245.

Musiek, F.E., Verkest, S.B., & Gollegly, K.M. (1988). Effects of neuromaturation on auditory-evoked potentials. In D.W. Worthington (Ed.), *Seminars in hearing* (Vol. 9, pp. 1–14). New York: Thieme Medical Publishers.

Musiek, F., Weider, D., & Mueller, R. (1982). Audiological findings in Charcot-Marie-Tooth disease. *Archives of Otolaryngology, 108*, 595–599.

Naatanen, R. (1992). *Attention and brain function.* Hillsdale, NJ: Lawrence Erlbaum.

Nabelek, A.K., & Donahue, A.M. (1986). Comparison of amplification systems in an auditorium. *Journal of the Acoustical Society of America, 79*, 2078–2082.

Nabelek, A.K., & Nabelek, I.V. (1994). Room acoustics and speech perception. In J. Katz (Ed.), *Handbook of clinical audiology* (4th ed., pp. 624–637). Baltimore: Williams & Wilkins.

Nabelek, A.K., & Pickett, J. (1974a). Monaural and binaural speech perception through hearing aids under noise and reverberation with normal and hearing-impaired listeners. *Journal of Speech and Hearing Research, 17*, 724–739.

Nabelek, A.K., & Pickett, J. (1974b). Reception of consonants in a classroom as affected by monaural and binaural listening, noise, reverberation, and hearing aids. *Journal of the Acoustical Society of America, 56*, 628–639.

Nabelek, A.K., & Robinson, P.K. (1982a). Monaural and binaural speech perception in reverberation with normal and hearing-impaired listeners. *Journal of Speech and Hearing Research, 17*, 724–739.

Nabelek, A.K., & Robinson, P.K. (1982b). Monaural and binaural speech perception through hearing aids under noise and reverberation with normal and hearing-impaired listeners. *Journal of Speech and Hearing Research, 17*, 724–739.

National Joint Committee on Learning Disabilities. (1991). Learning disabilities: Issues on definition. *Asha, 33*(Suppl. 5), 18–20.

Neely, J.G., Thompson, A.M., & Gower, D.J. (1991). Detection and localization of heat shock protein 70 in the normal guinea pig cochlea. *Hearing Research, 52*, 403–406.

Neff, W. (1961). Neuromechanisms of auditory discrimination. In W. Rosenblith (Ed.), *Sensory communication* (pp. 259–278). New York: John Wiley and Sons.

Neisser, U. (1967). *Cognitive psychology*. New York: Appleton, Century, Crofts.

Neisser, U. (1976). *Cognition and reality.* San Francisco: W.H. Freeman.

Nejime, Y., Arisuka, T., Imamura, T., Ifukube, T., & Matsushima, J. (1996). A portable digital speech-rate converter for hearing impairment. *Transactions on Rehabilitation Engineering, 2*, 73–83.

Nellum-Davis, P. (1993). Clinical practice issues. In D.E. Battle (Ed.), *Communication disorders in multicultural populations* (pp. 306–316). Boston: Andover Medical Publishers.

Neuman, A., & Hochberg, I. (1983). Children's perception of speech in reverberation. *Journal of the Acoustical Society of America, 73*(6), 2145–2149.

Neuss, D., Blair, J., & Viehweg, S. (1991). Sound field amplification: Does it improve word recognition in a background of noise for students with minimal hearing impairments. *Educational Audiology Monograph, 2*, 43–52.

Newhoff, M., Cohen, M.J., Hynd, G.W., Gonzalez, J.J., & Riccio, C.A. (1992, November). *Etiological, educational and behavioral correlates of ADHD and language disabilities*. Presented at the annual convention of the American Speech-Language-Hearing Assocation, San Antonio, TX.

Niccum, N. , Rubens, A., & Speaks, C. (1981). Effects of stimulus material on the dichotic listening performance of aphasic patients. *Journal of Speech and Hearing Research, 24*, 526–534.

Nicholas, M., Obler, L., Albert, M., & Goodglass, H. (1985). Lexical retrieval in healthy aging. *Cortex, 21*, 595–606.

Nicholson, C.D. (1990). Pharmacology of nootropics and metabolically active comounds in relation to their use in dementia. *Pyschopharmacology, 101*(2), 147–159.

Nickerson, R.S. (1986). *Reflections on reasoning*. Hillsdale, NJ: Lawrence Erlbaum.

Nieder, P.C., & Nieder, I. (1970). Antimasking effect of crossed olivocochlear bundle stimulation with loud clicks in guinea pigs. *Experimental Neurology, 28*, 179–188.

Ninio, A. (1980). Picture-book reading in mother-infant dyads belonging to two sub-groups in Israel. *Child Development, 51*, 587–590.

Nippold, M.A. (1988). The literate lexicon. In M. Nippold (Ed.), *Later language development* (pp. 29–47). Boston: College-Hill Press.

Nippold, M.A. (1991). Evaluating and enhancing idiom comprehension in language-disordered students. *Language, Speech, and Hearing Services in Schools, 22*, 100–106.

Nippold, M.A., & Fey, S.H. (1983). Metaphoric understanding in preadolescents having history of language acquisition difficulties. *Language, Speech, and Hearing Services in Schools, 14*, 171–180.

Nittrouer, S. (1996). Discriminability and perceptual weighting of some acoustic cues to speech perception by 3-year olds. *Journal of Speech and Hearing Research, 39*, 278–297.

Nittrouer, S., & Boothroyd, A. (1990). Context effects in phoneme and word recognition by young children and older adults. *Journal of the Acoustical Society of America, 87*(6), 2705–2715.

Noback, C.R. (1985). Neuroanatomical correlates of central auditory function. In M.L. Pinheiro & F.E. Musiek (Eds.), *Assessment of central auditory dysfunction: Foundations and clinical correlates* (pp. 7–21). Baltimore: Williams & Wilkins.

Nober, L., & Nober, E. (1975). Auditory discrimination of learning disabled children in quiet and classroom noise. *Journal of Learning Disabilities, 8*, 656–677.

Nodar, R., & Kinney, S. (1980). The contralateral effects of large tumors on brain stem auditory evoked potentials. *Laryngoscope, 90*, 1762–1768.

Noffsinger, D., Olsen, W.O., Carhart, R., Hart, C.W., & Sahgal, V. (1972). Auditory and vestibular aberrations in multiple sclerosis. *Acta Otolaryngologica, 303*(Suppl.), 1–63.

Norris, J.A., & Damico, J.S. (1990). Whole language in theory and practice: Implications for language intervention. *Language, Speech, and Hearing Services in Schools, 21*(4), 212–220.

Nozza, R., Wagner, E., & Crandall, M. (1988). Binaural release for masking for speech sounds in infants, preschoolers and adults. *Journal of Speech and Hearing Research, 31*, 212–218.

Nuru, N. (1993). Multicultural aspects of deafness. In D.E. Battle (Ed.), *Communication disorders in multicultural populations* (pp. 287–308). Boston: Andover Medical Publishers.

Obert, A., & Cranford, J. (1990). Effects of neocortical lesions on the P300 component of the auditory evoked resonse. *American Journal of Otology, 11*, 447–453.

Obrzut, J.E., & Hynd, G.W. (Eds.). (1991). *Neuropsychological foundations of learning disabilities*. San Diego: Academic Press.

Oh, S., Kuba, T., Soyer, A., Choi, I., Bonikowski, F., & Viter, J. (1981). Lateralization of brain stem lesions by brain stem auditory evoked potentials. *Neurology, 31*, 14–18.

Oliver, D.L., & Morest, D.K. (1984). The central nucleus of the inferior colliculus in the cat. *Journal of Comparative Neurology, 222*, 237–264.

Oliver, D.L., Potashner, S., Jones, D., & Morest, D. (1983). Selective labeling of spiroganglion and granule cells with D-asparatate in the auditory system of the cat and guinea pig. *Journal of Neuroscience, 3*, 455–472.

Olsen, W. (1977, November). *Performance of temporal lobectomy patients with dichotic CV test materials*. Presented at the Annual Convention of the American Speech-Language-Hearing Association, Chicago, IL.

Olsen, W., & Kurdziel, S. (1978, November). *Berlin and Katz SSW test results for temporal lobe lesion patients*. Presented at the Annual Convention of the American Speech-Language-Hearing Association, San Francisco, CA.

Olsen, W.O., Noffsinger, D., & Carhart, R. (1976). Masking level differences encountered in clinical populations. *Audiology, 15*, 287–301.

Olsen, W.O., Noffsinger, D., & Kurdziel, S. (1975). Speech discrimination in quiet and in white noise by patients with peripheral and central lesions. *Acta Otolaryngologica, 80*, 375–382.

Olswang, L. (1990). Treatment efficacy research: A path to quality assurance. *Asha, 32*(1), 45–47.

Olswang, L.B., & Bain, B. (1994). Data collection: Monitoring children's treatment progress. *American Journal of Speech-Language Pathology, 3*(3), 55–66.

Osterhamel, P., Shallop, J., & Terkildsen, K. (1985). The effects of sleep on auditory brainstem response (ABR) and the middle latency response (MLR). *Scandinavian Audiology, 14*, 47–50.

Otterson, O., & Storm-Mathison, J. (1984). Glutamate- and GABA-containing neurons in the mouse and rat brain, as demonstrated with a new immunoytochemical technique. *Journal of Comparative Neurology, 229*, 374–392.

Owen, E. (1961). Intelligibility of words varying in familiarity. *Journal of Speech and Hearing Research, 4*(2), 113–129.

Palincsar, A.S., & Brown, A.L. (1984). Reciprocal teaching of comprehension fostering and comprehension monitoring activities. *Cognition and Instruction, 1*, 117–175.

Palincsar, A.S., & Brown, A.L. (1986). Interactive teaching to promote independent learning from text. *Reading Teacher, 39*, 771–771.

Palincsar, A.S., & Brown, A.L. (1987) Enhancing instructional time through attention to metacognition. *Journal of Learning Disabilities, 20*, 66–75.

Palincsar, A.S., Brown, A.L., & Campione, J.C. (1994). Models and practices of dynamic assessment. In G.P. Wallach & K.G. Butler (Eds.), *Language learning disabilities in school-age children and adolescents* (pp. 132–144). New York: Charles E. Merrill.

Pandya, D., & Seltzer, B. (1986). The topography of commissural fibers. In F. Lepore, M. Pitito, & H. Jasper (Eds.), *Two hemispheres in one brain: Functions of the corpus callosum* (pp. 47–74). New York: Alan R. Liss.

Paris, S.G., & Myers, M. (1981). Comprehension monitoring, memory, and study strategies of good and poor readers. *Journal of Reading Behavior, 13*, 5–22.

Paris, S.G., Newman, R.S., & McVey, K.A. (1982). Learning the functional significance of mnemonic actions: A microgenetic study of strategy acquisition. *Journal of Experimental Child Psychology, 34*, 490–509.

Paris, S.G., Wixson, K.K., & Palincsar, A.S. (1986). Instructional approaches to reading comprehension. In E.Z. Rothkopf (Ed.), *Review of research on education* (Vol. 13, pp. 91–218). Washington, DC: American Educational Research Association.

Parkinson, F.E., Rudolphi, K.A., & Fredholm, B.B. (1994). Propentofylline: A nucleoside transport inhibitor with neuroprotective effects in cerebral ischemia. *General Pharmacology, 25*(6), 1053–1058.

Pascual-Leone, A., Grafman, J., & Hallett, M. (1994). Modulation of cortical motor output maps during development of implicit and explicit knowledge. *Science, 263*, 1287–1292.

Patterson, R.D., Nimmo-Smith, I., Weber, D.L., & Milroy, R. (1982). The deterioration of hearing with age: Frequency selectivity, the critical ratio, the audiogram and speech threshold. *Journal of the Acoustical Society of America, 72*(6), 1788–1804.

Payne, K.T. (1986). Cultural and linguistic groups in the United States. In O.L. Taylor (Ed.), *Nature of communication disorders in culturally and linguistically diverse populations* (pp. 19–46). San Diego: College-Hill Press.

Pearl, R.A. (1982). LD children's attributions for success and failure: A replication with a labeled LD sample. *Learning Disability Quarterly, 5,* 173–176.

Pearson, P.D. (1982). *Asking questions about stories*. Ginn Occasional Papers. (No. 15). Columbus, OH: Ginn.

Pearson, P.D., & Fielding, L. (1982). Research update: Listening comprehension. *Language Arts, 59*(9), 617–629.

Pedersen, P.B., & Ivey, A. (1993). *Culture-centered counseling and interview skills*. Westport, CT: Praeger.

Penfield, W., & Perot, P. (1963). The brain's record of auditory and visual experience: A final summary and discussion. *Brain, 86*, 596–695.

Penfield, W., & Rasmussen, T. (1950). *The cerebral cortex of man.* New York: Macmillan.

Penfield, W., & Roberts, L. (1959). *Speech and brain mechanisms*. Princeton, NJ: Princeton University Press.

Pengilly, L. (1992). *Normative studies on the Auditory Duration Patterns Test.* Unpublished master's thesis. University of New Mexico, Albuquerque.

Penner, M.J. (1976). The effect of marker variability on the discrimination of temporal intervals. *Perception and Psychophysics, 19*, 466–469.

Pennington, B.F. (1991). *Diagnosing learning disorders: A neuropsychological framework.* New York: Guilford.

Pennington, B.F., Bennetto, L., McAleer, O., & Roberts, R.J. (1996). Executive functions and working memory: Theoretical and measurement issues. In G.R. Lyon & N.A. Krasnegor (Eds.), *Attention, memory, and executive function* (pp. 327–348). Baltimore: Paul H. Brookes.

Perfetti, C.A. (1985). *Reading ability.* New York: Oxford University Press.

Perfetti, C.A., & McCutchen, D. (1982). Speech processes in reading. *Speech and Language Advances in Basic Research and Practice, 7*, 237–269.

Peronnet, F., & Mickel, F. (1977). The asymmetry of auditory evoked potentials in normal man and patients with brain lesions. In J. Desmedt (Ed.), *Auditory evoked potentials in man: Psychopharmacology correlates of EPs* (pp. 130–141). Basel, Switzerland: Karger.

Pfeiffer, R.R. (1966). Classification of response patterns of spike discharges for units in the cochlear nucleus. Tone burst stimulation. *Experimental Brain Research, 1*, 220–235.

Pfingst, B., & O'Conner, T. (1981). Characteristics of neurons in auditory cortex of monkeys performing a simple auditory task. *Journal of Neurophysiology, 45*, 16–34.

Phillips, D. (1990). Neural representation of sound amplitude in the auditory cortex: Effects of noise masking. *Behavioral Brain Research, 37*, 197–214.

Phillips, D.P. (1993). Representation of acoustic events in the primary auditory cortex. *Journal of Experimental Psychology: Human Perception and Performance, 19*, 203–216.

Phillips, D.P. (1995). Central auditory processing: A view from auditory neuroscience. *The American Journal of Otology, 16*(3), 338–352.

Phillips, D., & Irvine, D. (1981). Responses of single neurons in physiologically defined area AI of cat cerebral cortex: Sensitivity to interaural intensity differences. *Hearing Research, 4*(9), 299–307.

Pichney, M.A., Durlach, N.I., & Braida, L.D. (1985). Speaking clearly for the hard of hearing. I: Intelligibility differences between clear and conversational speech. *Journal of Speech and Hearing Research, 28*, 96–103.

Pichney, M.A., Durlach, N.I., & Braida, L.D. (1986). Speaking clearly for the hard of hearing. II: Acoustic characteristics of clear and conversational speech. *Journal of Speech and Hearing Research, 29*, 434–446.

Pichora-Fuller, M.K., & Schneider, B.A. (1991). Masking-level differences in the elderly: A comparison of antiphasic and time-delay dichotic conditions. *Journal of Speech and Hearing Research, 34*, 1410–1422.

Pickett, L.M., & Pollack, I. (1963). Intelligibility of excerpts from fluent speech: Effects of rate of utterance and duration of excerpt. *Language and Speech, 6*, 151–165.

Pickles, J. (1985). Physiology of the cerebral auditory system. In M. Pinheiro, & F. Musiek (Eds.), *Assessment of central auditory dysfunction: Foundations and clinical correlates* (pp. 67–85). Baltimore: Williams & Wilkins.

Pickles, J. (1988). *An introduction to the physiology of hearing* (2nd ed.). New York: Academic Press.

Pickles, J.O., & Comis, S.D. (1973). Role of centrifugal pathways to cochlear nucleus in detection of signals in noise. *Journal of Neurophysiology, 36*(6), 1131–1137.

Pillsbury, H.C., Grose, J.H., & Hall, J.W. (1991). Otitis media with effusion in children: Binaural hearing before and after corrective surgery. *Archives of Otolaryngology—Head and Neck Surgery, 117*, 718–723.

Pillsbury, H.C., Grose, J.H., Coleman, W.L., Conners, C.K., & Hall, J.W. (1995). Binaural function in children with attention-deficit hyperactivity disorder. *Archives of Otolaryngology—Head and Neck Surgery, 121*, 1345–1350.

Pinheiro, M. (1977). Tests of central auditory function in children with learning disabilities. In R. Keith (Ed.), *Central auditory dysfunction* (pp. 223–256). New York: Grune & Stratton.

Pinheiro, M.L., & Musiek, F.E. (1985). Sequencing and temporal ordering in the auditory system. In M.L. Pinheiro & F.E. Musiek (Eds.), *Assessment of central auditory dysfunction: Foundations and clinical correlates* (pp. 219–238). Baltimore: Williams & Wilkins.

Pinheiro, M.L., & Musiek, F. (1985). *Assessment of central auditory dysfunction: Foundations and clinical correlates.* Baltimore: Williams & Wilkins.

Pinheiro, M.L., & Ptacek, P.H. (1971) Reversals in the perception of noise and pure tones. *Journal of the Acoustical Society of America, 49*, 1778–1782.

Pinheiro, M., & Tobin, H. (1969). Interaural intensity differences for intracranial lateralization. *Journal of the Acoustical Society of America, 46,* 1482–1487.

Pisoni, D.B. (1984). Acoustic-phonetic representations in word recognition. *Research on Speech Perception* (pp. 129–152). [Progress Report.] Bloomington: Department of Psychology, Indiana University.

Pisoni, D.B., & Luce, P.A. (1987). Acoustic-phonetic representations in word recognition. *Cognition, 25*, 21–52.

Polich, J. (1987). Task difficulty, probability and interstimulus interval as determinants of P300 from auditory stimuli. *Electroencephalography and Clinical Neurophysiology, 68*, 311–320.

Polich, J. (1989). Frequency, intensity and duration as determinants of P300 from auditory stimuli. *Journal of Electroencephalography and Clinical and Neurophysiology, 6*, 277–286.

Polich, J., Howard, L., & Starr, A. (1985). Aging effects on the P300 component of the event-related potential from auditory stimuli: Peak definition, variation and measurement. *Journal of Gerontology, 40*, 721–726.

Pollack, I., Rubenstein, H., & Decker, L. (1959). Intelligibility of known and unknown message sets. *The Journal of the Acoustical Society of America, 31*(3), 273–279.

Pons, T.P., Garraghty, P.E., Ommaya, A.K., Kaas, J.H., Taub, E., & Mishkin, M. (1991). Massive cortical reorganization after sensory deafferentation in adult macaques. *Science, 252*, 1857–1860.

Poplin, M.S. (1988a). Holistic/constructivist principles of the teaching/learning process: Implications for the field of learning disabilities. *Journal of Learning Disabilities, 21*, 401–416.

Poplin, M.S. (1988b). The reductionist fallacy in learning disabilities: Replicating the past by reducing the present. *Journal of Learning Disabilities, 21*, 389–400.

Portman, M., Sterkers, J., Charachon, R., & Chouard, C. (1975). *The internal auditory meatus: Anatomy, pathology, and surgery*. New York: Churchill Livingstone.

Pressley, M. (1982). Elaboration and memory development. *Child Development, 53*, 296–309.

Pressley, M., Borkowski, J.G., & O'Sullivan, J.T. (1984). Memory strategy instruction is made of this: Metamemory and durable strategy use. *Educational Psychologist, 19*, 94–107.

Pressley, M., Johnson, C.J., & Symons, S. (1987). Elaborating to learn and learning to elaborate. *Journal of Learning Disabilities, 20*, 76–91.

Pressley, M., & Levin, J.R. (1987). Elaborative learning strategies for the inefficient learner. In S.J. Ceci (Ed.), *Handbook of cognitive, social and neuropsychological aspects of learning disabilities* (Vol. 2, pp. 175–212). Hillsdale, NJ: Lawrence Erlbaum.

Preves, D.A. (1994). Future trends in hearing aid technology. In M. Valente (Ed.), *Strategies for selecting and verifying hearing aid fittings* (pp. 363–396). New York: Thieme Medical Publishers.

Prior, M., & Sanson, A. (1986). Attention deficit disorder with hyperactivity: A critique. *Journal of Child Psychology and Psychiatry, 27*, 307–319.

Prosser, S., Turrini, M., & Arslan, R. (1991). Effects of different noises on speech intelligibility in the elderly. *Acta Otolaryngologica, 476,* 167–176.

Ptacek, P.H., & Pinheiro, M.L. (1971). Pattern reversal in auditory perception. *Journal of the Acoustical Society of America, 49*, 493–498.

Quine, D., Regan, D., & Murry, T. (1983). Delayed auditory tone perception. *Canadian Journal of Neuroscience, 10*, 183–186.

Rajan, R. (1988). Effect of electrical stimulation of the crossed olivococlear bundle on temporary threshold shifts in auditory sensitivity. I. Dependence on electrical stimulation parameters. *Journal of Neurophysiology, 60*, 549–568.

Rajan, R., & Johnstone, B.M. (1983). Crossed cochlear influences on monaural temporary threshold shifts. *Hearing Research, 9*, 279–294.

Rajan, R., & Johnstone, B.M. (1988). Binaural acoustic stimulation exercises protective effects at the cochlea that mimics the effects of electrical stimulation of an auditory efferent pathway. *Brain Research, 459*, 241–255.

Rajan, R., & Johnstone, B.M. (1989). Contralateral cochlear descruction mediates protection from monaural loud sound exposures through the crossed olivococlear bundle. *Hearing Research, 39*, 263–278.

Rampp, D.L. (1976). *Classroom activities for auditory perceptual disorders.* Danville, IL: Interstate Printers and Publishers.

Rampp, D.L. (1980). *Auditory processing and learning disabilities.* Lincoln, NE: Cliffs Notes.

Rapin, I., Schimmel, H., & Cohen, M. (1972). Reliability in detecting auditory evoked responses (AER) for audiometry in sleeping subjects. *Electroencephalography and Clinical Neurophysiology, 32*, 521–528.

Rappaport, M., & Clifford, J. (1994). Comparison of passive P300 brain evoked potentials in normal and severely traumatically brain-injured subjects. *Journal of Head Trauma and Rehabilitation, 9*, 94–104.

Rapport, M.D., Denney, C., DuPaul, G.J., & Gardner, M.J. (1994). Attention deficit disorder and methylphenidate normalization rates, clinical effectiveness, and response prediction in 76 children. *Journal of the American Academy of Child and Adolescent Psychiatry, 33*, 882–893.

Rapport, M.D., Jones, J.T., DuPaul, G.J., Kelly, K.L., Gardner, M.J., Tucker, S.B., & Shea, M.S. (1987). Attention deficit disorder and methylphenidate: Group and single-subject analysis of dose effects on attention in clinic and classroom settings. *Journal of Clinical Child Psychology, 16*, 329–338.

Rauschecker, J.P., & Marler, P. (1987). Cortical plasticity and imprinting: Behavioral and physiological contrasts and parallels. In J.P. Rauschecker & P. Marler (Eds.), *Imprinting and cortical plasticity* (pp. 349–366). New York: John Wiley.

Ravizza, R., & Masterton, R. (1972). Contribution of neocortex to sound localization in opossum (Didelphis virginiana). *Journal of Neurophysiology, 35*, 344–356.

Ray, H., Sarff, L.S., & Glassford, J.E. (1984, Summer/Fall). Sound field amplification: An innovative educational intervention for mainstreamed learning disabled students. *The Directive Teacher*, pp. 18–20.

Recanzone, G.H., Allard, T.T., Jenkins, W.M., & Merzenich, M.M. (1990). Receptive-field changes induced by peripheral nerve stimulation in SI of adult cats. *Journal of Neurophysiology, 63*(5), 1213–1225.

Recanzone, G.H., Jenkins, W.M., Hradek, G.T., & Merzenich, M.M. (1992). Progressive improvement in discriminative abilities in adult owl monkeys performing a tactile frequency discrimination task. *Journal of Neurophysiology, 67*(5), 1015–1030.

Recanzone, G.H., Merzenich, M.M., & Jenkins, W.M. (1992). Frequency discrimination training engaging a restricted skin surface results in an emergence of a cutaneous response zone in cortical area 3a. *Journal of Neurophysiology, 67*(5), 1057–1070.

Recanzone, G.H., Merzenich, M.M., Jenkins, W.M., Grajski, K.A., & Dinse, H.R. (1992). Topographic reorganization of the hand representation in cortical area 3b of owl monkeys trained in a frequency-discrimination task. *Journal of Neurophysiology, 67*(5), 1031–1056.

Recanzone, G.H., Merzenich, M.M., & Schreiner, C.E. (1992). Changes in the distributed temporal response properties of SI cortical neurons reflect improvements in performance on a temporally based tactile discrimination task. *Journal of Neurophysiology, 67*(5), 1071–1091.

Recanzone, G.H., Schreiner, C.E., Hradek, G., Sutter, M., Beitel, R., & Merzenich, M. (1991). Functional reorganization of the primary auditory cortex in adult owl monkeys parallel improvements in performance in an auditory frequency discrimination task. *Society for Neuroscience Abstracts, 17*(213.2), 534.

Recanzone, G.H., Schreiner, C.E., & Merzenich, M.M. (1993). Plasticity in the frequency representation of primary auditory cortex following discrimination training in adult owl monkeys. *Journal of Neuroscience, 13*, 87–103.

Rees, N.S. (1973). Auditory processing factors in language disorders: The view from Procruste's bed. *Journal of Speech and Hearing Disorders, 38,* 304–315.

Rees, N.S. (1981). Saying more than we know: Is auditory processing disorder a meaningful concept? In R.W. Keith (Ed.), *Central auditory and language disorders in children* (pp. 94–120). Houston: College-Hill Press.

Rehm, L.P., Fuchs, C.Z., Roth, D.M., Kornblith, S.J., & Romano, J.M. (1979). A comparison of self-control and assertion skills treatments of depression. *Behavior Therapy, 10*, 429–442.

Reid, D.K., & Hresko, W.P. (1981). *A cognitive approach to learning disabilities*. New York: McGraw-Hill.

Reid, M.K., & Borkowski, J.G. (1987). Causal attributions of hyperactive children: Implications for training strategies and self-control. *Journal of Educational Psychology, 76*, 225–235.

Reid, R., Maag, J.W., & Vasa, S.F. (1993). Attention deficit hyperactivity disorder as a disability category: A critique. *Exceptional Children, 60*(3), 198–214.

Reutzel, D.R. (1985). Story maps improve comprehension. *The Reading Teacher, 38*, 400–404.

Revoile, S., Kozma-Spytek, L, Holden-Pitt, L., Pickett, J.M., & Droge, J. (1995). Acoustic-phonetic context considerations for speech recognition testing of hearing-impaired listeners. *Ear & Hearing, 16*, 254–262.

Reynolds, A. (1975). Development of binaural responses of units in the inferior colliculus of the neonate cat. Unpublished undergraduate paper, Department of Physiology, Monash University, Clayton Victoria, Australia.

Reynolds, B.A., & Weiss, S. (1992). Generation of neurons and astrocytes from isolated cells of the adult mammalian central nervous system. *Science, 225*, 1707–1710.

Reynolds, W. (1987). *Auditory Discrimination Test* (2nd ed.). Los Angeles: Western Psychological Services.

Rhode, W. (1985). The use of intracellular techniques in the study of the cochlear nucleus. *Journal of the Acoustical Society of America, 78,* 320–327.

Rhode, W. (1991). Physiological-morphological properties of the cochlear nucleus. In R. Altschuler, R. Bobbin, B. Clopton, & D. Hoffman (Eds.), *Neurobiology of hearing: The central auditory system* (pp. 47–78). New York: Raven Press.

Rholes, W.S., Blackwell, J., Jordan, C., & Walters, C. (1980). A developmental study of learned helplessness. *Developmental Psychology, 16*, 616–624.

Riccio, C.A., Hynd, G.W., Cohen, M.J., & Gonzalez, J. J. (1993). Neurological basis of attention deficit hyperactivity disorder. *Exceptional Children, 60*(2), 118–124.

Riccio, C.A., Hynd, G.W., Cohen, M.J., & Molt, L. (1996). The Staggered Spondaic Word Test: Performance of children with attention-deficit hyperactivity disorder. *American Journal of Audiology, 5*(2), 55–62.

Ringel, B.A., & Springer, C.J. (1980). On knowing how well one is remembering: The persistence of strategy use during transfer. *Journal of Experimental Child Psychology, 29*, 322–333.

Rintelmann, W. (1985). Monaural speech tests in the detection of central auditory disorders. In F.E. Musiek & M.L. Pinheiro (Eds.), *Assessment of central auditory dysfunction: Foundations and clinical correlates*. (pp. 173–200). Baltimore: Williams & Wilkins.

Roberts, J.E., Burchinal, M.R., Collier, A.M., Ramey, C.T., Koch, M.A., & Henderson, F.W. (1989). Otitis media in early childhood, and cognitive, academic, and classroom performance of the school-aged child. *Pediatrics, 83,* 477–485.

Roberts, J.E., & Medley, L.P. (1995). Otitis media and speech-language sequelae in young children: Current issues in management. *American Journal of Speech-Language Pathology, 4*, 15–24.

Robertson, D., & Irvine, D.R.F. (1989). Plasticity of frequency organization in auditory cortex of guinea pigs with partial unilateral deafness. *Journal of Comparative Neurology, 282*, 456–471.

Robin, D.A., Tomblin, J.B., Kearney, A., & Hugg, L.N. (1989). Auditory temporal pattern learning in children with speech and language impairments. *Brain & Language, 36*(4), 604–613.

Robin, D.A., Tranel, D., & Damasio, H. (1990). Auditory perception of temporal and spectral events in patients with focal left and right cerebral lesions. *Brain and Language, 39*, 539–555.

Robinette M. (1992). Clinical observations with patients with transient evoked otoacoustic emissions with adults. *Seminars in Hearing, 13*, 23–36.

Rodriguez, G.P., DiSarno, N.J., & Hardiman, C.J. (1990). Central auditory processing in normal-hearing elderly adults. *Audiology, 29*, 85–92.

Ronald, K., & Roskelly, H. (1985, March). *Listening as an act of composing.* Paper presented at the Annual Meeting of the Conference on College Composition and Communication, Minneapolis, MN.

Rose, J.E., Galambos, R., & Hughes, J.R. (1959). Microelectrode studies of the cochlear nuclei of the cat. *Johns Hopkins Hospital Bulletin, 104*, 211–251.

Rosenberg, G., & Blake-Rahter, P. (1995a). Inservice training for the classroom teacher. In C. Crandell, J. Smaldino, & C. Flexer, *Sound-field FM amplification* (pp. 149–190). San Diego: Singular Publishing Group.

Rosenberg, G., & Blake-Rahter, P. (1995b). Sound-field amplification: A review of the literature. In C.C. Crandell, J.J. Smaldino, & C. Flexer (Eds.), *Sound-field FM amplification* (pp. 107–123). San Diego: Singular Publishing Group.

Rosenzweig, M., & Postman, L. (1957). Intelligibility as a function of frequency of usage. *Journal of Experimental Psychology, 54*, 412–422.

Ross, M. (1992). *FM auditory training systems: Characteristics, selection and use.* Timonium, MD: York Press.

Ross, M., (1994). FM large-area listening systems. In M. Ross (Ed.), *Communication access for persons with hearing loss* (pp. 51–69). Baltimore: York Press.

Ross, M., Brackett, D., & Maxon, A.B. (1991). *Assessment and management of mainstreamed hearing-impaired children.* Austin, TX: Pro–Ed.

Ross, M., & Giolas, T. (1971). Three classroom listening conditions on speech intelligibility. *American Annals of the Deaf, 116*, 580–584.

Ross, M., Giolas, T., & Carver, D. (1973). Effect of three classroom listening conditions on speech intelligibility. A replication in part. *Language, Speech, and Hearing Services in Schools, 4*, 72–76.

Rosvold, H.E., Mirsky, A.F., Sarason, I., Bransome, E.D., & Beck, L.H. (1956). A continuous performance test of brain damage. *Journal of Consulting Psychology, 20*, 343–350.

Roush, J., & Tait, C. (1984). Binaural fusion, masking level difference and auditory brainstem responses in children with language learning disabilities. *Ear & Hearing, 5*, 37–41.

Royster, L.H., Royster, J.D., & Thomas, W.G. (1980). Representative hearing levels by race and sex in North Carolina industry. *Journal of the Acoustical Society of America, 68*(2), 551–566.

Rubel, E.W., Oesterle, E.C., & Weisleder, P. (1991). Hair cell regernation in the avian inner ear. *Ciba Foundation Symposium, 160*, 77–96.

Ruben, R.J. (1967). Development of the inner ear of the mouse: A radioautographic study of terminal mitoses. *Acta Otolaryngologica, 220*, 1–44.

Ruben, R.J. (1996). Introduction. In T.R. Van De Water, A.N. Popper, & R.R. Fay (Eds.), *Clinical aspects of hearing* (pp. 1–9). New York: Springer.

Rubens, A. (1986). Anatomical asymmetries of the human cerebral cortex. In S. Harnad & R. Doty (Eds.), *Lateralization in the nervous system* (pp. 597–610). New York: Academic Press.

Rumbaugh, D.M., & Washburn, D.A. (1996). Attention and memory in relation to learning: A comparative adaptation perspective. In G.R. Lyon & N.A. Krasnegor (Eds.), *Attention, memory, and executive function* (pp. 199–220). Baltimore: Paul H. Brookes.

Rumelhart, D.E. (1977). *Introduction to human information processing.* New York: John Wiley & Sons.

Rumelhart, D.E. (1980). Schemata: The basic building blocks of cognition. In R. Spiro, B. Bruce, & W. Brewer (Eds.), *Theoretical issues in reading comprehension* (pp. 33–58). Hillsdale, NJ: Lawrence Erlbaum.

Rumelhart, D.E. (1984). Understanding understanding. In J. Flood (Ed.), *Understanding reading comprehension* (pp. 1–20). Newark, DE: International Reading Association.

Rumelhart, D.E., McClelland, J.L., & The PDP Research Group. (Eds.). (1986). *Parallel distributed processing: Explorations in the microstructure of cognition* (Vol. 1). Cambridge, MA: The MIT Press.

Rutter, M., & Tuma, A.H. (1988). Diagnosis and classification: Some outstanding issues. In M. Rutter, A.H. Tuma, & I.S. Lann (Eds.), *Assessment and diagnosis in child psycopathology* (pp. 437–452). New York: Guilford Press.

Ryals, B.M., & Rubel, E.W. (1988). Hair cell regeneration after acoustic trauma in adult coturnix quail. *Science, 240*, 1774–1776.

Ryan, A.F. (1988). The relationship between metabolism and blood flow in the cochlea. In S. Jahn & J. Santos-Sacchi (Eds.), *Physiology of the ear* (pp. 317–326). New York: Raven Press.

Ryan, A.F., Bennett, T.M., Woolf, N.K., & Axelsson, A. (1994). Protection from noise-induced hearing loss by prior exposure to a nontraumatic stimulus: Role of the middle ear muscles. *Hearing Research, 72*, 23–28.

Ryan, A.F., Luo, L., Lieber, R.L., Woolf, N.K., & Axelsson, G.A. (1996). Role of the middle ear muscles in acoustic conditioning: Physiological and molecular studies. In R.J. Salvi, D. Henderson, F. Fiarino, & V. Colletti (Eds.), *Auditory system plasticity and regeneration* (pp. 155–164). New York: Thieme.

Ryan, E.B., Weed, K.A., & Short, E.J. (1986). Cognitive behavior modification: Promoting active, self-regulatory learning styles. In J.K. Torgesen & B.Y.L. Wong (Eds.), *Psychological and educational perspectives on learning disabilities* (pp. 367–398). San Diego: Academic Press.

Ryugo, D., & Weinberg, N. (1976). Corticofugal modulation of the medial geniculate body. *Experimental Neurology, 51*, 377–391.

Safer, D.J., & Allen, R.D. (1976). *Hyperactive children: Diagnosis and management.* Baltimore: University Park Press.

Sahley, T.L., Kalish, R.B., Musiek, F.E., & Hoffman, D. (1991). Effects of opioid drugs on auditory evoked potentials suggest a role of lateral efferent olivocochlear dynorphins in auditory function. *Hearing Research, 55,* 133–142.

Sahley, T.L., Musiek, F.E., & Nodar, R.H. (1996). Naloxone blockage of (-)pentazocine-induced changes in auditory function. *Ear & Hearing, 17*(4), 341–353.

Sahley, T.L., & Nodar, R.H. (1994). Improvement in auditory function following pentazocine suggests a role for dynorphins in auditory sensitivity. *Ear & Hearing, 15*(6), 422–431.

Salamy, A. (1978). Commissural transmission: Maturational changes in humans. *Science, 200*, 1409–1410.

Salamy, A., Mendelson, T., Tooley, W., & Chapline, E. (1980). Differential development of brainstem potentials in healthy and high risk infants. *Science, 210*, 553–555.

Salamy, M.C. (1976). Postnatal development of human brainstem potentials during the first year of life. *Electroenephalography and Clinical Neurophysiology, 40*, 418–426.

Salasoo, A., & Pisoni, D.B. (1985). Interaction of knowledge sources in spoken word identification. *Journal of Memory and Language, 24*, 210–231.

Saletu, B., Moller, H.J., Grunberger, J., Deutsch, H., & Rossner, M. (1990). Propentofylline in adult-onset cognitive disorders: Double-blind, placebo-controlled, clinical, psychometric and brain mapping studies. *Neuropsychobiology, 24*(4), 173–184.

Salvi, R.J., Henderson, D., Boettchner, F.A., & Powers, N.L. (1992). Functional changes in central auditory pathways resulting from cochlear disease. In J. Katz, N. Stecker, & D. Henderson (Eds.), *Central auditory processing: A transdisciplinary view* (pp. 47–60). St. Louis, MO: Mosby Year Book.

Salvi, R.J., Powers, N.L., Saunders, S.S., Boettcher, F.A., & Clock, A.E. (1992). Enhancement of evoked response amplitude and single unit activity after noise exposure. In A.L. Dancer, D. Henderson, R.J. Salvi, & R.P. Hamernik (Eds.), *Noise-induced hearing loss* (pp. 156–171). St. Louis: Mosby Year Book.

Sameroff, A.J. (1983). Developmental systems: Contexts and evolution. In P.H. Mussen (Series Ed.) and W. Kessen (Vol. Ed.), *Handbook of child psychology: Vol. 1. History, theory, and methods* (4th ed., pp. 237–294). New York: John Wiley.

Samuels, S.J. (1987). Factors that influence listening and reading comprehension. In R. Horowitz & S.J. Samuels (Eds.), *Comprehending oral and written language* (pp. 295–325). San Diego: Academic Press.

Sanchez-Longo, L.P., & Forster, F.M. (1958). Clinical significance of impairment of sound localization. *Neurology, 8,* 119–125.

Sanchez-Longo, L.P., Forster, F.M., & Auth, T.L. (1957). A clinical test for sound localization and its applications. *Neurology, 8*, 119–125.

Sanders, D. (1965). Noise conditions in normal school classrooms. *Exceptional Children, 31*, 344–353.

Sanders, D., & Goodrich, S. (1971). Relative contribution of visual and auditory components of speech intelligibility as a function of three conditions of frequency distortion. *Journal of Speech and Hearing Research, 14*(1), 154–159.

Sando, I. (1965). The anatomical interrelationships of the cochlear nerve fibers. *Acta Otolaryngologica, 59*, 417–436.

Sangal, J.M., Sangal, R.B., & Persky, B. (1995). Abnormal auditory P300 topography in attention deficit disorder predicts poor response to pemoline. *Clinical Electroencephalography, 26*(4), 204–213.

Saniga, R.D., & Carlin, M.F. (1991). Auditory dysfunction in voice disordered patients. *American Auditory Society Bulletin, 16*, 9–10, 22–23.

Sano, M., Bell, K., Marder, K., Stricks, L., Stern, Y., & Mayeux, R. (1993). Safety and efficacy of oral physostigmine in the treatment of Alzheimer disease. *Clinical Neuropharmacology, 16*(1), 61–69.

Sarff, L. (1981). An innovative use of free field amplification in regular classrooms. In R. Roeser & M. Downs (Eds.), *Auditory disorders in school children* (pp. 263–272.) New York: Thieme-Stratton.

Sarff, L., Ray, H., & Bagwell, C. (1981). Why not amplification in every classroom? *Hearing Aid Journal, 34*(10), 47–52.

Saul, L.J., & Davis, H. (1932). Action currents in the central nervous system: I. Action currents of the auditory tracts. *Archives of Neurology and Psychiatry, 28*, 1104–1116.

Saville-Troike, M. (1986). Anthropological considerations in the study of communication. In O.L. Taylor (Ed.), *Nature of communication disorders in culturally and linguistically diverse populations* (pp. 47–72). San Diego: College-Hill Press.

Saville-Troike, M. (1989). The ethnograpy of communication. New York: Basil Blackwell.

Savin, H.B. (1963). Word-frequency effect and errors in the perception of speech. *Journal of the Acoustical Society of America, 35*(2), 200–206.

Schaughency, E.A., & Hynd, G.W. (1989). Attentional control systems and the attention deficit disorders. *Learning and Individual Differences, 14,* 423–449.

Scheich, H. (1991). Auditory cortex: Comparative aspects of maps and plasticity. *Current Opinion in Neurobiology, 1*, 236–247.

Scherer, W.J., & Udin, S.B. (1989). N-Methy-D-Aspartate antagonists prevent interaction of binocular maps in Xenopus tectum. *Journal of Neuroscience, 9*(11), 3837–3843.

Scherg, M. (1982). Distortion of the middle latency auditory response produced by analog filtering. *Scandanavian Audiology, 11*, 57–69.

Scherg, M., & Von Cramon, D. (1986). Evoked dipole source potentials of the human auditory cortex. *Electroencephalography and Clinical Neurophysiology, 65*, 344–360.

Schiavetti, N., Sitler, R.W., Metz, D.E., & Houde, R.A. (1984). Prediction of contextual speech intelligibility from isolated word intelligibility measures. *Journal of Speech and Hearing Research, 27*, 623–626.

Schlaggar, B.L., & O'Leary, D.D.M. (1991). Potential of visual cortex to develop an array of functional units unique to somatosensory cortex. *Science, 252*, 1556–1560.

Schmidt, J.T. (1990). Long-term potentiation and activity-dependent retinotopic sharpening in the regenerating retinotectal projection of goldfish: Common sensitive period and sensitivity to NMDA blockers. *Journal of Neuroscience, 10*(1), 233–246.

Schneider, D. (1992). Audiologic management of central auditory processing disorders. In J. Katz, N. Stecker, & D. Henderson (Eds.), *Central auditory processing: A transdisciplinary view* (pp. 161–168). St. Louis: Mosby.

Schoeny, Z., & Talbott, R. (1994). Non-speech procedures in central testing. In J. Katz (Ed.) *Handbook of clinical audiology* (4th ed., pp. 212–221). Baltimore: Williams & Wilkins.

Schuknecht, H.T. (1974). *Pathology of the ear*. Cambridge, MA: Harvard University Press.

Schultz, M. (1964). Word familiarity influences in speech discrimination. *Journal of Speech and Hearing Research, 7*, 395–400.

Schumaker, J.B., Deshler, D.D., Alley, G.R., & Warner, M.M. (1983). Toward the development of an intervention model for LD adolescents. *Exceptional Education Quarterly, 4*(1), 45–74.

Schuman, E.M., & Madison, D.V. (1994). Locally distributed synaptic potentiation in the hippocampus. *Science, 263*, 532–536.

Schunk, D.H. (1982). Effects of effort attributional feedback on children's perceived self-efficacy and achievement. *Journal of Educational Psychology, 74*, 548–556.

Schwaber, M.K., Garraghty, P.E., & Kaas, J.H. (1994). Neuroplasticity of the adult primate auditory cortex following cochlear hearing loss. *American Journal of Otology, 14*(3), 252–258.

Schwartz, D.M. (1987). Neurodiagnostic audiology: Contemporary perspectives. *Ear & Hearing, 8*, 43–48.

Scott, D.M. (1986). Sickle–cell anemia and hearing loss. [Concerns for minority groups in communication disorders.] *ASHA Reports, 16*, 69–73.

Screen, R.M., & Anderson, N.B. (1994). *Multicultural perspectives in communication disorders*. San Diego: Singular Publishing Group.

Seidel, W.T., & Joschko, M. (1990). Evidence of difficulties in sustained attention in children with ADDH. *Journal of Abnormal Child Psychology, 18*, 217–229.

Seikel, J.A., Somers, E.K., & Chermak, G.D. (1996, April). *Behavioral signs of central auditory processing disorder and attention deficit hyperactivity disorder.* Paper presented at the annual convention of the American Academy of Audiology, Salt Lake City, UT.

Seligman, M., & Darling, R.B. (1990). *Ordinary families, special children: A systems approach to disability*. New York: Guilford.

Selnes, O.A. (1974). The corpus callosum: Some anatomical and functional considerations with special reference to language. *Brain and Language, 1,* 111–139.

Seltzer, B., & Pandya, D. (1978). Afferent cortical connections and archetectonics of the superior temporal sulcus and surrounding cortex in Rhesus monkey. *Brain Research, 149,* 1–24.

Semel, E., Wiig, E.H., & Secord, W.A. (1996). *Clinical evaluation of language fundamentals* (3rd ed.). San Antonio: Psychological Corporation.

Sergeant, J., & van der Meere, J. (1990). Convergence of approaches in localizing the hyperactivity deficit. In B.B. Lahey & A.E. Kazdin (Eds.), *Advances in clinical child psychology* (Vol. 13, pp. 207–245). New York: Plenum.

Shah, S., & Salamy, A. (1980). Brainstem auditory potential in myelin deficient mice. *Neuroscience, 5*, 2321–2323.

Shannon, R.V., Zeng, F.G., Kamath, V., Wygonski, J., & Ekelid, M. (1995). Speech recognition with primarily temporal cues. *Science, 270*, 303–304.

Shapiro, A.H., & Mistal, G. (1985). ITE–aid auditory training for reading– and spelling-disabled children. Clinical case studies. T*he Hearing Journal, 38*(2), 26–31.

Shapiro, A.H., & Mistal, G. (1986). ITE-aid auditory training for reading- and spelling-disabled children: A longitudinal study of matched groups. *The Hearing Journal, 39*(2), 14–16.

Sharp, M., & Orchik, D.J. (1978). Auditory function in sickle cell anemia. *Archives of Otolaryngology, 104*, 322–324.

Shaywitz, B.A., Fletcher, J.M., & Shaywitz, S.E. (1994a). Interrelationships between reading disability and attention deficit-hyperactivity disorder. In A.J. Capute, P.J. Accardo, & B.K. Shapiro (Eds.), *Learning disabilities spectrum* (pp. 107–120). Baltimore: York Press.

Shaywitz, S.E., Fletcher, J.M., & Shaywitz, B. (1994b). Issues in the definition and classification of attention deficit disorder. *Topics in Language Disorders, 14*(4), 1–25.

Shaywitz, S.E., & Shaywitz, B.A. (1988). Attention deficit disorder: Current perspectives. In J.F. Kavanaugh & T.J. Truss (Eds.), *Learning disabilities:*

Proceedings of the national conference (pp. 369–523). Parkton, MD: York Press.

Shehata-Dieler, W., Shimizu, H., Soliman, S., & Tusa, R. (1991). Middle latency auditory evoked potentials in temporal lobe disorders. *Ear & Hearing, 12*, 377–388.

Sherg, M. (1982). Distortion of the middle latency auditory response produced by analog filtering. *Scandinavian Audiology, 11*, 57–59.

Shriberg, L. (1983). Natural phonologic process approach. In W. Perkins (Ed.), *Phonologic-articulatory disorders* (pp. 3–9). New York: Thieme-Stratton.

Silva, P.A., Chalmers, D., & Stewart, I. (1986). Some audiological, psychological, educational and behavioral characteristics of children with bilateral otitis media with effusion: A longitudinal study. *Journal of Learning Disabilities, 19*, 165–169.

Silva, P.A., Kirkland, C., Simpson, A., Stewart, I.A., & Williams, S.M. (1982). Some developmental and behavioral problems associated with bilateral otitis media with effusion. *Journal of Learning Disabilities, 15,* 417–421.

Singer, W. (1995). Development and plasticity of cortical processing architectures. *Science, 270,* 758–764.

Skinner, M.W. (1978). The hearing of speech during language acquisition. *Otolaryngology Clinics of North America, 11*, 631–650.

Skinner, P. (1972). *Electroencephalic response audiometry.* Maico Audiological Library Series Report I.

Slavin, R.E. (1983). When does cooperative learning increase student achievement? *Psychological Bulletin, 94*, 429–445.

Slingerland, B.H. (1971). *A multi-sensory approach to language arts for specific language disability children: A guide for primary teachers.* Cambridge: Educators Publishing Service.

Sloan, C. (1980a). Auditory processing disorders and language development. In P.J. Levinson & C. Sloan (Eds.), *Auditory processing and language: Clinical and research perspectives* (pp. 101–116). New York: Grune & Stratton.

Sloan, C. (1980b). Auditory processing disorders in children: Diagnosis and treatment. In P.J. Levinson & C. Sloan (Eds.), *Auditory processing and language* (pp. 117–133). New York: Grune & Stratton.

Sloan, C. (1986). *Treating auditory processing difficulties in children.* San Diego: College-Hill Press.

Sloan, C. (1992). Language, language learning, and language disorder: Implications for central auditory processing. In J. Katz, N.A. Stecker, & D. Henderson (Eds.), *Central auditory processing: A transdisciplinary view* (pp. 179–186). St. Louis: Mosby Year Book.

Slowiaczek, L.M., Nusbaum, H.C., & Pisoni, D.B. (1987). Phonological priming in auditory word-recognition. *Journal of Experimental Psychology, 13*(1), 64–75.

Smith, B.B., & Resnick, D.M. (1972). An auditory test for assessing brain stem integrity: Preliminary report. *Laryngoscope, 82*, 414–424.

Smith, D., McConnell, J., Walter, T., & Miller, S. (1985). Effect of using an auditory trainer on the attentional, language, and social behaviors of autistic children. *Journal of Autism Developmental Disorders, 15*, 285–302.

Smith, M.D., Gould, D., Marsh, L., & Nichols, A. (1995). The metaphysics of ADHD: A unifying case scenario. *Seminars in Speech and Language, 16*(4), 303–313.

Smith, S. (1988). Progress on LTP at hippocampal synapses: A postsynaptic CA II plus trigger for memory storage? *Trends in Neuroscience, 11,* 112–114.

Smoski, W.J., Brunt, M.A., & Tannahill, J.C. (1992). Listening characteristics of children with central auditory processing disorders. *Language, Speech, and Hearing Services in Schools, 23*, 145–152.

Snider, V.E. (1989). Reading comprehension performance of adolescents with learning disabilities. *Learning Disability Quarterly, 12*, 87–96.

Sparks, R., Goodglass, H., & Nichel, B. (1970). Ipsilateral versus contralateral extinction in dichotic listening resulting from hemisphere lesions. *Cortex, 6*, 249–260.

Speaks, C.K. (1975). Dichotic listening: A clinical or research tool? In H. Sullivan (Ed.), *Proceedings of a symposium on central auditory processing disorders*. Omaha: University of Nebraska Medical Center.

Speaks, C.K., Gray, T., Miller, J., & Rubens, A. (1975). Central auditory deficits and temporal lobe lesions. *Journal of Speech and Hearing Disorders, 40*, 192–205.

Speaks, C.K., Niccum, N., & Van Tasell, D. (1985). Effects of stimulus material on dichotic listening performance on patients with sensorineural hearing loss. *Journal of Speech and Hearing Research, 28,* 16–25.

Speece, D., McKinney, J., & Appelbaum, M. (1985). Classification and validation of behavioral subtypes of learning disabled children. *Journal of Educational Psychology, 77*, 67–77.

Spence, K.W., & Norris, E.B. (1950). Eyelid conditioning as a function of the intertrial interval. *Journal of Experimental Psychology, 40*, 716–720.

Squire, L. R. (1987). Memory and brain. Oxford: Oxford University Press.

Squires, K., & Hecox, K. (1983). Electrophysiological evaluation of higher level auditory processing. *Seminars in Hearing, 4*, 415–432.

St. James-Roberts, I. (1979). Neurological plasticity, recovery from brain insult, and child development. *Advances in Child Development and Behavior, 14*, 253–319.

Stach, B.A. (1990). Hearing aid amplification and central processing disorder. In R.E. Sandlin (Ed.), *Handbook of hearing aid amplification* (Vol. 2, pp. 87–111). Boston: College-Hill Press.

Stach, B.A. (1992). Controversies in the screening of central auditory processing disorders. In F.H. Bess & J.W. Hall (Eds.), *Screening children for auditory function* (pp. 61–77). Nashville, TN: Bill Wilkerson Center Press.

Stach, B.A., Loiselle, L.H., & Jerger, J.F. (1987a). Clinical experience with personal FM assistive listening devices. *Hearing Journal, 40*, 24–30.

Stach, B.A., Loiselle, L.H., & Jerger, J.F. (1987b, November). *FM systems use by children with central auditory processing disorders*. Paper presented at the annual convention of the American Speech-Language-Hearing Association, New Orleans, LA.

Stach, B.A., Loiselle, L.H., & Jerger, J.F. (1991). Special hearing aid considerations in elderly patients with auditory processing disorders. *Ear & Hearing, 12*(6, Suppl.), 131S–138S.

Stach, B.A., Loiselle, L.H., Jerger, J.F., Mintz, S.L., & Taylor, C.D. (1987). Clinical experience with personal FM assistive listening devices. *Hearing Journal, 10*(5), 24–30.

Stach, B.A., Spretnjak, M.L., & Jerger, J. (1990). The prevalence of central presbycusis in a clinical population. *Journal of the American Academy of Audiology, 1*(2), 109–115.

Staley, T., Kalish, R., Musiek, F., & Hoffman, D. (1991). Effects of opioid drugs on auditory evoked potentials suggest a role of lateral olivocochlear dynorphins in auditory function. *Hearing Research, 55,* 133–142.

Stanovich, K.E. (1986). Cognitive process and the reading problems of learning disabled children: Evaluating the assumption of specificity. In J.K. Torgesen & B.L. Wong (Eds.), *Psychological and educational perspectives on reading disabilities* (pp. 87–131). New York: Academic Press.

Stanovich, K.E. (1993). The construct validity of discrepancy definitions of reading disability. In G.R. Lyon, D.B. Gray, J.F. Kavanaugh, & N.A. Krasnegor (Eds.), *Better understanding learning disabilities* (pp. 273–307). Baltimore: Paul H. Brookes.

Starch, D. (1912). Periods of work in learning. *Journal of Educational Psychology, 3*, 209–213.

Starr, A., & Achor, J. (1975). Auditory brainstem responses in neurological disease. *Archives of Neurology, 32*, 761–768.

Steel, K.P., & Brown, S.D.M. (1994). Genes for deafness. *Trends in Genetics, 10*, 428–435.

Steel, K.P., & Kimberling, W. (1996). Approaches to understanding the molecular genetics of hearing and deafness. In T.R. Van de Water, A.N. Popper, & R.R. Fay (Eds.), *Clinical aspects of hearing* (pp. 10–40). New York: Springer.

Sternberg, R. (1985). *Beyond I.Q.: A triarchic theory of intelligence.* New York: Cambridge University Press.

Stewart, J.L. (1986). Hearing disorders among the indigenous peoples of North America and the Pacific Basin. In O.L. Taylor (Ed.,) *Nature of communication disorders in culturally and linguistically diverse populations* (pp. 237–376). San Diego: College-Hill Press.

Stewart, J.L. (1990a). Current status of otitis media in the American Indian population. *Annals of Otology, Rhinology, and Laryngology, 99*(Suppl. 149), 20–22.

Stewart, J.L. (1990b). Otitis media in the first year of life in two Eskimo communities. *Annals of Otology, Rhinology, and Laryngology, 98*(3), 200–201.

Sticht, T.G., & James, J.H. (1984). Listening and reading. In P.D. Pearson (Ed.), *Handbook of reading research* (pp. 293–317). New York: Longman.

Stipek, D.J. (1981). Children's perceptions of their own and their classmates' ability. *Journal of Educational Psychology, 73*, 404–410.

Stipek, D.J., & Tannatt, L.M. (1984). Children's judgments of their own and their peers' academic competence. *Journal of Educational Psychology, 76*, 75–84.

Stockard, J., & Rossiter, V. (1977). Clinical and pathological correlates of brainstem auditory response abnormalities. *Neurology, 27*, 316–325.

Stokes, T.F., & Baer, D.M. (1977). An implicit technology of generalization. *Journal of Applied Behavior Analysis, 10*, 349–367.

Stone, C.A., & Wertsch, J.V. (1984). A social interactional analysis of learning disabilities remediation. *Journal of Learning Disabilities, 17*, 194–199.

Streitfeld, B. (1980). The fiber connections of the temporal lobe with emphasis on the Rhesus monkey. *International Journal of Neuroscience, 11*, 51–71.

Strominger, N.L, & Hurwitz, J.L. (1976). Anatomical aspects of the superior olivary complex. *Journal of Comparative Neurology, 170*, 485–497.

Strominger, N.L., & Strominger, A.L. (1971). Ascending brain stem projections of the anteroventral cochlear nucleus in the rhesus monkey. *Journal of Comparative Neurology, 143*, 217–232.

Strouse, A.L., Hall, J.W. III, & Burger, M.C. (1995). Central auditory processing in Alzheimer's disease. *Ear & Hearing, 16*(2), 230–238.

Stubblefield, J.H., & Young, C.E. (1975). Central auditory dysfunction in learning disabled children. *Journal of Learning Disabilities, 8*, 32–37.

Studdert-Kennedy, M. (1980). Speech perception. *Language and Speech, 23*, 45–66.

Subramaniam, M., Campo, P., & Henderson, D. (1991). The effect of exposure level on the development of progressive resistance to noise. *Hearing Research, 52*, 181–188.

Subramaniam, M., Henderson, D., Campo, P., & Spongr, V. (1992). The effect of "conditioning" on a high frequency traumatic exposure. *Hearing Research, 58*, 57–62.

Subramaniam, M., Henderson, D., & Spongr, V. (1993). Effect of low frequency "conditioning" on hearing loss from high frequency exposure. *Journal of the Acoustical Society of America, 93*, 952–956.

Sudakov, K., MacLean, P., Reeves, A., & Marino, R. (1971). Unit study of exteroceptive inputs to the claustrocortex in the awake sitting squirrel monkey. *Brain Research, 28*, 19–34.

Sue, D.W., & Sue, D. (1990). *Counseling the culturally different.* New York: John Wiley and Sons.

Suiter, M.L., & Potter, R.E. (1978). The effects of paradigmatic organization on recall. *Journal of Learning Disabilities, 11*, 247–250.

Sun, J.C., Bohne, B.A., & Harding, G.W. (1995). Age at the time of acoustical injury affects the magnitude of nerve-fiber regeneration. *Abstracts of the Eighteenth Midwinter Meeting of the Association for Research in Otolaryngology*, Abstr. 294, p. 74.

Sussman, J.E. (1991). Stimulus ratio effects on speech discrimination by children and adults. *Journal of Speech and Hearing Research, 34*, 671–678.

Sutton, S., Braren, M., Zubin, J., & John, E. (1965). Evoked potential correlates of stimulus uncertainty. *Science, 150*, 1187–1188.

Swanson, H.L. (1983). Relations among metamemory, rehearsal activity and word recall in learning disabled and nondisabled readers. *British Journal of Education Psychology, 53*, 186–194.

Swanson, H.L. (1987). Information processing theory and learning disabilities: A commentary and future perspective. *Journal of Learning Disabilities, 20*, 155–166.

Swanson, H.L. (1989). Strategy instruction: Overview of principles and procedures for effective use. *Learning Disability Quarterly, 12*, 3–15.

Swanson, H.L. (1993). Learning disabilities from the perspective of cognitive psychology. In G.R. Lyon, D.B. Gray, J.F. Kavanagh, & N.A. Krasnegor (Eds.), *Better understanding learning disabilities* (pp. 199–228). Baltimore: Paul H. Brookes.

Swanson, H.L. (1996). *Swanson Cognitive Processing Test (S-CPT)*. Austin, TX: Pro-Ed.

Swanson, H.L., & Cooney, J.B. (1991). Learning disabilities and memory. In B.Y.L. Wong (Ed.), *Learning about learning disabilities* (pp. 104–127). San Diego: Academic Press.

Swanson, J.M., Cantwell, D.P. Lerner, M., McBurnett, K., & Hanna, G. (1992). Effects of stimulant medication on learning in children with ADHD. In S.E. Shaywitz & B.A. Shaywitz (Eds.), *Attention deficit disorder comes of age* (pp. 293–321). Austin, TX: Pro-Ed.

Sweetow, R., & Reddell, R. (1978). The use of masking level differences in the identification of children with perceptual problems. *Journal of the American Audiological Society, 4*, 52–56.

Sweetow, R.W. (1986). Cognitive aspects of tinnitus patient management. *Ear and Hearing,* 7(6), 390–396.

Swinomish Tribal Mental Health Project. (1991). *A gathering of wisdoms: Tribal mental health: A cultural perspective*. LaConner, WA: Swinomish Tribal Community.

Swisher, L.P., & Hirsh, I.J. (1972). Brain damage and the ordering of two temporally successive stimuli. *Neuropsychologia, 10*, 137–152.

Szatmari, P., Boyle, M., & Offord, D.R. (1989). ADDH and conduct disorder: Degree of diagnostic overlap and differences among correlates. *Journal of the American Academy of Child and Adolescent Psychiatry, 28*, 865–872.

Takata, Y., & Nabelek, A.K. (1990) English consonant recognition in noise and in reverberation by Japanese and American listeners. *Journal of the Acoustical Society of America, 88*, 663–666.

Tallal, P. (1980a). Auditory processing disorders in children. In P.J. Levinson & C. Sloan (Eds.), *Auditory processing and language: clinical and research perspectives* (pp. 81–100). New York: Grune & Stratton.

Tallal, P. (1980b). Auditory temporal perception, phonics and reading disabilities in children. *Brain and Language, 9*, 1982–198.

Tallal, P. (1985). Neurophyschological research approaches to the study of central auditory processing. *Human Communications, 9*, 17–22.

Tallal, P., Miller, S., Bedi, G., Byma, G., Wang, X., Nagarajan, S.S., Schreiner, C., Jenkins, W.M., & Merzenich, M.H. (1996). Language comprehension in language-learning impaired children improved with acoustically modified speech. *Science, 271*, 81–84.

Tallal, P., Miller, S., & Fitch, R. (1993). Neurobiological basis of speech: A case for the preeminence of temporal processing. In P. Tallal, A. Galaburda, R. Llinas, & C. von Euler (Eds.), *Temporal information processing in the nervous system* (pp. 27–47). New York: New York Academy of Sciences.

Tallal, P., & Newcombe, F. (1978). Impairment of auditory perception and language comprehension in dysphasia. *Brain and Language, 5*, 13–24.

Tallal, P., & Piercy, M. (1973a). Defects of non-verbal auditory perception in children with developmental aphasia. *Nature, 241*, 468–469.

Tallal, P., & Piercy, M. (1973b). Developmental aphasia: Impaired rate of non-verbal processing as a function of sensory modality. *Neuropsychologia, 11,* 389–398.

Tallal, P., & Piercy, M. (1974). Developmental aphasia: Rate of auditory processing and selective impairment of consonant perception. *Neuropsychologica, 12*, 83–94.

Tallal, P., & Piercy, M. (1975). Developmental aphasia: The perception of brief vowels and extended consonants. *Neuropsychologia, 13*, 69–74.

Tallal, P., & Stark, R.E. (1981). Speech acoustic-cue discrimination abilities of normally developing and language impaired children. *Journal of the Acoustical Society of America, 69*, 568–578.

Tallal, P., & Stark, R.E. (1982). Perceptual/motor profiles of reading impaired children with or without concomitant oral language deficits. *Annals of Dyslexia, 32*, 163–176.

Tallal, P., Stark, R., & Curtiss, B. (1976). The relation between speech perception impairment and speech production impairment in children with developmental dysphasia. *Brain and Language, 3*, 305–317.

Tallal, P., Stark, R., Kallman, C., & Mellits, D. (1980). Perceptual constancy for phonemic categories: A developmental study with normal and language impaired children. *Applied Psycholinguistics, 1*, 49–64.

Tallal, P., Stark, R.E., & Mellits, D. (1985). Identification of language-impaired children on the basis of rapid perception and production skills. *Brain and Language, 25*, 314–322.

Tasaki, I. (1954). Nerve impulses in individual auditory nerve fibers of the guinea pig. *Journal of Neurophysiology, 17*, 97–122.

Taylor, E. (1986). The overactive child. *Clinics in Development Medicine*, No. 97. Philadelphia: J.B. Lippincott.

Taylor, O.L. (1986). Historical perspectives and conceptual framework. In O.L. Taylor (Ed.), *Nature of communication disorders in culturally and linguistically diverse populations* (pp. 1–17). San Diego: College-Hill Press.

Taylor, O.L., & Payne, K. (1983). Culturally valid testing: A proactive approach. *Topics in Lanugage Disorders, 3*, 8–20.

Teale, W.H. (1984). Reading to young children: Its significance for literacy development. In H. Goelman, A.A. Oberg & F. Smith (Eds.), *Awakening to literacy* (pp. 110–121). London: Heineman Educational Books.

Teele, D.W., Klein, J.O., & Rosner, B.A. (1989). Epidemiology of otitis media during the first seven years of life in children in greater Boston. *Journal of Infectious Diseases, 160*, 83–94.

Terrell, B.Y. (1993). Multicultural perspectives: Are the issues and questions different? *Asha, 35*(11), 51–52.

Terrell, B.Y., & Hale, J.E. (1992). Serving a multicultural population: Different learning styles. *American Journal of Speech-Language Pathology, 1*(2), 5–8.

Thatcher, R. (1991). Maturation of the human frontal lobes: Physiological evidence for staging. *Developmental Neuropsychology, 7*, 397–419.

Thomas, A., & Pashley, B. (1982). Effects of classroom training on LD students' task persistence and attributions. *Learning Disability Quarterly, 5*, 133–144.

Thompson, M., & Abel, S. (1992). Indices of hearing in patients with central auditory pathology. II: Choice response time. *Scandinavian Audiology, 21*, 17–22.

Thornton, A., Mendel, M., & Anderson, C. (1977). Effects of stimulus frequency and intensity on the middle components of the averaged electroencephalic response. *Journal of Speech and Hearing Research, 20*, 81–94.

Tierney, R.J., & Cunningham, J.W. (1984). Research on teaching reading comprehension. In P.D. Pearson (Ed.), *Handbook of reading research* (pp. 609–655). New York: Longman.

Tillman, T.W., & Carhart, R. (1966). *An expanded test for speech discrimination utilizing CNC monosyllabic words* (Northwestern University Auditory Test No. 6) (Tech. Rep. SAM-TR-66-55). Brooks AFB, TX: USAF School of Aerospace Medical Division (AFSC).

Tillman, T.W., & Jerger, J. (1959). Some factors affecting the spondee threshold in normal hearing subjects. *Journal of Speech and Hearing Research, 2*, 141–146.

Tobin, H. (1985). Binaural interaction tasks. In M.L. Pinheiro & F.E. Musiek (Eds.), *Assessment of central auditory dysfunction: Foundations and clinical correlates* (pp. 151–171). Baltimore: Williams & Wilkins.

Torgesen, J.K. (1979). Factors related to poor performance on rote memory tasks in reading-disabled children. *Learning Disability Quarterly, 2*, 17–23.

Torgesen, J.K. (1980). Conceptual and educational implications of the use of efficient task strategies by learning disabled children. *Journal of Learning Disabilities, 13*, 364–371.

Torgesen, J.K. (1988). Applied research and metatheory in the context of contemporary cognitive theory. *Journal of Learning Disabilities, 21*, 271–274.

Torgesen, J.K. (1994). Issues in the assessment of executive function: An information-processing perspective. In G.R. Lyon (Ed.), *Frames of reference for the assessment of learning disabilities* (pp. 143–162). Baltimore: Paul H. Brookes.

Torgesen, J.K. (1996). A model of memory from an information processing perspective: The special case of phonological memory. In G.R. Lyon & N.A.

Krasnegor (Eds.), *Attention, memory, and executive function* (pp. 157–184). Baltimore: Paul H. Brookes.

Torgesen, J.K., & Houck, G. (1980). Processing deficiencies in learning disabled children who perform poorly on the digit span task. *Journal of Educational Psychology, 72*, 141–160.

Torigoe, R., Hayashi, T., Anegawa, S., Harada, K., Toda, K., Maeda, K., & Katsuragi, M. (1994). The effect of propentofylline and pentoxifylline on cerebral blood flow using 1231–IMP SPECT in patients with cerebral arteriosclerosis. *Clinical Therapeutics, 16*(1), 65–73.

Toscher, M.M., & Rupp, R.R. (1978). A study of the central auditory processes in stutterers using the synthetic sentence identification (SSI) test battery. *Journal of Speech and Hearing Research, 21*, 779–792.

Trainor, L.J., & Trehub, S.E. (1989). Aging and auditory temporal sequencing: Ordering the elements of repeating tone patterns. *Perception and Psychophysics, 45*, 417–426.

Treat, N.J., Poon, L.W., Fozard, J.L., & Popkin, S.J. (1977, August). *Toward applying cognitive skill training to memory problems.* Paper presented at the meeting of the American Psychological Association, San Francisco, CA.

Tsuchitani, C., & Boudreau, J.C. (1966). Single unit analysis of cat superior olive S-segment with tonal stimuli. *Journal of Neurophysiology, 29*, 684–697.

Tucci, D., Born, D., & Rubel, E. (1987). Changes in spontaneous activity in CNS morphology associated with conductive and sensorineural hearing loss in chickens. *Annals of Otology, Rhinology, and Laryngology, 96*, 343–350.

Tucci, D., & Rubel, D. (1985). Afferent influence on brainstem auditory nuclei of the chicken: Effects of conductive and sensorineural hearing loss on an magnocellularis. *Journal of Comparative Neurology, 238*, 371–381.

Tulving, E., & Schacter D.L. (1990). Priming and human memory. *Science, 247*, 301–306.

Turner, R. (1991). Making clinical decisions. In W. Rintelmann (Ed.), *Hearing assessment* (2nd ed., pp. 679–738). Austin, TX: Pro-Ed.

Tyler, L.K. (1984). The structure of the initial cohort: Evidence from gating. *Perception and Psychophysics, 36*, 417–427.

Tyler, L.K. (1992) *Spoken language comprehension: An experimental approach to disordered and normal processing.* Cambridge, MA: MIT Press.

Tyler, L.K. & Wessels, J. (1985). Is gating an on-line task? Evidence from naming latency data. *Perception and Psychophysics, 38*(3), 217–222.

Ungerleider, L.G. (1995). Functional brain imaging studies of cortical mechanisms for memory. *Science, 270*, 769–775.

United States Department of Education. (1990). *Digest of educational statistics*. Washington, DC: National Center for Educational Statistics (Report No. NCES-91-660).

United States Bureau of the Census. (1990). *Statistical abstract of the United States: 1990* (110th ed.). Washington, DC: Government Printing Office.

United States Department of Commerce, Bureau of the Census. (1991). *Census and you, 26*(4). Washington, DC: Government Printing Office.

Valasco, M., Valasco, F., & Valasco, M. (1989) Intracranial studies on potential generators of some vertex evoked potentials in man. *Stereotactic and Functional Neurosurgery, 53*, 49–73.

Van De Water, T.R., Staecker, H., Apfel, S.C., & Lefebvre, P.P. (1996). Regeneration of the auditory nerve: The role of neurotrophic factors. In T.R. Van De Water, A.N. Popper, & R.R. Fay (Eds.), *Clinical aspects of hearing* (pp. 41–85). New York: Springer.

Van Dijk, T.A. (1985). Semantic discourse analysis. In T.A. Van Dijk (Ed.), *Handbook of discourse analysis. Vol. 2: Dimensions of discourse* (pp. 103–136). London: Academic Press.

Van Engeland, H. (1993). Pharmacotherapy and behavior therapy—competition or cooperation? *Acta Paedopsychiatrica, 56*(2), 123–127.

Van Kleeck, A. (1994). Metalinguistic development. In G.P. Wallach & K.G. Butler (Eds.), *Language learning disabilities in school-age children and adolescents* (pp. 53–98). New York: Charles E. Merrill.

Van Noort, J. (1969). *The structure and connections of the inferior colliculus: An investigation of the lower auditory system*. Leiden: Van Corcum.

Van Tasell, D.J., Soli, S.D., Kirby, V.M., & Widin, G.P. (1987). Speech waveform envelope cues for consonant recognition. *Journal of the Acoustical Society of America, 82*(4), 1152–1161.

Vaughan, H., & Ritter, W. (1970). The sources of auditory evoked responses recorded from the human scalp. *Electroencephalography and Clinical Neurophysiology, 28*, 36–367.

Velasco, M., Velasco, F., Castaneda, R., & Sanchez, R. (1984). Effect of fentanyl and naloxone on human somatic and auditory-evoked potential components. *Neuropharmacology, 23*(3), 359–366.

Velasco, M., Velasco, F., & Velasco, A. (1989). Intracranial studies on potential generators of some vertex auditory evoked potentials in man. *Stereotactic and Functional Neurosurgery, 53*, 49–73.

Voeller, K.K. (1991). Toward a neurobiologic nosology of attention deficit hyperactivity disorder. *Journal of Clinical Neurology, 6*(Suppl.), S2–S8.

Von Bertalanffy, L. (1968). *General system theory: Foundations, development, applications*. New York: George Braziller.

Wada, S., & Starr, A. (1983). Generation of auditory brain stem responses III. Effects of lesions of the superior olive, lateral lemniscus and inferior colliculus on the ABR in guinea pig. *Electroencephalography and Clinical Neurophysiology, 56*, 352–366.

Waddington, M. (1974). *Atlas of cerebral angiography with anatomic correction*. Boston: Little, Brown.

Waddington, M. (1984). *Atlas of human intracranial anatomy*. Rutland, VT: Academy Books.

Wagner, R.K., & Torgesen, J.K. (1987). The nature of phonological processing and its causal role in the acquisition of reading skills. *Psychological Bulletin, 101*, 192–212.

Walley, A. (1988). Spoken word recogniton by young children and adults. *Cognitive Development, 3*, 137–165.

Warchol, M.E., Lambert, P.R., Goldstein, B.J., Forge, A., & Corwin, J.T. (1993). Regenerative proliferation in inner ear sensory epithelia from adult guinea pigs and humans. *Science, 259*, 1619–1622.

Ward, L.B. (1937). Reminiscence and rote learning. *Psychological Monographs, 49*(220).

Warr, B. (1980). Efferent components of the auditory system. *Annals of Otology, Rhinology, and Laryngology, 89*, 114–120.

Warr, W.B. (1966). Fiber degeneration following lesions in the anterior ventral cochlear nucleus of the cat. *Experimental Neurology, 14*, 453–474.

Warren, R.M. (1970). Perceptual restoration of missing speech sounds. *Science, 167*, 392–393.

Warren, R.M. (1981). Multiple meanings of "phoneme" (articulatory, acoustic, perceptual, graphemic) and their confusions. In N.J. Lass (Ed.), *Speech and language: Advances in basic research and practice* (Vol 9, pp. 285–311). New York: Academic Press.

Warren, R.M. (1982) *Auditory perception: A new synthesis*. New York: Pergamon Press.

Warren, R.M. (1984). Perceptual restoration of obliterated sounds. *Psychological Bulletin, 96*(2), 371–383.

Warren, R.M., & Warren, R.P. (1970). Auditory illusions and confusions. *Scientific American, 223*, 30–36.

Washburn, D.A. (1993). The stimulus movement effect: Allocation of attention or artifact? *Journal of Experimental Psychology: Animal Behavior Processes, 19*, 1–10.

Watson, C.S., & Foyle, D.C. (1985). Central factors in the discrimination and identification of complex sounds. *Journal of the Acoustical Society of America, 78*, 375–380.

Watson, C.S., & Gengel, R.W. (1969). Signal duration and signal frequency in relation to auditory sensitivity. *Journal of the Acoustical Society of America, 46*, 989–997.

Watson, M., & Rastatter M. (1985). The effects of time compression on the auditory processing abilities of learning disabled children. *The Journal of Auditory Research, 25*, 167–173.

Watson, T. (1964). The use of hearing aids by hearing impaired pupils in ordinary schools. *The Volta Review, 66*, 741–744.

Weaver, C. (1985). Parallels between new paradigms in science and in reading and literary theories: An essay review. *Research in the Teaching of English, 19*(3), 298–316.

Weaver, C. (1993). Understanding and educating students with attention deficit hyperactivity disorder: Toward a system theory and whole language perspective. *American Journal of Speech-Language Pathology, 2*(3), 78–89.

Webster, D. (1971). Projection of the cochlea to cochlear nuclei in Merriam's kangaroo rat. *Journal of Comparative Neurology, 143*, 323–340.

Webster, D. (1983). A critical period during post natal auditory development in mice. *International Journal of Pediatric Otorhinolaryngology, 6*, 107–118.

Webster, D. (1988a). Conductive hearing loss affects growth of the cochlear nuclei over an extended period of time. *Hearing Research, 32*, 185–192.

Webster, D. (1988b). Sound amplification begets central effects of neonatal conductive hearing loss. *Hearing Research, 32*, 192–195.

Webster, D., & Webster M. (1977). Neonatal sound deprivation affects brainstem auditory nuclei. *Archives of Otolaryngology, 103*, 392–396.

Webster, J.C., & Snell, K.B. (1983). Noise levels and the speech intelligibility of teachers in a classroom. *Journal of the Academy of Rehabilitative Audiology, 16*, 234–255.

Weinberger, N.M., & Diamond, D.M. (1987). Physiological plasticity in auditory cortex: Rapid induction by learning. *Progress in Neurobiology, 29*, 1–55.

Weiss, M.R. (1987). Use of an adaptive noise canceler as an input preprocessor for a hearing aid. *Journal of Rehabilitation Research and Development, 24*(4), 93–102.

Wells, G. (1985). Preschool literacy-related activities and success in school. In D.R. Olson, N. Torrance, & A. Hildyard (Eds.), *Literacy, language, and learning* (pp. 229–255). Cambridge: Cambridge University Press.

Welsh, M.C., & Pennington, B.F. (1988). Assessing frontal lobe functioning in children: Views from developmental psychology. *Developmental Neuropsychology, 4*, 199–230.

Wenthold, R., Huie, D., Altschuler, R., & Reeks, K. (1987). Glycine immunoreactivity localized in the cochlear nucleus and superior olivary complex. *Neuroscience, 22*, 897–912.

Werner, L.A. (1992). Interpreting developmental psychoacoustics. In L.A. Werner & E.W. Rubel (Eds.), *Developmental psychoacoustics* (pp. 47–88). Washington, DC: American Pyschological Association.

Westby, C.E., & Cutler, S.K. (1994). Language and ADHD: Understanding the bases and treatment of self-regulatory deficits. *Topics in Language Disorders, 14*(4), 58–76.

Wetherby, A.M., Koegel, R.L., & Mendel, M. (1981). Central nervous system dysfunction in echolaic autistic individuals. *Journal of Speech and Hearing Research, 24*, 420–429.

Wever, E.G., & Bray, C.W. (1930). Auditory nerve impulses. *Science, 71*, 215.

Whitfield, I.C. (1967). *The auditory pathway*. Baltimore: Williams & Wilkins.

Whitman, T.L., Burgio, L., & Johnson, M.B. (1984). Cognitive behavioral interventions with mentally retarded children. In A. Meyers & W.E. Craighead (Eds.), *Cognitive behavior therapy with children* (pp. 193–227). New York: Plenum Press.

Wiederhold, M.L. (1986). Physiology of the olivocochlear system. In R.A. Altschuler, D.W. Hoffman, & R.P. Bobbin (Eds.), *Neurobiology of hearing: The cochlea* (pp. 349–370). New York: Raven Press.

Wiens, J.W. (1983). Metacognition and the adolescent passive learner. *Journal of Learning Disabilities, 16*, 144–149.

Wiig, E.H., & Secord, W. (1985). *Test of Language Competence*. San Antonio, TX: The Psychological Corporation.

Wiig, E.H., & Semel, E.M. (1984). *Language assessment and intervention for the learning disabled*. Columbus, OH: Charles E. Merrill.

Wiig, E.H., Semel, E.M., & Crouse, M.A.B. (1973). The use of morphology by high risk and learning disabled children. *Journal of Learning Disabilities, 6*(7), 457–465.

Willeford, J.A. (1977). Assessing central auditory behavior in children: A test battery approach. In R. Keith (Ed.), *Central auditory dysfunction* (pp. 43–72). New York: Grune & Stratton.

Willeford, J.A. (1980). Central auditory behaviors in learning disabled children. *Seminars in Speech, Language and Hearing, 1*, 127–140.

Willeford, J.A. (1985). Assessment of central auditory disorders in children. In M.L. Pinheiro & F.E. Musiek (Eds.), *Assessment of central auditory dysfunction* (pp. 239–257). Baltimore, MD: Williams & Wilkins.

Willeford, J.A., & Billger, J. (1978). Auditory perception in children with learning disabilities. In J. Katz (Ed.), *Handbook of clinical audiology.* (2nd ed., pp. 410–425). Baltimore: Williams & Wilkins.

Willeford, J.A., & Burleigh, J.M. (1985). *Handbook of central auditory processing disorders in children*. Orlando, FL: Grune & Stratton.

Williams, J., & Carey, A.L. (1995). Impact of the Americans with disabilities act on audiologists. In R.S. Tyler & D.J. Schum (Eds.), *Assistive devices for persons with hearing impairment* (pp. 1–9). Boston: Allyn and Bacon.

Willott, J.F. (1991). *Aging in the auditory system*. San Diego: Singular Publishing Group.

Willott, J.F. (1996). Anatomic and physiologic aging: A behavioral neuroscience perspective. *Journal of the American Academy of Audiology, 7*, 141–151.

Willott, J.F., Aitken, L.M., & McFadden, S.L. (1993). Plasticity of auditory cortex associated with sensorineural hearing loss in adult mice. *Journal of Comparative Neurology, 329*(3), 402–411.

Willott, J.F., & Lu, S.M. (1982). Noise-induced hearing loss can alter neural coding and increase excitability in the central nervous system. *Science, 216*, 1331–1332.

Wilson, C.C., Lanza, J.R., & Barton, J.S. (1988). Developing higher level thinking skills through questioning techniques in the speech and language setting. Language, *Speech, and Hearing Services in Schools, 19*, 428–431.

Wilson, R. (1994). Word recognition with segmented-alternated CVC words: Compact disc trials. *Journal of the American Academy of Audiology, 5*, 255–258.

Wilson, R., & Margolis, R. (1991). Acoustic reflex measurements. In W. Rintelmann (Ed.), *Hearing assessment* (2nd ed., pp. 247–319). Austin, TX: Allyn & Bacon.

Wilson, U. (1983). Nursing care of American Indian patients. In M. Orque, B. Bloch, & L. Monrroy (Eds.), *Ethnic nursing care: A multicultural approach* (pp. 271–295). St. Louis: C.V. Mosby.

Winer, J.A. (1984). The human medial geniculate body. *Hearing Research, 15*, 225–247.

Winer, J.A. (1985). The medial geniculate body of the cat. *Advances in Anatomy, Embryology, and Cell Biology, 86*, 1–98.

Wingfield, A., Goodglass, H., & Smith, K. (1994). Does memory constrain utilization of top-down information in spoken word recognition? Evidence from normal aging. *Language and Speech, 37*, 221–235.

Wingfield, A., Poon, L.W., Lombardi, L., & Lowe, D. (1985). Speed of processing in normal aging: Effects of speech rate, linguistic structure, and processing time. *Journal of Gerontology, 40*, 579–585.

Wingfield, A., & Stine, E.A.L. (1992). Age differences in perceptual processing and memory for spoken language in everyday memory and aging. In R.L. West & J.S. Sinnot (Eds.), *Everyday memory and aging* (pp. 101–123). New York: Springer Velag.

Winslow, R., & Sachs, M. (1987). Effect of electrical stimulation of the crossed olivocochlear bundle on auditory nerve responses to tones in noise. *Journal of Neurophysiology, 57*, 1002–1021.

Witelson, S. (1986). Wires of the mind: Anatomical variation in the corpus callosum in relation to hemispheric specialization and integration. In F. Lepore, M. Ptito, & H. Jasper (Eds.), *Two hemispheres in one brain: Functions of the corpus callosum*. New York: Alan R. Liss.

Wong, B.Y.L. (1982). Strategic behaviors in selecting retrieval cues in gifted, normal achieving and learning disabled children. *Journal of Learning Disabilities, 15*, 33–37.

Wong, B.Y.L. (1987). How do the effects of metacognitive research impact on the learning disabled individual? *Learning Disability Quarterly, 10*, 189–195.

Wong, B.Y.L. (1991). The relevance of metacognition to learning disabilities. In B.Y.L. Wong (Ed.), *Learning about learning disabilities* (pp. 232–261). San Diego: Academic Press.

Wong, B.Y.L., & Jones, W. (1982). Increasing metacomprehension in learning-disabled and normally-achieving students through self-questioning training. *Learning Disability Quarterly, 5*, 228–240.

Woodcock, R. (1976). *Goldman, Fristoe, Woodcock auditory skills test battery technical manual*. Circle Pines, MN. American Guidance and Service.

Woods, D., Clayworth, C., & Knight, R. (1985). Middle latency auditory evoked potentials following cortical and sub-cortical lesions. *Electroencephalography and Clinical Neurophysiology, 61*, 55.

Woods, D., Clayworth, C., Knight, R., Simpson, G., & Naeser, A. (1987). Generators of middle and long latency auditory evoked potentials: Implications from studies of patients with bitemporal lesions. *Electroencephalography and Clinical Neurphysiology, 68*, 132–148.

Woolsey, C. (1960). Organization of cortical auditory system: A review and synthesis. In G. Rasmussen & W. Windell (Eds.), *Neuromechanics of the auditory and visibility systems* (pp. 165–180). Springfield, IL: Charles C. Thomas.

Wren, C.T. (1983). *Language and learning disabilities: Diagnosis and remediation*. Rockville, MD: Aspen.

Wright, H.N. (1968). The effect of sensori-neural hearing loss on threshold-duration function. *Journal of Speech and Hearing Research, 11*(4), 842–852.

Yacobacci-Tam, B. (1987). Interacting with the culturally different family. In D.A. Atkins (Ed.), *Families and their hearing-impaired children* (pp. 46–59). *Volta Review, 89*(5), Washington, DC: Alexander Graham Bell Assocation for the Deaf.

Yacullo, W., & Hawkins, D. (1987). Speech recognition in noise and reverberation by school-age children. *Audiology, 26*, 235–246.

Yakovlev, P.I., & Lecours, A.R. (1967). Myelogenetic cycles of regional maturation of the brain. In A. Minkiniwski (Ed.), *Regional development of the brain in early life* (pp. 3–70). Oxford: Blackwell Press.

Yaqub, B., Gascon, G., Al-Nosha, M., & Whitaker, H. (1988). Pure word deafness (acquired verbal auditory agnosia) in an Arabic-speaking patient. *Brain, 111*, 457–466.

Yost, W.A., & Moore, M.J. (1987). Temporal changes in a complex spectral profile. *Journal of the Acoustical Society of America, 81*, 1896–1905.

Young, M.L., & Protti-Patterson, E. (1984). Management perspectives of central auditory problems in children: Top-down and bottom-up considerations. *Seminars in Hearing, 5*(3), 251–261.

Yozawitz, A., Bruder, G., Sutton, S., Sharpe, L., Gurland, B., Fleiss, J., & Costa, L. (1979). Dichotic perception: Evidence for right hemisphere dysfunction in affective psychosis. *British Journal of Psychiatry, 135*, 224–237.

Yuzon, E. (1994). FM personal listening systems. In M. Ross (Ed.), *Communication access for persons with hearing loss* (pp. 73–101). Baltimore: York Press.

Zametkin, A.J., Nordahl, T., Gross, M., King, A.C., Semple, W.E., Rumsey, J., Hamburger, S., & Cohen, R.M. (1990). Cerebral glucose metabolism in adults with hyperactivity of childhood onset. *New England Journal of Medicine, 323*, 1361–1366.

Zentall, S.S. (1985). A context for hyperactivity. In K.D. Gadow & I. Bailer (Eds.), *Advances in learning and behavioral disabilities* (Vol. 4, pp. 273–343). Greenwich, CT: JAI Press.

Zerlin, S., & Naunton, R. (1974). Early and late average electroencephalic responses to low sensation levels. *Audiology, 13*, 366–378.

Zwicker, E., & Wright, H.N. (1963). Temporal summation for tones in narrow-band noise. *Journal of the Acoustical Society of America, 35*, 691–699.

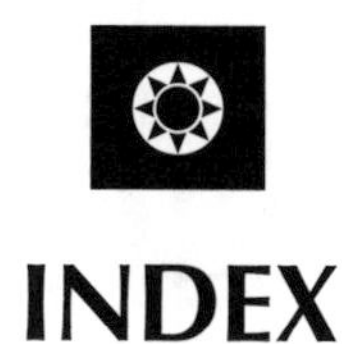

INDEX

B

C

D

E

F

G

I

L

M

N

O

P

R

S

T

V

W